Daniel Kondziella • Gunhild Waldemar

Neurology at the Bedside

Second Edition

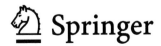 Springer

Daniel Kondziella
Department of Neurology
Rigshospitalet, University of
Copenhagen
Copenhagen
Denmark

Gunhild Waldemar
Department of Neurology
Rigshospitalet, University of
Copenhagen
Copenhagen
Denmark

ISBN 978-3-319-55990-2   ISBN 978-3-319-55991-9   (eBook)
DOI 10.1007/978-3-319-55991-9

Library of Congress Control Number: 2017943485

Printed on acid-free paper

This Springer imprint is published by Springer Nature
The registered company is Springer International Publishing AG
The registered company address is: Gewerbestrasse 11, 6330 Cham, Switzerland

Disclaimer

Medicine, including neurology, is an ever-changing field. As new research and clinical experience extends our knowledge, revisions of diagnostic procedures, treatment protocols, and drug therapy may become necessary. While the authors have made considerable efforts to describe generally accepted practices and to confirm the accuracy of the data, they are not responsible for errors or omissions or for any consequences from application of the information in this publication. To the fullest extent of the law, neither the authors nor the publisher assumes any liability for any damage and/or injury to persons or property arising from this book. The application of the information in this book remains the professional responsibility of the practitioner. In particular, the reader is urged to confirm the accuracy of the information relating to drug therapy by checking the most current product information provided by the drug manufacturer and by consulting other pharmaceutical literature to verify the recommended dose, the method and duration of administration, as well as possible contraindications and drug side effects. The treating physician is responsible for the decision on dosages and the best available treatment for each individual patient.

Contents

Abbreviations

ACA	Anterior cerebral artery
ACE	Addenbrooke's cognitive examination
AChR	Acetylcholine receptor
AComA	Anterior communicating artery
ACTH	Adrenocorticotropic hormone
AD	Alzheimer's disease
ADC	Apparent diffusion coefficient
ADEM	Acute demyelinating encephalomyelitis
ADHD	Attention deficit hyperactivity disorder
AED	Antiepileptic drug
AICA	Anterior inferior cerebellar artery
AIDP	Acute inflammatory demyelinating polyneuropathy
AIE	Autoimmune encephalitis
AION	Anterior ischemic optic neuropathy
ALS	Amyotrophic lateral sclerosis
AMAN	Acute motor axonal neuropathy
AMPA	α-amino-3-hydroxy-5-methyl-4-isoxazolepropionic acid
AMSAN	Acute motor sensory axonal neuropathy
ANA	Antinuclear antibody
ANCA	Antineutrophil cytoplasmic antibodies
ARAS	Ascending reticular activating system
ARUBA	A randomized trial of unruptured brain arteriovenous malformations
AV	Arteriovenous
AVM	Arteriovenous malformations
BAEP	Brainstem auditory evoked potentials
BECTS	Benign partial epilepsy of childhood with centrotemporal spikes
BPPV	Benign paroxysmal positional vertigo
BRBNS	Blue rubber bleb nevus syndrome
bvFTD	Behavioral variant frontotemporal dementia
C9ORF72	Chromosome 9 open reading frame 72
CAA	Cerebral amyloid angiopathy
CADASIL	Cerebral autosomal dominant arteriopathy with subcortical infarcts and leukoencephalopathy
CARASIL	Cerebral autosomal recessive arteriopathy with subcortical infarcts and leukoencephalopathy

CAE	Childhood absence epilepsy
CAG	Cytosine, adenine, guanine
CASPR2	Contactin-associated protein-like 2
CBD	Corticobasal degeneration
CBF	Cerebral blood flow
CDT	Carbohydrate-deficient transferrin
CEA	Carotid endarterectomy
CES	Clinical exome sequencing
CGH	Comparative genomic hybridization
CIDP	Chronic inflammatory demyelinating polyneuropathy
CIPM	Critical illness polyneuropathy and myopathy
CIS	Clinically isolated syndrome
CJD	Creutzfeldt-Jakob disease
CK	Creatine kinase
CLIPPERS	Chronic lymphocytic inflammation with pontine perivascular enhancement responsive to steroids
CMAP	Compound muscle action potentials
CMT	Charcot-Marie-Tooth disease
CN	Cranial nerve
CNS	Central nervous system
CO	Carbon monoxide
CO_2	Carbon dioxide
COHb	Carboxyhemoglobin
COMT	Catechol-O-methyltransferase
CPAP	Continuous positive airway pressure
CPEO	Chronic progressive external ophthalmoplegia
CPP	Cerebral perfusion pressure
CRP	C-reactive protein
CSF	Cerebrospinal fluid
CT	Computed tomography
CTA	Computed tomography angiography
DADS	Distal acquired demyelinating symmetric polyneuropathy
DAI	Diffuse axonal injury
DAP	3,4-Diaminopyridine
DAT scan	Dopamine transporter scanning
DBS	Deep brain stimulation
DECIMAL	Decompressive craniectomy in malignant middle cerebral artery infarction
DESTINY	Decompressive surgery for the treatment of malignant infarction of the middle cerebral artery
DLB	Dementia with Lewy bodies
DMD	Duchenne muscular dystrophy
DMPK	Dystrophia myotonica-protein kinase
DoC	Disorders of consciousness
DRPLA	Dentatorubral-pallidoluysian atrophy
DTI	Diffusion tensor imaging
DWI	Diffusion-weighted MRI
DYT	Dystonia

EEG	Electroencephalography
EFNS	European federation of neurological societies
EMG	Electromyography
eMCS	Emerged from minimal conscious state
EVT	Endovascular therapy
FCMS	Foix-Chavany-Marie syndrome
FDG	Fludeoxyglucose
FLAIR	Fluid-attenuated inversion recovery
FMD	Fibromuscular dysplasia
FMR1	Fragile X mental retardation 1
fMRI	Functional magnetic resonance imaging
FOUR	Full outline of unresponsiveness
FSH	Facioscapulohumeral muscular dystrophy
FTD	Frontotemporal dementia
FXTAS	Fragile X-associated tremor/ataxia syndrome
g	Gram
GABA	Gamma-aminobutyric acid
GAD	Glutamic acid decarboxylase
GBS	Guillain-Barré syndrome
GCS	Glasgow Coma Scale
GHB	Gamma-hydroxybutyrate
GI	Gastrointestinal
GluT1	Glucose transporter type 1
h	Hour
HAART	Highly active antiviral therapy
HAMLET	Hemicraniectomy after middle cerebral artery infarction with life-threatening edema trial
HaNDL	Headache with neurological deficits and CSF lymphocytosis
HAS-BLEED	Hypertension, abnormal renal/liver function, stroke, bleeding history or predisposition, labile INR, elderly, drugs/alcohol
HD	Huntington's disease
Hg	Hectogram
HNPP	Hereditary neuropathy with liability to pressure palsies
HSP	Hereditary spastic paraparesis
HSV	Herpes simplex virus
HTLV-1	Human T-lymphotropic virus type 1
i.a.	Intra-arterial
IBM	Inclusion body myositis
ICA	Internal carotid artery
IC-EC	Intracranial-extracranial
ICH	Intracerebral hemorrhage
ICP	Intracranial pressure
ICU	Intensive care unit
Ig	Immunoglobulin
IIH	Idiopathic intracranial hypertension
ILAE	International League Against Epilepsy
IM	Intramuscularly
INO	Internuclear ophthalmoplegia

INR	International normalized ratio
IRIS	Immune reconstitution inflammatory syndrome
IV	Intravenously
IVIG	Intravenous immunoglobulin
IVT	Intravenous thrombolysis
JAE	Juvenile absence epilepsy
JC	John Cunningham (virus)
JME	Juvenile myoclonic epilepsy
kg	Kilogram
KSS	Kearns-Sayre syndrome
L	Liter
LACS	Lacunar syndromes
LEMS	Lambert-Eaton myasthenic syndrome
LG1	Leucine-rich glioma-inactivated 1
LHON	Leber's hereditary optic neuropathy
LMN	Lower motor neuron
MADSAM	Multifocal acquired demyelinating sensory and motor neuropathy
MAG	Myelin-associated glycoprotein
MAO-B	Monoamine B
MAP	Median arterial pressure
MAPs	Compound muscle action potentials
max	Maximally
MCA	Middle cerebral artery
MCI	Mild cognitive impairment
MCS	Minimal conscious state
MCV	Motor conduction velocity
MELAS	Mitochondrial encephalomyopathy with lactic acidosis and stroke-like episodes
MEP	Motor evoked potential
mEq	Milliequivalent
MERFF	Myoclonic epilepsy with ragged red fibers
MERS	Mild encephalitis/encephalopathy with a reversible splenial lesion
mg	Milligram
MG	Myasthenia gravis
mGluR5	Metabotropic glutamate receptor 5
MGUS	Monoclonal gammopathy of unknown significance
MLF	Medial longitudinal fasciculus
MLPA	Multiplex ligation-dependent probe amplification
MLST	Multiple sleep latency test
mm	Millimeter
MMN	Multifocal motor neuropathy
MMNCB	Multifocal motor neuropathy with conduction block
mmol	Millimole
MMSE	Mini-Mental State Examination
MND	Motor neuron disease
MNGIE	Mitochondrial neurogastrointestinal encephalopathy

MOG	Myelin oligodendrocyte glycoprotein
MR	Magnetic resonance
MRC	Medical Research Council
MRI	Magnetic resonance imaging
MRS	Magnetic resonance spectroscopy
mRS	Modified Rankin Scale
MS	Multiple sclerosis
MSA	Multisystem atrophy
ms	Millisecond
MSUD	Maple syrup urine disease
MUPs	Motor unit potentials
MuSK	Muscle-specific kinase
NARP	Neuropathy, ataxia, and retinitis pigmentosa
NBIA	Neurodegeneration with brain iron accumulation
NCS	Nerve conduction studies
NFL	Neurofilament
NFLE	Nocturnal frontal lobe epilepsy
NIHSS	National Institute of Health Stroke Scale
NINDS	National Institute of Neurological Disorders and Stroke
NMDA	N-Methyl-D-aspartate
NMO	Neuromyelitis optica
NOAC	Novel (or non-vitamin K antagonist) oral anticoagulants
NPH	Normal pressure hydrocephalus
NREM	Non-rapid eye movement
NSAID	Nonsteroidal anti-inflammatory drugs
OCD	Obsessive compulsive disorder
OMIM	Online Mendelian Inheritance in Man
p.o.	Per oral
PACS	Partial anterior circulation syndromes
PCA	Posterior cerebral artery
PCommA	Posterior communicating artery
PCR	Polymerase chain reaction
PD	Parkinson's disease
PDE-5	Phosphodiesterase type 5
PET	Positron-emission tomography
PFO	Patent foramen ovale
PICA	Posterior inferior cerebellar artery
PLED	Periodic lateralized epileptiform discharges
PLMT	Painful legs and moving toes
PML	Progressive multifocal leukoencephalopathy
PNES	Psychogenic nonepileptic seizures
PNET	Primitive neuroectodermal tumors
PNFA	Progressive nonfluent aphasia
PNS	Peripheral nervous system
POCS	Posterior circulation syndromes
POEMS	Polyneuropathy, organomegaly, endocrinopathy, M protein, and skin changes
PRES	Posterior reversible encephalopathy syndrome

PROMM	Proximal myotonic myopathy
PSP	Progressive supranuclear palsy
RCVS	Reversible cerebral vasoconstriction syndrome
REM	Rapid eye movement
RIS	Radiologically isolated syndrome
RLS85	Reaction Level Scale 85
RVCL	Retinal vasculopathy with cerebral leukodystrophy
SAH	Subarachnoidal hemorrhage
SC	Subcutaneously
SCA	Spinocerebellar ataxias
SCA1	Spinocerebellar ataxia type 1
SCA2	Spinocerebellar ataxia type 2
SCLC	Small cell lung cancer
SD	Semantic dementia
SIADH	Syndrome of inadequate antidiuretic hormone secretion
SLE	Systemic lupus erythematosus
SMA	Spinal muscular atrophy
SNAPs	Sensory (nerve) action potentials
SOD1	Copper-zinc superoxide dismutase
SPECT	Single photon emission computed tomography
SSA	Sjögren syndrome type A antibody
SSB	Sjögren syndrome type B antibody
SSEP	Somatosensory evoked potentials
SSPE	Subacute sclerosing panencephalitis
SSRI	Selective serotonin reuptake inhibitor
STICH	Surgical Trial in Intracerebral Hemorrhage
STIR	Short tau inversion recovery
SUNCT	Short-lasting unilateral neuralgiform headache attacks with conjunctival injection and tearing
SUNA	Short-lasting unilateral neuralgiform headache with cranial autonomic symptoms
SVP	Spontaneous venous pulsations
SWI	Susceptibility-weighted imaging
TAC	Trigeminal autonomic cephalalgias
TACS	Total anterior circulation syndromes
TBE	Tick-borne encephalitis
TCA	Tricyclic antidepressant
TEE	Transesophageal echocardiography
TENS	Transepidermal nerve stimulation
TGA	Transient global amnesia
TIA	Transitory ischemic attack
TMS	Transcranial magnetic stimulation
TPO	Thyroid peroxidase
TTE	Transthoracic echocardiography
TTR-FAPs	Transthyretin familial amyloid polyneuropathies
UMN	Upper motor neuron
UWS	Unresponsive wakefulness syndrome
vCJD	Variant form of Creutzfeldt-Jakob disease

VDRL	Venereal Disease Research Laboratory
VEP	Visual evoked potentials
VGCC	Voltage-gated calcium channel
VGKC	Voltage-gated potassium channel
VN	Vestibulocochlear nerve
VOR	Vestibulo-ocular reflex
VOR	Volume of interest
VS	Vegetative state
VZV	Varicella zoster virus
w	Week
WMSN	Wartenberg's migrant sensory neuritis
×	Times
μg	Microgram
μmol	Micromol
μV	Microvolt

List of Cases

What to Expect from This Book (and What Not to)

1

Abstract

Neurologists take pride in their clinical bedside skills, perhaps even more so than other physicians. Good clinical mentorship is mandatory in order to develop such skills; however, due to an ever-increasing need for more efficient working structures, the time and dedication that mentorship requires may not always be available. The authors have therefore written this book for neurology residents who are looking for a personal clinical mentor, guiding them through the entire patient encounter: from a comprehensive history and an efficient clinical examination to a thorough differential diagnosis, ancillary investigations, and finally treatment options.

Keywords

Clinical skills • Clinical neurology • Examination • Differential diagnosis • Examination • Mentorship • Neuroanatomy • Patient history • Treatment

Few things in medicine are as fascinating as watching an experienced neurologist perform a history and bedside examination to generate a differential diagnosis prior to any laboratory investigations. Good clinical skills are mandatory when it comes to placing the patient on the right diagnostic track and to interpreting laboratory results correctly. These skills are acquired through regular training, in-depth theoretical knowledge, and good mentorship. The neurology trainee is responsible for the first two aspects, while good clinical mentorship requires a dedicated consultant who may not always be available.

Neither a traditional textbook nor a pocket manual, the aim of this book is to act as a clinical mentor and provide information otherwise difficult to look up in the usual reference sources. It tries to answer the sort of questions neurology trainees typically would ask their consultants.

- How do I distinguish clinically between myasthenia gravis and Lambert-Eaton myasthenic syndrome?
- What is the differential diagnosis of a rapidly progressive dementia if the initial workup is negative?

© Springer International Publishing AG 2017
D. Kondziella, G. Waldemar, *Neurology at the Bedside*, DOI 10.1007/978-3-319-55991-9_1

- Which anatomical lesions can lead to Horner's syndrome?
- Which neurophysiological features distinguish axonal from demyelinating polyneuropathy?
- How do I treat autonomic dysreflexia in a patient with chronic spinal injury?

To this end, the approach of *the present book reflects the course of the neurological consultation*. The history, bedside examination, and generation of a working diagnosis are discussed first, followed by a review of laboratory investigations and medical treatment (Fig. 1.1).

Like any clinical mentor, this book demands an active effort and commitment from you. It is assumed that you have at least a superficial knowledge of neurology and that you will consult a good reference source if needed.

Chapters 2 and 3 review the relevant neuroanatomy from a clinical point of view and provide the tools to obtain an efficient clinical history and bedside examination. These chapters can be read straightforwardly from the first to the last page.

Chapter 4 is somewhat more complicated and demands greater flexibility. The chapter's aim is twofold.

First, using a specific clinical syndrome as its case, it intends to teach the reader how to approach differential diagnosis in a structured manner. This is the bird's-eye view. Although there are hundreds of etiologies to a given polyneuropathy, most can be diagnosed using a simple three-step approach. Headache can be classified into primary and secondary headache syndromes, the latter of which can be further divided into intracranial and extracranial disorders and so on.

Second, this chapter provides a comprehensive differential diagnosis of most of the disorders encountered in neurological practice. Due to space limitations, the background information is limited, but the chances are minimal that a patient, even at tertiary care level, has a neurological diagnosis not covered by this chapter.

Chapter 5 provides a short overview of the main laboratory investigations performed in neurology with emphasis on the clinical aspects.

Chapter 6 offers a reference of medical, surgical, and other treatment options for most neurological conditions. Again, this chapter is written from a clinical mentor's point of view. It suggests the medication and dosage that may be chosen for a given condition but assumes that the reader is familiar with the pharmacodynamic and pharmacokinetic data, contraindications, and side effects. The main focus of this chapter is to guide the residents on call. Thus, the emphasis is on treatment of cerebrovascular disorders and epilepsy. Neurorehabilitation, counseling, and regular follow-up, which should be an integral part of neurological management, will not be covered.

The authors are grateful for any comments and suggestions for improving future editions. Also, they hope that upon completion of your neurology training, you will know most of the content of this publication like the back of your hand.

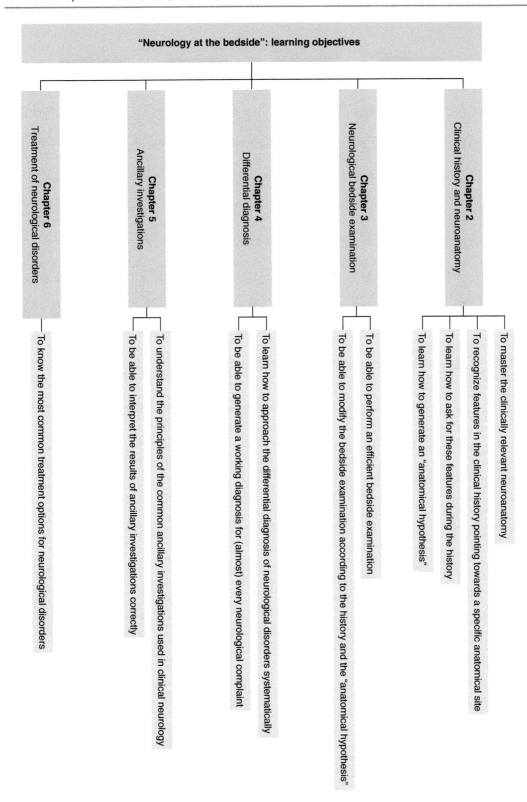

Fig. 1.1 Summary of chapter learning objectives

Clinical History and Neuroanatomy: "Where Is the Lesion?"

2

Abstract

The first step in the management of the neurological patient is to localize the lesion. While taking the history, the neurologist generates an anatomical hypothesis, which subsequently can be confirmed or rejected during the bedside examination. Following this, a working diagnosis is established and ancillary tests are chosen accordingly. Although the anatomy of the nervous system is highly complex, distinct anatomical entities have characteristic features. For instance, the hallmark of a myopathy is symmetric proximal weakness without sensory disturbances. Fatigability together with proximal weakness, including bulbar and oculomotor features, is typical for a disorder of the neuromuscular junction. In contrast, diseases of peripheral nerves, the brachial and lumbosacral plexus, as well as nerve roots usually lead to both motor and sensory deficits. Further, injury to the spinal cord is associated with a triad of paraparesis, a sensory level of the trunk, and sphincter disturbances. Brainstem processes often produce ipsilateral cranial nerve deficits and contralateral sensorimotor signs. While damage of the cerebellar hemispheres causes ataxia and intention tremor of the ipsilateral extremity, lesions of the midline region mainly lead to gait ataxia and truncal instability. Movement disorders due to disease involving the basal ganglia can be divided into hypo- and hyperkinetic disorders. Lesions involving the subcortical white matter frequently induce visual field deficits, complete hemiplegia, and dense numbness. Impairment of higher cognitive function, incomplete hemiparesis (sparing the leg), and epileptic seizures are common signs of cortical disease. This chapter reviews the relevant neuroanatomy from a clinical viewpoint and provides the reader with the tools to perform a competent clinical history.

Keywords

Basal ganglia • Brachial plexus • Lumbosacral plexus • Brainstem • Cerebellum • Cortex • Cranial nerves • Muscle • Nerve roots • Neuromuscular synapse • Peripheral nerves • Spinal cord • Subcortical white matter • Thalamus

The neurological history differs from the history in other medical specialties insofar as it is primarily anatomy based. When examining a new patient, the first question a neurologist attempts to answer is, "Where is the lesion?" The main principle is *to use the history to generate an anatomical hypothesis and to use the bedside examination to confirm this hypothesis.* Following this, other features of the history, such as epidemiological data and the speed of symptom development, are taken into account in order to answer the next question, "What is the lesion?" Thereafter, the neurologist forms a differential diagnosis and a working diagnosis and then accordingly orders the most relevant laboratory tests. Strictly adhering to this schema allows for a safe and rapid diagnostic procedure. Obviously, in many cases, the experienced neurologist uses a shortcut called instant pattern recognition to reach a diagnosis. Yet, when confronted with a difficult diagnostic problem, nothing is more useful than to return to the bedside and take a more detailed history. Also, the history is more likely to lead to the correct diagnosis than the physical examination. Therefore, as a rule, more time should be devoted to the history compared to the bedside examination.

In order to obtain a neurological history, it is helpful to divide the complexity of the nervous system's anatomy into small manageable entities (Fig. 2.1). From peripheral to central, these include:

- Muscle
- Neuromuscular synapse
- Peripheral nerves
- Brachial and lumbosacral plexus
- Nerve roots
- Spinal cord
- Cranial nerves (CNs)
- Brainstem
- Cerebellum
- Subcortical gray matter such as the thalamus and basal ganglia
- Subcortical white matter
- Cortex

The subcortical white matter and the cortex can be further differentiated into:

- Frontal lobes
- Temporal lobes
- Parietal lobes
- Occipital lobes

Many diseases can be classified according to which of these entities they affect. For instance, myasthenia gravis (MG) is a disease of the neuromuscular synapse, while Alzheimer's diesease (AD) and epilepsy are mainly disorders of cortical function. Importantly, each anatomical unit has a specific symptomatology that can be elicited during the history. The neurologist can therefore "examine" the patient from the muscle to the cortex solely by performing a good neurological history. The essential anatomical and clinical features are summarized in the following pages and in Table 2.1.

Although it is of preeminent importance not to push the patient into reporting the symptoms that one is trying to elicit, the history must be meticulous and detailed. A useful clinical rule is that after finishing the history, one should have a clear and detailed idea of what has happened and be able to fully visualize the sequence of events. The focus should be on the principal symptoms and signs; the neurologist should not let minor findings and uncertain clinical data distract from the greater picture. (Admittedly, this is not easy without experience.) If the patient has many different and seemingly unrelated complaints, it is useful to ask what bothers him most and then concentrate on this complaint.

Taking a history is difficult in patients with a disorder that affects the level of consciousness, communication skills, and/or cognitive function, e.g., due to amnesia, aphasia, impaired judgment, lack of insight, and confabulation. A patient with AD, for instance, may not be able to explain his symptoms or the course of the disease; if he can, it might well be that not all of the information can be taken at face value. Likewise, the aphasic patient following a left middle cerebral artery (MCA) occlusion may have difficulties under-

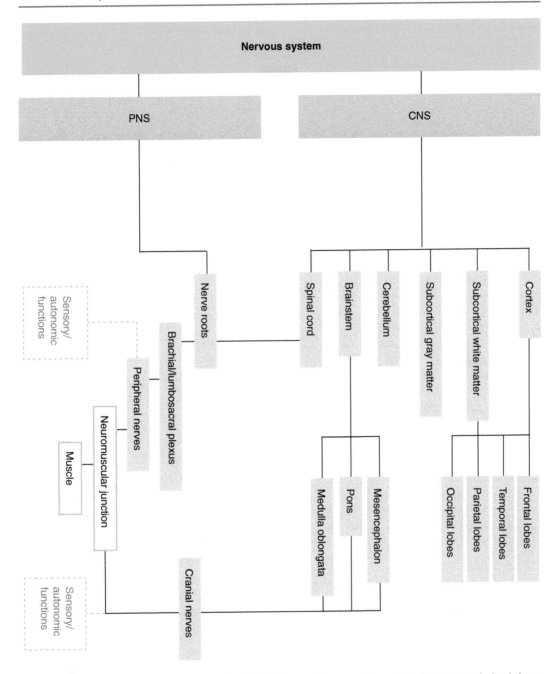

Fig. 2.1 The nervous system's anatomy can be divided into small manageable entities. Each anatomical unit has a specific symptomatology that can be elicited during the history

standing the examiner's questions, or he may well understand but be unable to formulate an appropriate answer. Further, a patient with a frontal brain tumor may have become so apathetic and indifferent that he might not complain at all despite an obvious inability to perform basic activities of daily living. In contrast, a patient with locked-in syndrome due to a large pontine infarct following a basilar artery thrombosis is awake and may fully understand the examiner but

Table 2.1 Summary of key anatomic features for history taking and bedside examination

Muscle: Proximal, symmetric weakness; no sensory symptoms

Neuromuscular junction: Fatigability; proximal, symmetric (or asymmetric) weakness; no sensory symptoms

Peripheral nerve: Sensory symptoms; distal, asymmetric weakness (except for symmetric polyneuropathy); normal or decreased muscle tone; hyporeflexia; eventually atrophy and fasciculations; motor and sensory deficits correlate to peripheral nerve distribution; sympathetic function (sweating) may be disturbed

Brachial plexus, lumbosacral plexus: Sensory symptoms; often distal greater than proximal weakness; normal or decreased muscle tone; hyporeflexia; eventually fasciculations and atrophy; motor and sensory deficits are neither consistent with a single peripheral nerve distribution nor with a specific dermatome/myotome; sympathetic function (sweating) may be disturbed; radiculopathic pain is common

Nerve root: Sensory symptoms; distal greater than proximal weakness; normal or decreased muscle tone; hyporeflexia; possibly atrophy and occasionally fasciculations; motor and sensory deficits associated with specific dermatome/myotome; radiculopathic pain; sympathetic function normal

Spinal cord:

Complete or near-complete transection or myelitis: Triad of paraparesis (spastic below site of lesion), sensory level, and sphincter disturbances

Anterior cord syndrome: Dissociated sensory loss with preserved vibration and proprioception but impaired perception of pain and temperature; paraparesis

Dorsal cord syndrome: Impairment of vibration and proprioception

Brown-Séquard syndrome (=hemitransection): Ipsilateral paresis; ipsilateral loss of vibration and proprioception; contralateral loss of pain and temperature

Syringomyelia (most often enlargement of cervicothoracic central cord): Dissociated sensory loss with bilateral impaired perception of pain and temperature; later bilateral paresis due to injury to nucleus of second motor neuron

Brainstem and cranial nerves: The brainstem includes (a) mesencephalon, (b) pons, and (c) medulla oblongata and consists of (x) all long afferent and efferent tracts, (y) vegetative centers (e.g., respiration), and the ARAS (arousal) and (z) nuclei of CN III–XII (mesencephalon III–V, pons V–VIII, medulla oblongata V and IX–XII). Thus, brainstem reflexes can be used to locate the lesion on a vertical axis (e.g., pupillary reflex, in, CN II, out, III; corneal and eyelash reflexes, in, V, out, VII; vestibulo-cephalic reflex and VOR, in, VIII, out, III and VI; and gag reflex, in, IX, out, X). Lesions often lead to ipsilateral CN and contralateral long tract signs, e.g., ipsilateral, peripheral (!) facial palsy, and contralateral hemiparesis. (However, if lesions affect the site above the nucleus of the facial nerve, there may be a contralateral, central facial palsy.) Other typical brainstem symptoms are, e.g., dysphagia, diplopia, and dysarthria (but not dysphasia, which is a cortical phenomenon)

Cerebellum: Cerebellar hemispheric lesions lead to ipsilateral (!) cerebellar ataxia and intention tremor. Cerebellar midline lesions lead to gait and truncal ataxia (without severe ataxia of the extremities)

Subcortical gray matter: Consists of basal ganglia, thalamus, and hypothalamus; deficit of dopamine functions leads to parkinsonism (tremor, bradykinesia, rigidity, postural instability) and dopamine hyperfunction to, e.g., chorea

Subcortical white matter: Visual field deficits, dense numbness, complete hemiparesis, executive dysfunction, and decreased psychomotor speed

Cortex: Impairment of higher cognitive function, including amnesia, aphasia, apraxia, visuospatial deficits, and neglect; epileptic seizures; incomplete hemiparesis sparing the leg; frontal lobe (executive dysfunction, personality impairment, hemiparesis due to lesions of the supplemental motor area and primary motor cortex, nonfluent or motor dysphasia); temporal lobe (auditory hallucinations due to lesions of the primary auditory cortex, memory disturbance with damage to the hippocampal formation, rising epigastric sensation and automatisms with temporal lobe seizures, fluent or sensory dysphasia); parietal lobe (visuospatial disorientation, sensory hemisymptoms due to lesions of the sensory cortex); and occipital lobe (visual hallucinations and cortical blindness with damage to primary visual cortex)

has lost all efferent motor control except for a few eye movements. Similarly, patients with terminal amyotrophic lateral sclerosis (ALS) or fulminant Guillain-Barré syndrome (GBS) may be anarthric and unable to communicate verbally. In all these situations, prior to taking a formal history, it is the duty of the neurologist to evaluate the cognitive capabilities of the patient and to find appropriate means of communication, e.g., by establishing a reliable code for locked-in patients to indicate yes and no using blinking or vertical eye movements. Also, it is of utmost importance to ensure that all other sources, e.g., spouses, family, friends, nurses, ambulance personnel, and patient notes, are taken into account to establish a history that is as detailed and as accurate as possible.

2.1 Muscle

The hallmark of a generalized myopathy is *proximal symmetric weakness without sensory symptoms*. For assessment of proximal weakness of the lower extremities, ask the patient about difficulties rising from a chair, getting out of bed, climbing stairs, or leaving the car without using his arms to pull himself up. In order to rise from a sitting position, a patient with severe weakness of the hips and thighs may have to flex his trunk at the hips, put his hands on his knees, and push his trunk upward by working his hands up his thighs. To discover upper extremity weakness, ask about problems working with the arms above the shoulder girdle. For instance, the patient may be unable to lift a child or a heavy bag, hang laundry on a clothesline, or wash his hair in the shower. Note that delicate hand movements usually do not present any difficulties, which is why writing, turning a key in the keyhole, or manipulating small buttons are not problematic. A patient with severe myopathy has a characteristic stance and gait pattern with marked lumbar lordosis. Also, when standing, the patient places his feet wide apart to increase the base of support, while his gait is characterized by the pelvis tilting from side to side because of bilateral weakness of the gluteus medius muscles. Thus, the patient "straddles as he stands and waddles as he walks."[1]

Importantly, the neurologist needs to rule out sensory symptoms. A myopathy may be painful, but a clear complaint of sensory symptoms is not compatible with a myopathic syndrome.

Hereditary myopathies may lead to involvement of cardiac muscle as well; thus, it is mandatory to ask for signs of cardiomyopathy and cardiac arrhythmias.

Other signs of muscle disease include:

- Scapular winging, e.g., *limb-girdle muscular dystrophy* and *facioscapulohumeral muscular dystrophy* (FSH).
- Orofacial weakness, e.g., FSH and *myotonic dystrophy*.
- Ptosis, e.g., *mitochondrial disease*, oculopharyngeal muscular dystrophy, and myotonic dystrophy.
- Gowers' sign. In order to rise from the ground, children with, e.g., *Duchenne muscular dystrophy (DMD)*, may have to assume a four-point position by fully extending the arms and legs and then working each hand alternately up the corresponding thigh.
- Muscle hypertrophy, e.g., the athletic appearance in *myotonia congenita.*
- Pseudohypertrophy of muscles, e.g., enlargement of the calves due to replacement of muscle cells by fat tissue as seen in DMD.
- Muscle contractures. Boys with DMD, for instance, may have to walk on their toes because of contractures of the gastrocnemius muscles.
- Distal weakness, e.g., hand weakness in myotonic dystrophy, weakness and atrophy of finger flexors and wrist flexors in *inclusion body myositis (IBM)*, and weakness of the thumbs and index fingers in *late-adult type 1 distal myopathy* (Welander or the Swedish type of distal myopathies).
- Myotonia. A patient with *myotonic dystrophy* may complain of difficulties releasing his hand after a handshake. Patients with *myotonia congenita* exhibit very stiff, awkward movements after resting. Movements become smoother after a few minutes, the so-called warm-up phenomenon.
- Pseudomyotonia. This is seen in *paramyotonia congenita of von Eulenburg*. In contrast to myotonia, pseudomyotonia becomes worse with exercise. Typically, cold temperatures increase symptoms, e.g., patients may complain about delayed eye opening and facial rigidity in the winter.
- Local atrophy, e.g., temporalis muscle atrophy in myotonic dystrophy; atrophy of finger flexors, wrist flexors, and quadriceps muscles in

---

[1]Samual A. K. Wilson, 1878–1937; British neurologist and describer of hepatolenticular degeneration (Wilson's disease).

IBM; and limb-girdle atrophy in limb-girdle muscular dystrophy and FSH.

- Progressive external ophthalmoplegia is encountered in mitochondrial disorders. Extramuscular manifestations of mitochondrial disorders include diabetes, hearing loss, a short stature, and dysfunction of the heart, kidneys, and liver.
- Exercise intolerance with or without subsequent rhabdomyolysis and myoglobinuria is seen in *glycogen storage disorders* such as McArdle disease and *lipid storage disorders* such as CPT II deficiency ("Has your gym teacher in school been angry with you because he thought you were lazy?" "Does your urine look like cola after you have been exercising?"). Characteristically, in lipid storage myopathy, myalgia occurs after exercise. In glycogen storage disorders, in contrast, myalgia tends to occur *during* exercise. After a few minutes of prolonged exercise, patients may experience a characteristic "second wind," and the pain may disappear due to metabolic adaptation of the muscles to enhance fat oxidation.
- Periodic weakness induced by hypo- or hyperkalemia, e.g., severe generalized but transitory weakness in *potassium-related channelopathies*.
- Skeletal deformities such as high palate, elongated facial appearance, pes cavus, chest deformities, and hip luxations are seen with *congenital myopathies*, e.g., nemaline myopathy, central core disease, and centronuclear myopathy. Patients with congenital myopathies usually present as "floppy babies" after birth, but the deficits often stabilize in later life, leading to relatively mild functional impairment. A history of severe myopathic weakness during childhood, improving and stabilizing during adolescence, and nasal speech because of a high palate are the main clues to the diagnosis of a congenital myopathy.
- Respiratory muscle weakness, e.g., *Pompe's disease*, leading to dyspnea, but also to more unusual presentations such as confusion or headache because of hypercapnia.

It is important to remember, however, that despite the large amount of space reserved in neurological textbooks for rare muscle diseases, the commonly encountered myopathies in general clinical practice are *drug-induced myopathies* (e.g., steroids, statins) and inflammatory myopathies (e.g., *polymyositis, dermatomyositis*). These are all characterized by the signs mentioned at the beginning of this chapter: proximal, symmetric weakness without sensory symptoms.

2.2 Neuromuscular Junction

Similar to myopathies, a disorder of the neuromuscular junction is characterized by *proximal weakness without sensory symptoms*. However, the hallmark of neuromuscular junction disorders such as MG is muscular *fatigability*. The symptoms therefore are of a waxing and waning nature. Symptoms may be better in the morning and worse in the evening; for instance, diplopia commonly increases during the afternoon. Yet it is generally of little use to ask about greater fatigability in the evening—who would say no? Instead, what needs to be elicited in the history is the following sequence: During a specific muscular activity, weakness develops. After a while weakness becomes so severe that the patient is forced to take a break, after which muscular strength normalizes. The activity is taken up again with normal or near-normal power, but after a while decreasing strength makes another break necessary, and so on. Examples include patients with masticatory weakness who cannot eat a whole meal without having to stop several times and patients whose speech becomes progressively dysarthric during a conversation, forcing them to pause often to regain their voice.

Weakness in most neuromuscular junction disorders is so proximal that it affects nuchal, facial, pharyngeal, and external ocular muscles. Consequently, head drop,[2] decreased facial expression, dysphagia, dysarthria, and ophthalmoplegia may develop. The smile of a myasthenic patient is highly characteristic. The face

---

[2]A patient with a recent history of head dropping has a high likelihood of having myasthenia gravis, but other differential diagnoses to keep in mind include amyotrophic lateral sclerosis (motor neuron disease), isolated neck extensor myopathy (including radiation-induced myopathy following neck radiation for malignancy), and multiple system atrophy (neurodegenerative disorder with atypical parkinsonism).

can be completely motionless except for half-raised corners of the mouth (it has been suggested that Leonardo's Mona Lisa has a myasthenic facial expression). Facial weakness may send highly negative social signals to someone not familiar with the disease. Symptoms in *MG* are often somewhat more asymmetric than in a myopathy; e.g., ptosis and ophthalmoplegia can be much worse on one side than the other.

Dyspnea is seen with affection of the respiratory muscles and acute respiratory failure is the most dreaded complication. MG tends to affect young women or elderly men. In the latter, outcome is sometimes still rather poor.

A history of bulbar symptoms arising in several individuals from the same household or who have shared a meal is highly suggestive of *botulism* (see Case 2.1 and Chap. 4). *Lambert-*

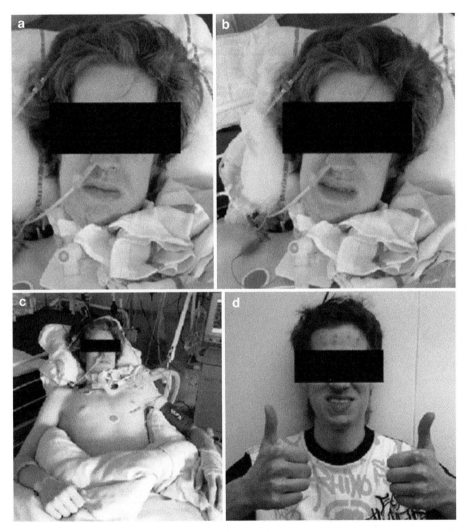

Case 2.1 Botulism. A 16-year-old male developed diarrhea 2 days after ingestion of spoiled canned tofu, followed the next day by double vision, impaired swallowing, and weakness in the arms and legs. Neurological examination revealed external ophthalmoplegia, bilateral facial palsy, (**a**, **b**; the patient tries to smile) anarthria, proximal tetraparesis, and absent tendon reflexes (**c**). Of note, loss of pupillary reflexes was seen not earlier than on the fifth day of admission. The patient was fully awake and communication was possible by sign language (thumbs up, thumbs down). The initial differential diagnosis included botulism and GBS. A lumbar puncture revealed normal protein and cell count. Analysis for anti-GQ1b antibodies, suggestive of Miller-Fisher syndrome, was negative. Electromyography and nerve conduction studies, including repetitive nerve stimulation and single fiber studies, were reported twice as normal but later revealed a neuromuscular transmission defect. Following a positive mouse bioassay test for botulism toxin, a diagnosis of botulism was made. One year later, the patient had made a full recovery (**d**)

Eaton myasthenic syndrome (LEMS), in contrast, seldom leads to bulbar symptoms. The usual presentation of LEMS is with generalized proximal upper and lower limb weakness and signs of autonomic dysregulation such as a dry mouth. Therefore, LEMS patients often carry a bottle of water with them. If these symptoms occur in a smoker, a diagnosis of small cell lung cancer is highly likely.

2.3 Peripheral Nerves, the Plexus, and Spinal Nerve Roots

In contrast to muscle or neuromuscular junction disorders, *weakness* is usually *combined with sensory symptoms* in diseases of the peripheral nerves, the plexus, and the nerve roots (Fig. 2.2). In addition, symptoms tend to be more asymmet-

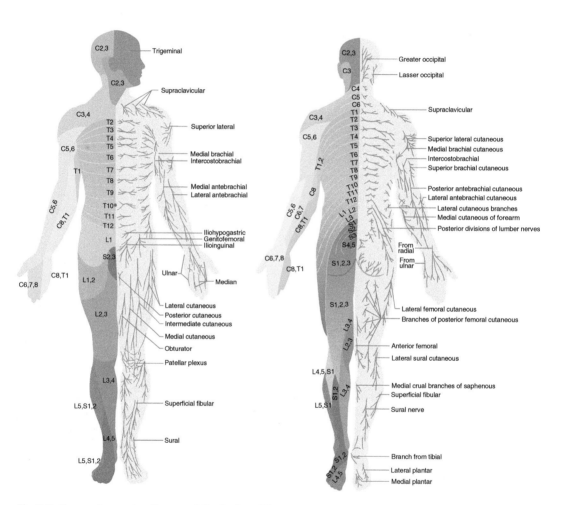

Fig. 2.2 Sensory innervation. Segmental distribution of the cutaneous nerves and typical dermatome distribution of the human body

ric (with the important exception of a symmetrical polyneuropathy) and more distal. Since the lower motor neuron (LMN) is affected, motor weakness is characterized by normal or decreased muscle tone, hyporeflexia, and eventually muscle atrophy and fasciculations.[3]

- The characteristic features of a mononeuropathy include sensory and muscular symptoms attributable to an individual peripheral nerve (e.g., carpal tunnel syndrome with compression of the median nerve at the wrist).
- The hallmark of a nerve root lesion is a combination of sensory and muscular symptoms derived from a specific dermatome and myotome (e.g., radiating pain in the L5 dermatome and weakness of dorsiflexion of the great toe in a L5 root disc herniation).
- The hallmark of a plexus lesion is that it comprises sensory and muscular symptoms that do correspond neither to a dermatome nor a myotome nor to a lesion of a single nerve. Plexus lesions therefore tend to have a more complex symptomatology than peripheral nerve lesions. Also, plexus and peripheral nerve

lesions may impair sympathetic function, such as sweating, in contrast to nerve root lesions.

While it is often difficult to differentiate between peripheral nerve, plexus, and root lesions by the history alone, there is a very characteristic feature of root lesions—and to a lesser extent of plexus lesions—that does not occur in peripheral nerve disorders. This feature is radiculopathic pain. A patient with radiculopathic pain usually has a history of chronic neck or lumbar pain acutely exacerbated by severe, electric shock-like pain that radiates down the arm or leg. Described differently, a sharp sudden pain, often evoked by abrupt cervical or lumbar movements, shoots from the neck and shoulders into the hands or from the lumbar spine into the feet. Pain from a peripheral lesion, in contrast, is more distal and localized. Carpal tunnel syndrome may lead to pain in the entire arm, but the pain clearly does not originate from the neck. Thus, the simple question "Do you feel sharp, sudden pain coming from your neck and radiating down your arm?" differentiates a C6/7 radiculopathy from carpal tunnel syndrome.

Some words of comfort: Although the anatomy of the peripheral nervous system (PNS) can be rather intimidating, the vast majority of clinically relevant features are due to lesions of only a few PNS structures. In the upper extremities, these include five nerve roots, the upper and the lower brachial plexus, and six peripheral nerves and in the lower extremities, three nerve roots and the cauda equina, the lumbosacral plexus, and eight peripheral nerves (Fig. 2.3). Knowing the signs and symptoms associated with lesions at these anatomical sites enables the categorization of the great majority of peripheral nerve disorders.[4]

---

[3] From the primary motor cortex in the cerebrum to the great toe, there are only two motor neurons. Thus, in a six-foot-tall man, these upper and lower motor neurons measure three feet each on average. "Corticospinal tract," "pyramidal tract," "first motor neuron," and "central motor neuron" are often used synonymously (but not 100% correctly) for "upper motor neuron" (UMN). Likewise, "second motor neuron," "alpha motor neuron," and "peripheral motor neuron" are frequently used instead of "lower motor neuron" (LMN). The UMN cell bodies are found in the motor cortex. The LMN cell bodies are situated in the ventral horns in the spinal cord and in the motor cranial nerve nuclei in the brainstem. Damage to the UMN is "supranuclear"; damage to the LMN "infranuclear." UMN weakness is characterized by spasticity, hyperreflexia, Babinski sign, and a typical pattern of weakness distribution that will be discussed later. LMN weakness is associated with hyporeflexia, decreased muscle tone, atrophy, and fasciculations.

---

[4] "Aids to the examination of the peripheral nervous system" by O'Brien M. (Saunders Ltd. 5th ed.) is a tremendously helpful pocket manual.

Fig. 2.3 Peripheral nervous system. Although the anatomy of the PNS is complicated, the great majority of patients will have symptoms and signs that can be attributed to lesions of only a few PNS structures

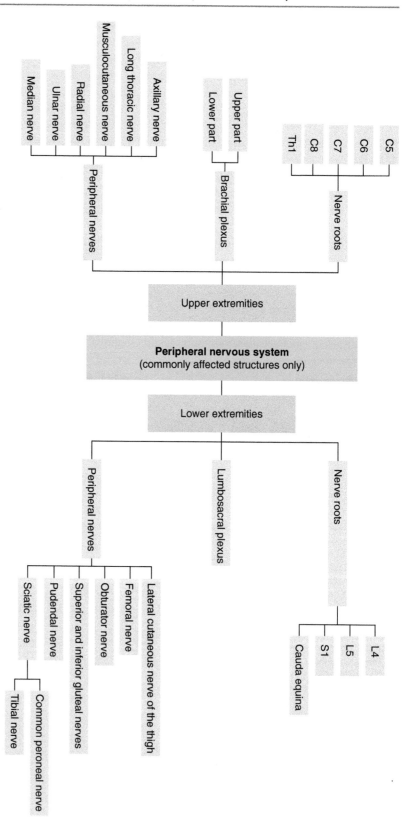

2.3.1 Peripheral Nerves

As mentioned above, peripheral nerve lesions generally cause a sensory deficit that may or may not be accompanied by a motor deficit. This distinguishes them from primary lesions of the muscle or of the neuromuscular junction, which never cause a sensory deficit. Also, symptoms in peripheral nerve disorders tend to be distal, and they are usually asymmetric (with the important exception of distal symmetric polyneuropathies). Since the lower motor neuron is affected, weakness is "flaccid"—thus, muscle tone is normal or decreased, and there is hyporeflexia and eventually atrophy and fasciculations. The motor and sensory deficits follow the distribution of the affected peripheral nerve.

Many peripheral nerve disorders have a typical history. Complaints involving walking on cushions, pins, and needles and burning sensations in the feet, particularly in a patient with alcoholism or diabetes mellitus, are typical of *distal symmetric polyneuropathy*. Only in severe cases are the hands affected, usually when hypesthesia and paresthesia in the lower extremities have reached half way up to the knees. (This represents the "length-dependent" pattern of axonal degeneration. Rarely, in especially severe cases of polyneuropathy, the truncal nerves can be affected as well—this leads to hypesthesia in the middle of the abdominal wall, where the most distal branches of the cutaneous nerves meet, an area that roughly corresponds to the rectus abdominis. In contrast to a sensory level associated with spinal cord lesions, sensation is intact in the back and the waist.) A painful neuropathy with prominent distal dysesthesias (burning feet syndrome) is seen with *small fiber disease*.[5] A complaint about not being able to walk in the dark, in contrast, is characteristic for the sensory ataxia of *large fiber disease*.[6] These patients cannot go to the bathroom at night without having to turn on the light. The gait unsteadiness is of the so-called stamp and stick type; the patients may need a walking aid and stamp their feet on the ground in order to activate all the remaining proprioceptive nerve fibers. Besides sensory ataxia, examination reveals a positive Romberg's sign, hypo- or areflexia, distal weakness, and atrophy of the small muscles of the feet.

Symmetric polyneuropathy, distal wasting, pes cavus, clawed toes, and palpable peripheral nerves point toward *hereditary polyneuropathy*. This is usually due to *Charcot-Marie-Tooth (CMT) disease* or a related disorder but is also seen in a few other conditions, e.g., Friedreich's ataxia.

The most common cause of acute neuromuscular weakness in the developed world is *GBS*. In Europe and North America, the most common variant of GBS is *acute inflammatory demyelinating polyneuropathy* (AIDP). AIDP is essentially a poly*radiculo*neuropathy (which is why high protein, leaking from inflamed nerve roots, is found in the cerebrospinal fluid (CSF)). Patients usually present with progressive ascending weakness with areflexia affecting the limbs more or less symmetrically. Symptoms are maximally expressed after 2 weeks in 50% of patients and after 4 weeks in 90%. Hyperacute onset with quadriplegia within 48 h or less is not uncommon, and in these patients reflexes may be initially preserved. Facial diplegia, respiratory failure, and autonomic dysfunction such as cardiac arrhythmias and labile blood pressure are frequent. Sensory symptoms and neuropathic pain are usual complaints but tend to be much less significant than motor paralysis. Red flags indicating that the diagnosis is wrong include persistent asymmetric weakness, early bladder and bowel paralysis, and a sensory level suggesting a spinal cord lesion. More than half of GBS

---

[5]Pain and temperature are transmitted by thin type III sensory fibers and unmyelinated type IV fibers. Both fiber types have very small diameters (0.2–5 μm). In contrast, proprioception and vibration are transmitted by large-diameter myelinated type Ia, Ib, and II sensory fibers (6–20 μm).

[6]Ataxia due to lost proprioception is called sensory ataxia and must be distinguished from ataxia of cerebellar and vestibular origin. Characteristically, and in contrast to cerebellar ataxia, visual information can compensate for sensory ataxia.

patients have a history of gastrointestinal (GI) and upper respiratory tract infection or vaccination 1–3 weeks prior to symptom onset. *GBS variants* are numerous. Among the more important are pharyngeal-cervical-brachial paresis, oculopharyngeal weakness, pure sensory GBS, pure autonomic failure, ataxic GBS, and the Miller-Fisher syndrome. The last variant mentioned is associated with GQ1b antibodies and consists of the triad of ophthalmoplegia, ataxia, and areflexia, although oligosymptomatic and overlapping syndromes exist. In contrast to AIDP, paralysis in the Miller-Fisher syndrome is usually descending. Axonal variants (acute motor axonal neuropathy (AMAN) and acute motor sensory axonal neuropathy (AMSAN)) represent only 3–5% of GBS cases in the Western world but are much more common in the Far East and South America. *GBS mimics* include diphtheric polyneuropathy (beware of a history of recent pharyngitis in patients without diphtheria vaccination) and porphyric polyneuropathy (classically associated with abdominal pain, psychosis, and dark urine). Nerve conduction studies reveal demyelinating features in the former and axonal features in the latter.

More or less symmetric ascending sensorimotor paralysis with hypo- or areflexia that develops during a period of 8 weeks or more is typical of *chronic inflammatory demyelinating polyneuropathy* (CIDP). Differentiation between GBS and CIDP is important for prognosis and treatment. While CIDP can be treated with steroids, GBS cannot. In contrast to GBS, multiple CN involvement, life-threatening dyspnea, and acute autonomic dysfunction are very rare with CIDP. The list of differential diagnoses for CIDP is long. Relapsing GBS, subacute GBS, alcoholism, nutritional deficiencies, paraneoplastic conditions, heavy metal poisoning, and certain drugs such as amiodarone, cisplatin, isoniazid, and nitrofurantoin may all give rise to a similar clinical picture that develops within a few weeks or months.

Monoclonal gammopathies (IgM, IgA, and IgG) are found in 10% of patients with idiopathic neuropathy. *Polyneuropathy associated with a monoclonal gammopathy* may be the presenting features of a plasma cell dyscrasia or may be related to a monoclonal gammopathy of unknown significance (MGUS). In addition, IgM-MGUS polyneuropathies can be associated with autoantibody activity against peripheral nerve glycoproteins such as myelin-associated glycoprotein (MAG). MGUS polyneuropathies typically affect patients over the age of 50, men roughly twice as often as women. A minority of patients with polyneuropathy associated with a monoclonal gammopathy have significant motor involvement and are clinically indistinguishable from those with CIDP, while in the majority of patients, the condition is chronic, mainly sensory and only slowly progressive, distal, and symmetric.

Mononeuritis multiplex is a form of asymmetric polyneuropathy in which several peripheral nerves are affected at the same time or subsequently. In full-blown mononeuritis multiplex, the patient complains of multiple motor and sensory symptoms in the extremities, which may often be rather painful. With time, mononeuritis multiplex may involve so many peripheral nerves that it simulates a peripheral polyneuropathy. The differential diagnosis includes metabolic (diabetes), immunologic (rheumatoid arthritis, sarcoidosis, systemic lupus erythematosus (SLE), amyloidosis), infectious (HIV, leprosy, neuroborreliosis), malignant (leukemia, lymphoma), and vasculitic disorders (Churg-Strauss vasculitis, polyarteritis nodosa, Wegener granulomatosis). Vasculitic neuropathies also occur without systemic manifestations; characteristically, they often include the sciatic nerve.

Multifocal motor neuropathy (MMN) is a predominantly distal, mainly upper limb, asymmetrical pure motor neuropathy. The male–female ratio is 2.5:1. A typical patient would be a middle-aged man with progressive (asymmetric) weakness in his arms, but normal sensation and who is concerned about having *amyotrophic lateral sclerosis* (ALS). In contrast to ALS, profound muscle atrophy is usually absent. Severe bilateral arm palsy in either MMN or ALS with preserved power in the legs occasionally leads to the "man-in-the-barrel syndrome," where the arms hang uselessly at the patient's side as if his trunk were trapped in a barrel. Another characteristic clinical feature that may be observed in a patient with ALS is dissociated atrophy of intrinsic hand muscles, known as the *ALS split hand*. The split-hand phenomenon refers to preferential wasting of the thenar muscles with relative sparing of the hypothenar muscles. Although the exact mechanisms remain elusive, it is a highly specific diagnostic sign in early ALS (Case 2.2). The clinical presentation and differential diagnosis of ALS, a disorder affecting the lower as well as the upper motor neuron (UMN), are discussed in Chap. 4.

In *hereditary neuropathy with liability to pressure palsies* (HNPP), motor symptoms typically predominate over sensory symptoms. Patients often complain that after trivial compression of the extremities, the subsequent numbness and dysesthesia last from days to months rather than minutes. Also, there is a tendency that minor or moderate compression of peripheral nerves, such as may occur when carrying heavy weights during housework and other trivial activities, leads to episodes of focal palsies. Childbirth, for instance, can give rise to a palsy of the lumbosacral plexus. When weakness is secondary to limb compression during sleep, the weakness will typically be noticed when the patient wakes up in the morning. The attacks in HNPP are usually of sudden onset and painless. Typically affected nerves are those

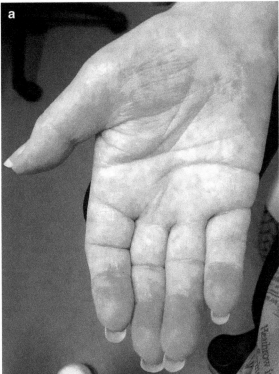 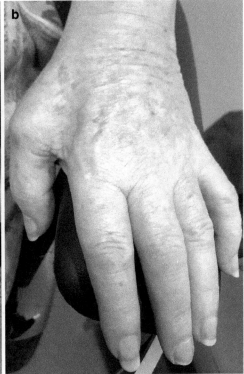

Case 2.2 Split-hand sign in amyotrophic lateral sclerosis. A 73-year-old female was referred for progressive weakness, which had started 3 years earlier in her right hand. Subsequently, her right leg became involved, followed by her left extremities. Despite cervical and lumbar decompressive surgery, she had started using a walking stick and then a walking frame 2 years and 12 months, respectively, prior to admission. At the time of referral, she was confined to a wheel chair. Swallowing had become increasingly difficult during the previous 3 months. Examination revealed dysphagia, a pronounced jaw jerk, and marked atrophy and fasciculations in all four extremities. Cognition and sensory functions were intact. Of note, dissociated atrophy of intrinsic hand muscles was noted. The ALS split hand refers to preferential wasting of the thenar muscles (abductor pollicis brevis (**a**) and first dorsal interosseous muscles (**b**)), with relative preservation of the hypothenar muscles (lateral abductor digiti minimi muscles). Both cortical and peripheral mechanisms have been suggested, but the origin of the split-hand sign remains poorly understood. Nevertheless, it is a useful diagnostic sign in early ALS with a high degree of specificity

associated with a specific anatomic vulnerability, e.g., in the arms, the radial (humerus), median (carpal tunnel), and ulnar (cubital tunnel) nerves, and in the legs, the peroneal nerve (compression at the fibular neck). But HNPP may also affect more uncommon nerves; e.g., it may lead to recurrent, sometimes bilateral, peripheral facial palsies, usually after the patient has rested his face on a hard surface. Mononeuropathies are initially followed by recovery, although patients with repeated episodes may have lasting neurologic abnormalities. A less common manifestation of HNPP is that of a more or less symmetric, slowly progressive polyneuropathy. With this subtype, high arches and hammertoes are common, which may lead to a misdiagnosis of CMT disease. At symptom onset, HNPP patients are typically in their 20s or 30s but, occasionally, patients may become symptomatic earlier or later in life. HNPP is inherited in an autosomal dominant fashion, so there is often a positive family history, but spontaneous mutations are well described.[7] Apart from entrapment neuropathy, electrophysiological examination typically shows a background demyelinating polyneuropathy, suggesting the correct diagnosis.

Sensory ganglionitis, also termed sensory neuronopathy, is due to inflammation of the sensory root ganglia. With the involvement of large-diameter ganglionic neurons, the main symptoms include a severe sensory ataxia of the arms and legs. With arms elevated and eyes closed, the patient may show typical pseudo-athetoid movements of the fingers. (This is simply because the patient does not know the exact position of the fingers.) With affection of small-diameter neurons, symmetric or asymmetric numbness, paresthesias, and burning pain occur and frequently involve the face or the trunk early in the development of sensory ganglionitis. (This is the so-called pseudo-syringomyelia distribution or the numb-chin syndrome, which is very characteristic for a sensory neuronopathy.) There are four major forms of noninfectious sensory ganglionitis:

- Acute sensory neuronopathy syndrome (often postinfectious; young and old, women and men are equally affected; this is a sensory variant of GBS)
- Subacute paraneoplastic sensory neuronopathy (e.g., occurring in middle-aged men with small cell lung cancer)
- Subacute sensory neuronopathy associated with Sjögren syndrome (usually affecting middle-aged women)
- Chronic ataxic neuropathy associated with paraproteinemia or polyclonal gammopathy with or without known autoantibodies (typically affecting the elderly, mostly men)

The most common infectious cause of sensory ganglionitis is herpes zoster due to reactivation of a dormant ganglionic varicella zoster virus (VZV), typically manifesting with an extremely painful rash in the affected dermatome.

Another sensory neuropathy is *Wartenberg's migrant sensory neuritis* (WMSN), in which the site of the lesion is much more peripheral. WMSN is a harmless, rare disorder of unknown etiology. It involves multiple cutaneous nerves and has a highly characteristic history, which is the clue to the diagnosis. An ordinary movement of a limb (e.g., stretching in bed, turning a key, putting on socks) induces a sudden brief pain in the distribution of a cutaneous nerve followed by sensory loss in the distribution of this nerve. Sensory loss may persist for several weeks. A complaint of motor symptoms is not compatible with this disorder. Different cutaneous nerves are affected at different times. WMSN may thus have a relapsing-remitting character, which is why it is a useful differential diagnosis to multiple sclerosis (MS). (See Case 3.13 for illustration.)

Another condition that deserves to be mentioned is the syndrome of *painful legs and moving toes* (PLMT). Although it remains poorly understood, PLMT is an easily recognized and distinct clinical entity. Patients complain about severe burning pain in the legs and more or less constant involuntary movements of the toes (occasionally also of the fingers). The movements are suggestive of both chorea and dystonia. The most frequent etiologies are cryptogenic and

---

[7] Similar to CMT disease type 1A, HNPP is due to mutation of the *PMP22* gene. HNPP is caused by a deletion or nonsense mutation of the *PMP22* gene in chromosome 17p11.2, the same region that is duplicated in CMT 1A.

peripheral neuropathies, followed by trauma and radiculopathies. PLMT responds poorly to treatment, and quality of life can be severely compromised because of debilitating pain.

2.3.1.1 Mononeuropathies of the Upper Extremities

The most common causes of mononeuropathies in the upper extremities are nerve entrapment and trauma.

In the upper extremities, a lesion of the *axillary nerve* (*C5/C6*) may lead to a weakness of shoulder abduction and sensory loss over the outer aspect of the upper arm.

Isolated lesions of the *musculocutaneous nerve* (*C5/6*) are usually secondary to a fracture of the humerus. They lead to wasting of the biceps brachii muscle, the brachialis, and coracobrachialis muscles and to weakness of flexion of the supinated forearm. Rupture of the biceps brachii muscle tendon may sometimes simulate wasting of the biceps brachii muscle, but differentiation between these two conditions is usually possible with careful inspection.

Rucksack palsy is compression of the *long thoracic nerve* (*C5–7*) leading to a posterior shoulder or scapular burning type of pain and scapular winging due to weakness of the serratus anterior muscle. This is seen with sports injuries or in soldiers and backpackers carrying heavy weights on their backs for a prolonged period, hence the name rucksack palsy. Paralysis of the long thoracic nerve and the serratus anterior muscle is the most frequent neuropathic cause of scapular winging, leading to medial winging of the scapula. Lateral winging, in contrast, is generated by trapezius and rhomboid muscle paralysis due to injury to the *spinal accessory* (*CN XI*) and *dorsal scapular nerves* (*C4–6*), respectively.

Paresis of the *radial nerve* (*C5–8*) is often encountered in patients who have consumed large amounts of alcohol and have slept with the back of their arms compressed by the back of a bench or a similar object. It is thus also known as Saturday night palsy and leads to a drop hand, an inability to actively extend the fingers, and numbness of the back of the hand and wrist. Another variety of this syndrome is called Honeymoon

palsy, which occurs in a patient whose bed partner has slept on the affected arm. Radial nerve is also seen with humeral fracture. Although exceedingly rare in the developed world nowadays, a classic cause of bilateral hand drop due to radial motor neuropathy is lead poisoning.[8]

Compression of the *ulnar nerve* (*C8/T1*) provokes a tingling sensation in the little finger, half of the ring finger, and the ulnar half of the hand and is usually due to entrapment or trauma at the elbow in the cubital tunnel (colloquially called the funny bone). Importantly, ulnar nerve injury does not lead to sensory symptoms above the wrist. (Sensory disturbances above the wrist on the ulnar aspect of the forearm therefore suggest a lesion of the lower brachial plexus or of the C8/T1 nerve roots.) With long-standing nerve compression, a claw hand may develop. The fact that a distal lesion at the wrist, despite affecting fewer muscles, leads to more pronounced clawing than a proximal lesion is called the ulnar paradox.

Median nerve (*C6–T1*) entrapment as seen in carpal tunnel syndrome is the most common of all nerve entrapment syndromes. A typical patient may complain about pins and needles in the thumb, index, and ring finger and in the medial aspects of the palm, but in practice, the patient may state that the entire hand and even the arm are involved. The condition can be rather painful. Symptoms usually awaken the patient at night and disappear when the hand is shaken and massaged. Later, symptoms also occur during daytime; especially dorsiflexion of the hand, e.g., during bicycling, may aggravate the symptoms. With long-standing median nerve entrapment, atrophy of the thenar muscle develops and the thumb drops back in the plane of the other digits, which leads to the so-called ape hand. Lightly tapping over the nerve at the wrist may elicit a typical sensation of tingling or pins and needles in the distribution of the nerve (Tinel's sign). The so-called reverse Phalen's test is a provocative examination maneuver during which the patient

---

[8]Lead poisoning also leads to microcytic anemia, abdominal pain, and gingival discoloration at the interface of the teeth and gums. Exposure to lead may be due to lead paint found in older housings or glazed ceramic coffee mugs.

is asked to maintain full wrist and finger extension for 2 min, thereby increasing pressure in the carpal tunnel. Paresthesias in the distribution of the median nerve make carpal tunnel syndrome diagnosis likely. A variety of conditions predisposes to carpal tunnel syndrome, e.g., pregnancy, trauma, rheumatoid arthritis, acromegaly, and hypothyroidism.

2.3.1.2 Mononeuropathies of the Lower Extremities

Meralgia paresthetica is due to compression of the *lateral cutaneous nerve of the thigh (L2/3)* beneath the inguinal ligament and affects men more often than women. The patient complains of numbness and burning pain over the anterolateral aspect of the thigh, but since the entrapped nerve is purely sensory, muscle power is normal. Examination reveals impaired or altered sensation in the same area, but there is no motor weakness or wasting and the knee jerk is preserved, distinguishing it from radiculopathy. Sometimes symptoms are caused by tight trousers, and a history of recent weight gain or weight loss is common. Obesity and pregnancy may be contributing factors, and certain habitual postures (e.g., sitting or prolonged standing for an obese person) may be particularly uncomfortable.

Injury to the *femoral nerve (L2–4)* leads to weakness of extension of the lower leg. In longstanding cases, there are wasting of the quadriceps muscle and failure of knee fixation. The patient may complain that the knee seems to give way and that climbing stairs is impossible. If the nerve is damaged proximal to the origin of the branches to the iliacus and psoas muscle, hip flexion is affected as well. In contrast to L3 radiculopathy, thigh adduction (mediated by the obturator nerve) is spared. A sensory deficit can be found on the anterior aspect of the thigh and the ventromedial aspect of the calf (supplied by the saphenous nerve). The most common cause of an isolated femoral neuropathy is diabetes mellitus. Femoral neuropathy is also seen with pelvic tumors, after surgery for hernia repair, appendectomies, hysterectomies, and similar operations in the pelvis. A hematoma in the iliopsoas muscle is a frequent cause of femoral neuropathy in patients

with anticoagulation or hemophilia. These patients complain about acute pain in the groin and characteristically assume a posture of flexion and lateral rotation of the hip.

The *obturator nerve (L2–4)* may be damaged by the fetal head or forceps during prolonged delivery. Other common causes include pelvic tumors, fractures, and obturator hernia. Thigh adduction is affected and sensory loss is found on the medial aspect of the distal thigh.

Lesions of the *superior (L4–S1)* and *inferior (L5–S2) gluteal nerves*, seen with misplaced intragluteal injections, direct trauma, or injury during childbirth, evoke a characteristic gait disturbance. When walking, the patient typically bends his trunk away from the affected side in order to compensate for mild weakness of the hip abductors. This phenomenon is called the Duchenne limp. With severe abductor paresis, lateral bending of the trunk is insufficient to prevent pelvic tilt toward the normal side (Trendelenburg's sign). If abductor paresis is bilateral, the patient has a typical waddling gait.

The *sciatic nerve (L4–S3)* is the largest peripheral nerve in the body. Prior to its division into the tibial and common peroneal nerve, the sciatic nerve supplies the skin and the muscles of the back of the thigh (e.g., the knee flexors). Its tibial and peroneal nerve branches innervate all the muscles below the knee as well as the skin of the foot and the outer and dorsal aspects of the lower leg. Sciatic nerve lesions thus provoke a variety of combinations of tibial and common peroneal nerve palsies. When the nerve is proximally injured, knee flexion may be impaired as well. Partial sciatic nerve lesions are more common than complete sciatic paralysis and tend to affect peroneal-innervated muscles more than tibial ones. Common causes of sciatic nerve damage include pelvic fracture, hip dislocation, misplaced injections into the lower gluteal regions, pressure from a toilet seat during a period of alcohol intoxication ("toilet seat palsy"), sitting in the lotus position ("yoga paralysis"), and lying flat on a hard surface for a prolonged time. The last cause mentioned is sometimes encountered in slender drug addicts or cachectic patients who are bedridden. Stab and gunshot wounds causing sciatic nerve lesions are fortunately rare.

The *common peroneal nerve (L4–S2)* emerges within the poplitea and turns around the fibular head—a common area of compression—where it divides into the superficial and the deep peroneal nerves. A lesion of the superficial branch affects the peroneus muscles and thereby elevation of the lateral edge of the foot (eversion). It also leads to sensory disturbances at the lateral aspect of the distal leg and the dorsum of the foot. Of note, elevation of the medial aspect of the foot (inversion) is spared, since this is mediated by the tibial nerve. Indeed, preserved inversion of the foot (together with preserved abduction of the hip) is the main clinical finding that distinguishes a peroneus lesion from a L5 radiculopathy. The deep peroneal nerve mediates dorsiflexion of the foot and toes and innervates the skin in a small zone between digits I and II. Peroneal nerve damage leads to a drop foot and the typical steppage gait. The patient must flex the hip and lift the knee in order that the foot, which cannot be dorsiflexed, can clear the ground. Peroneal nerve impairment may arise spontaneously or follow prolonged pressure at the fibular head due to, e.g., leg crossing, tight casts, activities in the kneeling position, and improper positioning during anesthesia. In patients with apparently spontaneous drop foot, a history of significant weight loss is not uncommon. Shrinkage of the subcutaneous fat tissue, usually protecting the nerve, is probably a causative factor. Common traumatic causes of foot drop include fracture of the fibular head (e.g., due to a skiing accident) and knee dislocation.

The *tibial nerve (L4–S3)* mediates inversion of the foot, flexion of the toes, and sensation of the sole of the foot. Isolated tibial nerve damage is uncommon because the tibial nerve is rather well protected in the poplitea. It may occur following hemorrhaging in the knee or after direct trauma, such as a knife stab. Baker cysts are a rare cause of peroneal or tibial nerve compression. Tarsal tunnel syndrome is due to compression of the tibial nerve beneath the flexor retinaculum in the tarsal tunnel. It leads to pain and pins and needles in the foot and sometimes the leg. Another condition that provokes pain in the foot, mostly in the forefoot, is metatarsalgia.

It may be primarily a problem of the joints and bones of the metatarsals, or it may be due to a neurinoma of the plantar nerve branches (Morton's neuroma). Muscle power is preserved in tarsal tunnel syndrome and metatarsalgia.

The *pudendal nerves (S2–4)* innervate the external genitalia as well as the sphincter of the anus and bladder. Stretching of the nerves during prolonged childbirth can result in incontinence and perianal sensory disturbances. The latter is also sometimes encountered in bicyclists after prolonged rides on hard saddles. Dysfunction of the nerve is usually temporary in the latter conditions, whereas with pelvic surgery or a tumor, the pudendal nerves may be damaged permanently.

2.3.2 Brachial Plexus and Lumbosacral Plexus

As with peripheral nerve and nerve root lesions, motor weakness due to a plexus lesion is typically accompanied by sensory deficits, and symptoms are unilateral. Since it is the second motor neuron that is affected, there may be normal or decreased muscle tone, hyporeflexia, fasciculations, and atrophy. The hallmark of a plexus lesion is that motor and sensory deficits follow neither the distribution of a single peripheral nerve nor a specific dermatome/myotome. The patient with a lesion of the plexus may complain of strong pain in the shoulder or hip with or without radiation into the extremities. In contrast to a lesion of the nerve root, plexus pathology may impair sympathetic function. This is because the fibers from the sympathetic trunk join the sensory and motor fibers distally to the nerve roots. As a consequence, decreased sweating within a localized area may be seen with a plexus or peripheral nerve lesion, but not with nerve root compression.

Plexus lesions are rather rare; this is especially true for lesions of the lumbosacral plexus, which is well protected. The three most serious disorders resulting in painful plexopathies are due to trauma, malignancy, and radiation injury. The most common painful plexopathy, which has an excellent prognosis, is brachial neuritis.

For all practical purposes, lesions of the brachial plexus (C5–T1) can be divided into upper and lower plexus syndromes. A lesion of the *upper brachial plexus (C5–C7)*, or Erb palsy, can be encountered in infants after traumatic delivery. Upper brachial plexus palsies acquired in adult life are usually due to trauma, e.g., because of a *motorcycle accident*. They result in the loss of the lateral rotators of the shoulder, arm flexors, and hand extensor muscles. Thus, the patient's arm hangs by his side and is rotated inward, and the dorsum of the slightly flexed hand faces forward, which is known as the characteristic waiter's tip position.

A lesion of the *lower brachial plexus (C8–T1)* is sometimes called Klumpke paralysis. Sudden upward pulling of the elevated arm stretches the lower brachial plexus. Symptoms include paralysis of intrinsic hand muscles, which may lead to a claw hand and hypesthesia in the ulnar aspect of the forearm. Involvement of sympathetic fibers from the T1 nerve roots results in ptosis, miosis, and anhidrosis (Horner's syndrome). Again, frequent causes in adults are motorcycle accidents and, in infants, complicated deliveries. However, malignancy is frequent as well, e.g., a smoker with shoulder pain, numbness in the lower arm, and ulnar weakness, and a unilateral Horner's syndrome most likely has a tumor of the lung apex, termed *Pancoast tumor* (Case 2.3).

Plexus neuritis (also called Parsonage-Turner syndrome, neuralgic amyotrophy, or brachial neuritis) manifests with severe sudden-onset shoulder pain, often awakening the patient during the night. Weakness, atrophy, and fasciculations typically develop when the pain subsides after some hours or days. (Occasionally, weakness may also manifest right from the beginning.) Often the condition affects muscles served by the upper brachial plexus, and elevating the arm above the shoulder may become impossible. However, all arm and shoulder muscles may be affected in isolation or in combination. A similar condition has been suggested as an explanation for sudden unilateral diaphragm weakness due to an isolated palsy of the ipsilateral phrenic nerve. The prognosis of plexus neuritis is usually good. In most cases weakness resolves after a few

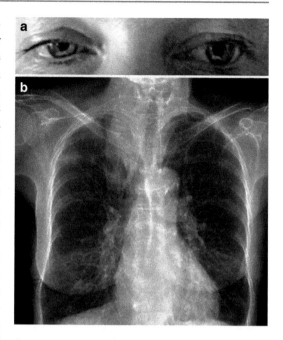

Case 2.3 Pancoast tumor. A 45-year-old female smoker complained of right-sided shoulder pain and numbness in the forearm that had lasted for 2 months. Examination revealed weakness of the ulnar muscles of the right hand and an ipsilateral Horner syndrome (**a**). The chest X-ray showed a right-sided tumor of the lung apex (**b**). Biopsy confirmed the diagnosis of a small cell carcinoma of the lung

months. Presumably of autoimmune origin and often occurring after an upper respiratory infection, the disorder has also been described after delivery, surgical operations, trauma, and many other conditions. In addition, there is an autosomal dominant form of recurrent plexus neuritis called *hereditary neuralgic amyotrophy*.

Lumbar and sciatic pains are some of the most frequently encountered syndromes in general practice and are usually caused by degenerative spinal disease affecting lumbosacral nerve roots, such as discopathy or stenosis of the intervertebral foramen. However, when local signs of spinal disease are absent in spite of leg weakness, sensory loss, and reflex asymmetry, when sweating is disturbed, or when the patient has a history of negative radiological examination of the spine, peripheral plexopathy becomes more likely. In adults *lumbosacral plexus (L1–S4)* pathology is probably more often than not due to a *malignancy*. Primary or metastatic visceral and extra-visceral tumors lead the list, but mass lesions due to Hodgkin's disease and other lymphoreticular and hematogenic disorders are also seen. Benign causes include, among others, *diabetic plexopathy*, *radiation plexopathy*, and spontaneous or iatrogenic *retroperitoneal hemorrhage*. Since the lumbosacral plexus lies deeply in the retroperitoneal space, trauma must be severe to affect the plexus and therefore almost always leads to pelvic fracture as well.

2.3.3   Spinal Nerve Roots

The ventral and dorsal spinal nerve roots form 31 pairs of spinal nerves (8 cervical, 12 thoracic, 5 lumbar, 5 sacral, and 1 coccygeal). Lesions of nerve roots, usually due to disc herniation and degenerative spine disease, occasionally due to

neuroma or schwannoma, typically provoke radiculopathic pain and sensory and motor symptoms. Weakness tends to be more pronounced distally than proximally. Muscle tone may be normal or slightly decreased. Physical examination reveals hyporeflexia or areflexia. Fasciculations are usually not a significant finding. The hallmark of a nerve root lesion is that the motor and sensory deficits are confined to a specific dermatome and myotome (Fig. 2.4).

Degenerative spine disease typically affects the spine where it is most mobile. Thus, lower lumbar (L4–S1) and lower cervical (C5–C8) nerve roots are most frequently damaged. Lesions of other nerve roots are rare. Most disc herniations affect the lower nerve root, e.g., a lateral L4/L5 disc protrusion typically leads to compression of the L5 nerve root, and a medial L4/L5 disc protrusion may compress the L5 nerve root

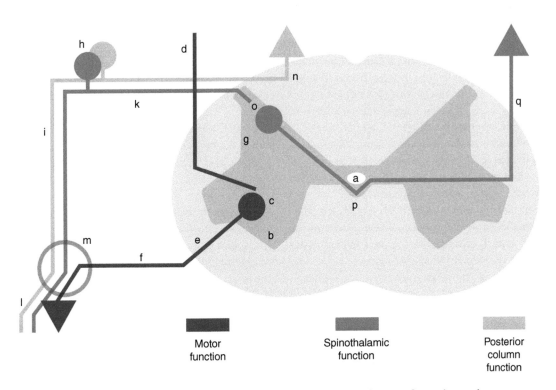

Motor function

Spinothalamic function

Posterior column function

Fig. 2.4 Normal spinal cord anatomy. (*a*) Central canal, (*b*) ventral horn, (*c*) lower motor neuron nucleus, (*d*) corticospinal tract, (*e*) lower motor neuron axon, (*f*) ventral nerve root, (*g*) dorsal column, (*h*) sensory ganglion, (*i*) sensory dendrite (dorsal nerve root), (*k*) sensory axon, (*l*) spinal nerve, (*m*) intervertebral foramen, (*n*) posterior col-

umn, (*o*) synapse between first and second sensory neuron, (*p*) commissura alba (contralateral spinothalamic pathway not shown), (*q*) spinothalamic tract. *Black*, motor pathway; *dark blue*, spinothalamic pathway; *light blue*, posterior column pathway

and also sacral nerve roots. In contrast, a far lateral disc herniation may occasionally affect the upper nerve root, e.g., a very laterally protruded L5/S1 disc may lead to compression of the L5 nerve root.

Lumbosacral disc herniation, which is the classic cause for sciatica, is more common than cervical disc herniation. A patient with lumbar nerve root compression typically complains about chronic lumbar pain exacerbated by sudden radiculopathic pain radiating down into the foot. Heavy weight lifting or other strenuous exercise preceding symptom onset for a few hours or days may or may not be reported. Coughing, defecation, and other forms of Valsalva maneuver typically increase the pain. However, it should be noted that degenerative spine disease as revealed by magnetic resonance imaging (MRI), for instance, is very common and often asymptomatic.

With damage to the *L5 nerve root*, examination may reveal a positive Lasègue's sign, a drop foot, paralysis of ankle dorsiflexion, and—in contrast to what is seen with a "simple" peroneal nerve lesion—impaired inversion of the foot and abduction of the thigh. With long-standing L5 nerve root damage, atrophy of the small dorsal foot muscles may occur.

With *S1 nerve root* compression, sensory disturbances occur in the lateral aspect of the leg and the foot. Plantar flexion may be impaired and the Achilles reflex will be diminished.

L3/4 disc herniation with *L4 nerve root* compression is somewhat less common and manifests with sensory disturbances on the anterior aspect of the thigh and the medial aspect of the leg, weakness of knee extension, and a diminished patellar reflex.

Cauda equina syndrome is due to damage to the lumbar and sacral nerve roots along their path within the spinal canal prior to their exit through the intervertebral foramina. The syndrome is often combined with conus medullaris syndrome, which will be discussed later in this chapter. Involvement of sacral nerve roots (S1–S4) leads to saddle anesthesia and sensory disturbances in the lateral aspect of the legs and the feet, bowel and bladder sphincter disturbances with urinary retention, and fecal incontinence, as well as erec-

tile dysfunction in males. If the lumbar roots are involved as well, there is paraparesis of the LMN type. Pain may or may not be present. A cauda equina syndrome may have *traumatic*, *degenerative* (e.g., spinal lumbar canal stenosis, median disc herniation, ankylosing spondylitis), *vascular* (e.g., epidural hematoma), *metastatic* (e.g., meningeal carcinomatosis, lymphoma), *inflammatory*, and *infectious* causes. A common infectious agent is *herpes simplex virus (HSV) II*, affecting the spinal nerve roots retrogradely. Women are at higher risk than men. The patient complains of sudden onset of urinary retention with or without saddle anesthesia. Power in the legs is usually normal. The patient is not necessarily aware of being infected with HSV II; indeed, cauda equina syndrome may manifest without visible genital herpes. Tactful questioning often reveals that the patient has a new sexual partner.

Analogous to lumbar spine disease, cervical spine pathology usually presents with chronic neck pain exacerbated with radiculopathic pain and paresthesias. Injury to the *C5 nerve root* leads to disturbed sensory function on the outer aspect of the shoulder and over the deltoid muscle. Abduction of the shoulder is impaired and the biceps reflex diminished.

C6 nerve root compression provokes radiating pain in the thumb and index finger and the radial aspect of the forearm. The biceps reflex will be lost or decreased, and there is weakness of arm flexion at the elbow.

Damage to the *C7 nerve root* impairs arm extension, affects the triceps reflex, and leads to pain and numbness in the second, third, and fourth finger and the dorsal aspect of the forearm.

Compression of the *C8 nerve root* also impairs arm extension at the elbow and diminishes the triceps reflex, but sensory symptoms will typically be confined to the fourth and fifth finger and the ulnar aspect of the forearm.

2.4   Spinal Cord

Spinal cord anatomy is rather complex (Fig. 2.4). Damage to the spinal cord therefore leads to many different but highly specific symptom constellations. The following is a simplified and selective review of spinal cord anatomy that nevertheless provides all that is needed to understand the clinical syndromes associated with spinal cord lesions.

On a transversal section, the gray matter of the spinal cord has a butterfly appearance and is surrounded by white matter (Fig. 2.4). In the middle of the butterfly is the central canal (a) that communicates with the brain's ventricles. The hind wings of the butterfly correspond to the right and left ventral horns (b) in which the nuclei of the LMNs (c) reside. The axons from the UMNs are termed the corticospinal tract.[9] The corticospinal tract (d) descends in the lateral aspect of the spinal cord. The axons of the UMNs synapse with the LMNs in the ventral horn. The axons of the LMNs (e) leave the gray matter and form the ventral nerve root (f).

The forewings of the butterfly form the right and left dorsal horns (g) that receive sensory information. However, the cell body of the peripheral sensory neuron is located in the dorsal spinal root ganglion (h). This nerve cell, the first sensory neuron in a chain of three, is a pseudounipolar cell. This means that it has one very short axon that, still within the spinal ganglion, divides into a distal process (actually the dendrite (i)) that conveys sensory information from the periphery (skin, muscle, internal organs) and a proximal process (essentially, this is the axon (j)) that reaches the spinal cord via the dorsal nerve root. Distal to the sensory dorsal root ganglion, the dorsal root and the ventral root merge into the spinal nerve (k) that leaves the spine through the intervertebral foramen (l).

For all practical purposes, sensory information can be divided into sensation mediated by:

- Posterior column pathways (vibration, proprioception, and light touch)
- Spinothalamic tracts (pain, temperature, and crude touch)

The posterior column pathway (or, more correctly, the posterior column-medial lemniscus pathway) mediates vibration, proprioception, and fine touch. Upon entering the spinal cord via the dorsal nerve root, fibers that convey vibration and proprioception travel upward through the ipsilateral posterior column (m).[10] The spinothalamic pathway that conveys temperature, pain, and crude touch, in contrast, crosses over to the contralateral side at the same level the fibers enter the spinal cord (or one or two segments higher). The axons from the first sensory neuron (of the spinothalamic pathway) synapse with second sensory neurons in the ipsilateral dorsal horn (n). Then, the axons of the second-order neurons cross the midline just anterior to the central canal. Together with the contralateral pain and temperature fibers, they form a white cross of myelinated nerve fibers within the gray matter. This white cross can be seen under the microscope and is called the commissura alba (o). Having crossed the midline, the fibers ascend in the anterior-lateral aspect of the spinal cord; this is the spinothalamic tract (p).[11]

In conclusion:

- The spinothalamic pathway mediates pain and temperature and decussates at the level of the spinal cord. This pathway ascends in the white matter region that lies anterior and laterally to the butterfly.
- The posterior column-medial lemniscus pathway conveys vibration and proprioception. It ascends ipsilateral to the entry of the dorsal root and crosses the midline at the brainstem level.

---

[9]As stated earlier, the cell bodies of the UMNs are found in the primary motor cortex in the frontal lobe, located on the anterior wall of the central sulcus. The major part of the corticospinal tract crosses the midline at the pyramidal decussation of the medulla oblongata.

[10]The axons that build up the posterior column pathway synapse in the medulla oblongata with second-order sensory neurons, the cell bodies of which are found in the gracile nucleus and the cuneate nucleus. The axons of the second sensory neurons cross the midline at the level of the medulla and form the contralateral medial lemniscus pathway. They synapse in the thalamus with third-order neurons, the axons of which end in the parietal lobe's postcentral gyrus, the primary sensory cortex.

[11]Axons forming the spinothalamic tract synapse in the thalamus with third-order neurons which send their axons to the primary sensory cortex.

- The corticospinal tract decussates also at the brainstem level and descends laterally to the butterfly and synapses with the peripheral motor neuron in the frontal horn.

Sympathetic fibers leave the thoracolumbar spinal cord (T1–L2) via different routes compared to sensory and motor fibers. They also join the spinal nerves distally via the sympathetic trunk. This is why nerve root compression does not impair sweating, in contrast to what may be seen with a lesion of the plexus or a peripheral nerve.

Note that the anatomical site of a spinal cord lesion may differ from the clinical level found during bedside examination. This is due to certain features of the spinal vascular supply and the topography of the motor and sensory pathways. There are cases of paraparetic patients operated on for an asymptomatic cervical spinal stenosis who later were found to suffer from thoracic meningioma. Complete neuroimaging of the spinal cord helps avoid such mistakes.

2.4.1 Complete or Near-Complete Transection of the Spinal Cord

Complete or near-complete transection of the spinal cord (Fig. 2.5), as seen with *trauma, tumor, hemorrhage, vascular malformations,* and *infectious and autoimmune myelitis* (e.g., *neuromyelitis optica (NMO)*), leads to the pathognomonic triad:

- Paraparesis (or tetraparesis)
- Sphincter disturbances
- Sensory disturbances below a "sensory level" on the trunk

It is of utmost importance to identify this triad in both the history and bedside examination in every patient suspected of harboring a spinal cord lesion (Case 2.4). Transection of the spinal cord at the cervical level leads to tetraparesis and, if the C3–C5 level is involved, diaphragm palsy and acute dyspnea ("C three, four, and five

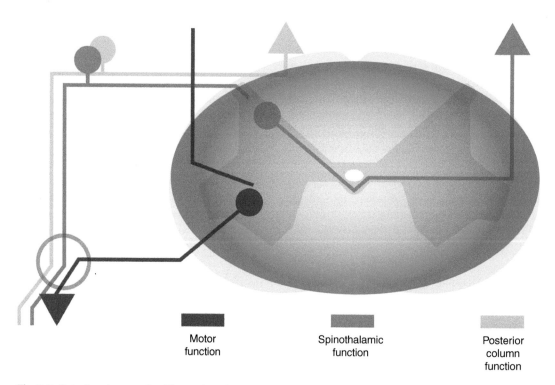

| Motor function | Spinothalamic function | Posterior column function |

Fig. 2.5 Spinal cord transection. Traumatic and nontraumatic spinal cord transections lead to a classical triad of paraparesis, a sensory level on the trunk and sphincter disturbances (*black*, motor pathway; *dark blue*, spinothalamic pathway; *light blue*, posterior column pathway

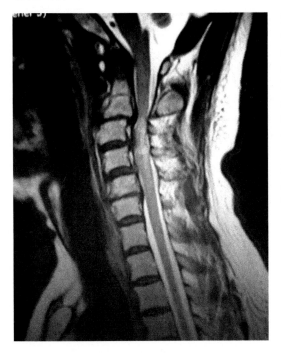

Case 2.4 Compressive cervical medullopathy in Down syndrome. A 49-year-old male with Down syndrome and associated Alzheimer's disease fell off the swing while playing on a playground. He was unable to get up from the ground as his legs gave way. The neurologist on call noticed hyperreflexia in all extremities, bilateral extensive toes, and urinary retention. The patient was unable to participate in a detailed sensory examination, but sensation for pain and temperature seemed decreased below the clavicles. Emergency MRI showed a cervical compressive medullopathy. The patient underwent emergency spinal surgery. Compression of the cervical spinal cord due to atlantoaxial instability (or, as in this case, slightly below this level) is a well-known complication of trisomy 21 (as is progressive cognitive decline due to early onset Alzheimer pathology), which is caused by the triplication of the amyloid precursor protein gene (*APP* located on chromosome 21)

keep the diaphragm alive."). Levels below T1 lead to paraparesis only. During the first phase of severe spinal injury following the traumatic event ("spinal shock"), muscle tone is lost, the weakness is flaccid, and there is hypo- or areflexia. (Note, however, that with incomplete spinal cord injury, hyperreflexia may be found immediately after the injury.) When the spinal shock resolves after days or weeks, weakness usually becomes spastic below the lesion because the corticospinal tract is disrupted. Thus, UMN signs including increased muscle tone, spastic-

ity, hyperreflexia, and extensor plantar reflexes develop. There is one important exception to this rule. At the very level of the spinal cord lesion, the ventral horn and thus the cell bodies of the LMNs are also damaged. Therefore, LMN signs such as flaccid weakness, decreased reflexes, atrophy, and fasciculations may develop at precisely this level. However, the clinical level of the spinal cord damage resulting in motor weakness is best established by assessing the presence or absence of weakness in key muscles. In the upper extremities, these include:

- C5 elbow flexion
- C6 wrist extension
- C7 elbow extension
- C8 long finger flexion
- T1 finger abduction

And in the lower extremities:

- L2 hip flexion
- L3 knee extension
- L4 ankle dorsiflexion
- L5 great toe extension
- S1 ankle plantar flexion

With acute para- or tetraparesis, symptoms will usually be so obvious that a detailed history of motor function is not necessary. However, with subacute or slower development, the most common complaints are stiffness of the legs, decreased walking distance, and dragging of one or both feet.

The patient is usually aware of a clear sensory level, but in cases where sensory disturbances are less pronounced, he may only report a band-like sensation on the trunk. The site of the sensory level corresponds to the uppermost dermatome that is functionally affected by the injury. This usually (but not always) reflects the site of the anatomical lesion. A sensory level corresponds to:

- T4 dermatome if involving the breast nipples
- T10 dermatome if involving the umbilicus
- L1 dermatome if involving the inguinal ligaments

As with muscles of the extremities, the sphincters tend to be paralyzed during the phase of spinal shock. In mild spinal cord injuries, bladder sphincter disturbance is usually more pronounced than anal sphincter dysfunction, resulting in urinary retention. Later, bladder sphincter and detrusor muscles become spastic and urinary urgency may develop. Voluntary anal contraction must always be assessed in the patient with acute spinal cord injury, and its presence or absence should be documented in the charts. With severe spinal cord injuries, temporary paralysis of the GI tract usually occurs. Sexual dysfunction, including erectile dysfunction, is another frequent symptom; all patients with spinal cord injury need empathetic guidance and help with their sexuality.

With chronic spinal cord injury above TH6, painful stimuli in the body below the transection level may lead to acute massive vasoconstriction of the mesenterical vessels and arterial hypertension. This is due to massive uninhibited

sympathetic discharge. Characteristically, the patient is "cold and pale" below the lesion and "red and hot" above. This is called *autonomic dysreflexia* and represents a true medical emergency. Since patients with chronic injury to the cervical or upper thoracic spinal cord usually have very low blood pressure, even blood pressure readings with apparently normal values (e.g., 130/80 mmHg) may be associated with life-threatening hypertensive encephalopathy. Chapter 6 discusses the treatment of autonomic dysreflexia.

2.4.2   Brown-Séquard Syndrome

Hemitransection of the spinal cord is called Brown-Séquard syndrome and denotes a lesion affecting the right or left half of the spinal cord (Fig. 2.6). Classical hemitransection is usually only encountered after *knife stabs* or *gunshots*, but less complete hemitransection may be seen

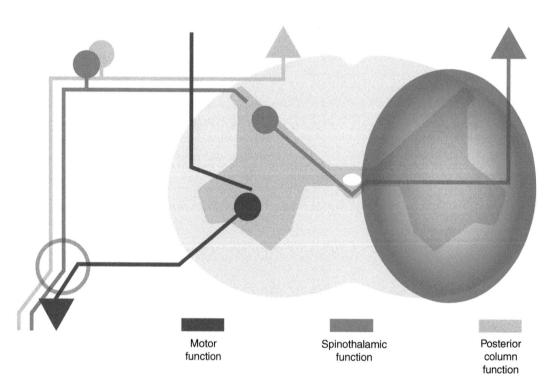

| Motor function | Spinothalamic function | Posterior column function |

Fig. 2.6 Brown-Séquard syndrome (spinal cord hemitransection). Spinal cord hemitransection is associated with injury to the ipsilateral motor pathway (*black*), the ipsilateral posterior column pathway (*light blue*), and the contralateral spinothalamic pathway (*dark blue*)

with, e.g., an *epidural tumor or hemorrhage* and lateral cord compression.

- Motor function will be lost below and ipsilateral to the lesion; thus, a right-sided truncal hemitransection leads to paresis of the right leg. Again, below the lesion weakness is usually spastic, whereas at the level of the lesion, there will be LMN palsy.
- Since the ipsilateral dorsal column is affected, vibration and position sense are impaired in the ipsilateral leg.
- Pain and temperature sense will be affected in the contralateral side of the trunk and the leg due to damage of the spinothalamic tract crossing at the spinal level.

Rephrased, examination of the ipsilateral leg will reveal motor paresis and decreased sensation for vibration and position sense but normal pain and temperature sensation: the contralateral leg,

in contrast, will have intact motor function and normal sensation for vibration and proprioception but disturbed sensation for pain and temperature. This is termed dissociated sensory loss. (Thus, spinothalamic tract sensation is affected, but dorsal column sensation is intact—and vice versa.) Dissociated sensory loss is a highly characteristic sign of spinal cord pathology.

2.4.3 Anterior Cord Syndrome

Infarction of the anterior spinal artery is usually due to occlusion of the artery of Adamkiewicz or of one or several of the many smaller feeding arteries and may occur spontaneously or secondary to, e.g., *aortic dissection* and *thoracic surgery*. It leads to the anterior cord syndrome (Fig. 2.7). Since the spinal anterior artery supplies the ventral two-thirds of the spinal cord, there is dissociated sensory loss with preserved

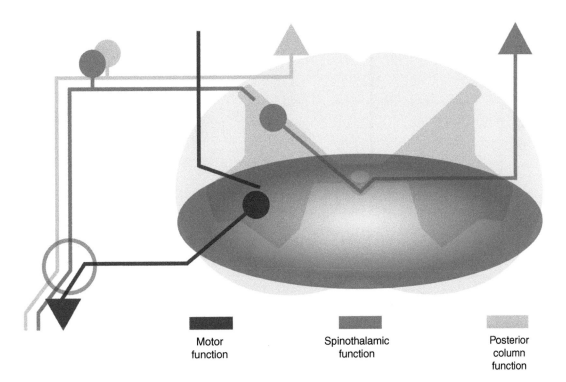

Motor function   Spinothalamic function   Posterior column function

Fig. 2.7 Anterior cord syndrome. With damage to the anterior spinal cord, usually due to infarction of the anterior spinal artery, the ventral two-thirds of the spinal cord will be damaged, leaving the vibration sense and proprioception intact (*black*, motor pathway; *dark blue*, spinothalamic pathway; *light blue*, posterior column pathway)

vibration sense and proprioception but impaired perception of pain and temperature below the affected level. In addition, the patient has a paraparesis with LMN signs at the level of the lesion and upper motor signs below it.

Compressive cervical myelopathy may occasionally affect the anterior horns selectively and lead to bibrachial diplegia of the LMN type. This is another differential diagnosis of the man-in-the-barrel syndrome. Mechanical compression of the spinal cord can be temporary and may be overlooked with MRI in neutral position, e.g., cervical flexion myelopathy associated with an intradural cyst. Spinal cord compression during neck flexion is also well described in *Hirayama disease* (juvenile muscular atrophy of the distal upper extremity), a self-limiting, distal, brachial mono- or diplegia due to segmental anterior horn cell lesion, typically affecting young people, frequently of Asian origin. Sensory symptoms do not occur. The hallmark of this disease is anterior displacement of the cervical spinal cord against the vertebral bodies during neck flexion, visualized only on MRI in flexed position.

2.4.4 Dorsal Cord Syndrome

Dorsal cord syndrome (Fig. 2.8) is characterized by impairment of vibration and proprioception in the legs. Sensation of pain and temperature and motor function are preserved. The most characteristic sign of this syndrome is sensory ataxia. The patient may complain of being unable to walk in the dark or to stand with eyes closed (Romberg's sign). A manifestation of neurosyphilis, *tabes dorsalis* is a classic example of tertiary syphilis. It is exceedingly rare in the developed world nowadays, although syphilis itself is on the rise again. *Subacute combined degeneration* due to *vitamin B12 deficiency* and *copper deficiency myelopathy* have a predilection for the dorsal columns as well but also affect the corticospinal

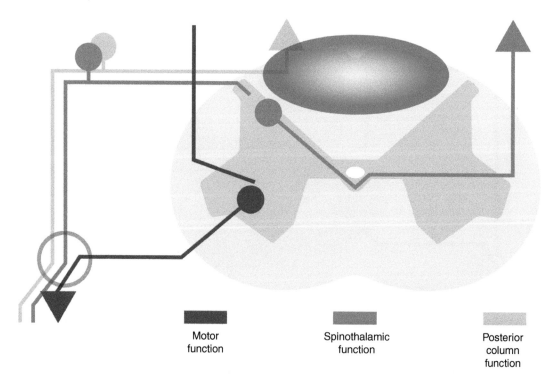

Motor function   Spinothalamic function   Posterior column function

Fig. 2.8 Dorsal cord syndrome. Posterior column function is impaired, but spinothalamic and motor pathways usually stay intact (*black*, motor pathway; *dark blue*, spinothalamic pathway; *light blue*, posterior column pathway) (Color figure online)

tracts, thus leading to a combination of decreased sensation for vibration and position sense and spastic leg weakness. Another example of dorsal cord dysfunction is the useless hand of Oppenheim, occasionally encountered with MS. Whereas power and cutaneous sensation are preserved, loss of proprioception induced by a plaque in the dorsal columns makes the hand more or less useless.

2.4.5 Syringomyelia

Syringomyelia indicates the presence of a fluid-filled cavity (syrinx) within the spinal cord (Fig. 2.9). This cavity can expand and elongate over time, damaging the spinal cord. Syringomyelia in its classic presentation is due to enlargement of the central canal of the cervical and thoracic cord, also termed hydromyelia. Extracanalicular syrinxes, in contrast, are associated with, e.g., cystic spinal tumors or may be seen following absorption of a spinal hemorrhage. The pathophysiology is not well understood. Syringomyelia may arise *spontaneously* and is often an incidental finding on MRI of the spine. Secondary causes include *spinal trauma, hemorrhage, tumor, and myelitis*. Syringomyelia is also frequently encountered in patients with congenital hydrocephalus and the Arnold-Chiari syndrome. Symptomatic syringomyelia has a typical clinical presentation. For unknown reasons, when the central canal dilates, it affects the ventral horn first. The first structures to be damaged are the myelinated fibers of the spinothalamic pathways that cross immediately ventral to the central canal. This is the commissura alba referred to earlier (Fig. 2.4). Since syringomyelia normally affects the cervicothoracic spine, patients present with loss of pain and temperature perception in the hands. They often have a history of painless wounds and injuries to the hands.

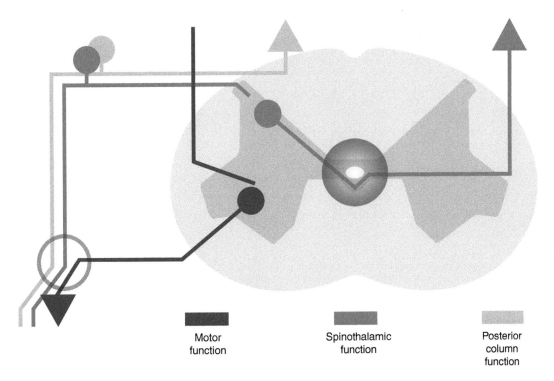

Motor function   Spinothalamic function   Posterior column function

Fig. 2.9 Syringomyelia. The anterior white commissure (*commissura alba*) is a bundle of nerve fibers that cross the midline of the spinal cord just anterior to the central canal. This structure is typically damaged early in cases of syringomyelia, leading to characteristic bilateral impairment of pain and temperature sensation (*black*, motor pathway; *dark blue*, spinothalamic pathway; *light blue*, posterior column pathway) (Color figure online)

Only later does the syrinx involve the whole of the ventral horns and then LMN signs develop, including atrophy, fasciculations, and deformities of both the hands and arms. Continuing enlargement of the syrinx may then damage the ventral horns of the thoracic spinal cord and lead to weakness and atrophy of the truncal musculature and to scoliosis. Bulbar signs such as dysarthria, dysphagia, and tongue paresis can occur with extension of the syrinx into the medulla oblongata. This condition is called *syringobulbia*.

2.4.6 Central Cord Syndrome

Acute traumatic central cord syndrome is usually caused by severe hyperextension of the neck. It is often associated with hemorrhaging in the central part of the spinal cord, destroying the axons of

the inner part of the corticospinal tract serving the arms. The outer part of the corticospinal tract devoted to the motor control of the legs, however, is not severely damaged. Thus, examination reveals bilateral paresis of the arms with more or less preserved power in the legs. It follows that the central cord syndrome is another cause for the man-in-the-barrel syndrome. In addition to the distal, more than proximal, arm weakness, bladder dysfunction and patchy sensory loss below the level of the lesion are seen. The prognosis is related to the degree of axonal damage, but long-term outcome is favorable in many patients.

2.4.7 Conus Medullaris Syndrome

Conus medullaris syndrome is due to a lesion in the lowermost part of the spinal cord (Case 2.5).

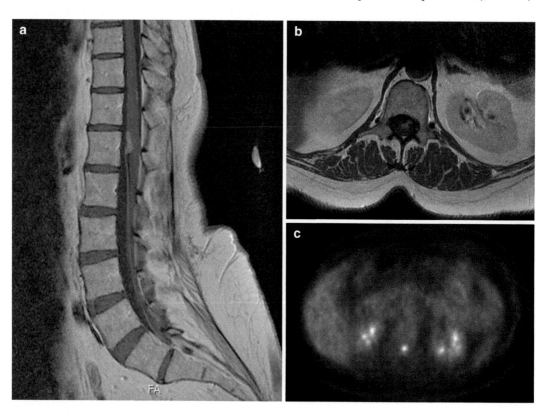

Case 2.5 Conus medullaris metastasis. A 51-year-old woman had received surgery, chemotherapy, and radiation for a non-small cell lung cancer (NSCLC). Two years later, she experienced slight urinary retention and perineal hypoesthesia. MRI revealed a contrast-enhancing lesion in the conus medullaris (**a**, sagittal T1 weighted; **b**, axial T1 weighted; both images following IV gadolinium). This process was hypermetabolic as shown by PET (**c**; note that high signal from the kidneys is a normal feature and due to tracer accumulation in the urine). Lumbar puncture revealed a mild lymphocytic pleocytosis. As CSF microscopy revealed only reactive inflammatory cells, a biopsy was performed which confirmed that this was an NSCLC metastasis

It leads to sphincter impairment of the bladder and bowel, saddle anesthesia, and sexual dysfunction. With a pure conus medullaris syndrome, e.g., due to a MS plaque, a metastasis or an *infectious or postinfectious process*, power in the legs will be normal. In practice, however, it is often combined with a cauda equina syndrome, which was discussed earlier.

2.5   Brainstem

The brainstem, from cranial to caudal, can be divided into three parts:

- Mesencephalon (or midbrain)
- Pons
- Medulla oblongata

The brainstem contains the following structures:

- All sensory pathways coming from the body (afferent pathways) and all motor and autonomic pathways destined for the body (efferent pathways)
- The nuclei of CN III–XII[12]
- Autonomic centers (e.g., respiration, circulation)
- The ARAS, mediating arousal
- The nuclei of the monoaminergic neurons (substantia nigra/dopamine, locus ceruleus/norepinephrine, raphe nuclei/serotonin)

The CN nuclei are organized numerically from cranial to caudal (Fig. 2.10):

- CN III and IV nuclei are found in the mesencephalon.
- The nuclei of CN V, VI, VII, and VIII are located in the pons.
- The medulla oblongata contains the CN nuclei of IX, X, XI, and XII.

---

[12]CN I and CN II do not possess nerve nuclei.

Although somewhat simplified, this list serves all practical purposes. A notable exception is the trigeminal nerve (CN V). As stated above, its motor nucleus is in the pons, but the sensory trigeminal nerve nuclei reside within the entire brainstem (midbrain, pons, and medulla).

The vertical organization of the CN nuclei has clinical significance insofar as CN palsies, and loss of brainstem reflexes can be used to define the site of a lesion on a cranial-caudal and left-right axis.

- Cranial-caudal axis. Brainstem lesions with impairment of the *pupillary reflex* involve the mesencephalon (afferent, CN II; efferent, CN III). The *corneal reflex* is located in the pons (afferent, CN V; efferent, CN VII); *the vestibulo-cephalic reflex and vestibulo-ocular reflex* (VOR) involve both the pons and mesencephalon (afferent, CN VIII; efferent, CN III and VI); and the *gag and cough reflexes* are mediated by the medulla oblongata (afferent, CN IX; efferent, CN X).
- Left-right axis. Brainstem lesions often lead to *crossed deficits with ipsilateral CN deficits and contralateral long tract signs* (Fig. 2.10). The latter is due to the fact that most brainstem lesions affect the corticospinal tract above its decussation in the medulla oblongata, and they affect the spinothalamic tract after it crosses the midline at the spinal cord level. Consequently, a patient with a right-sided pontine hemorrhage may present with right-sided facial palsy (CN VII) and a left-sided hemiparesis and/or hemihypesthesia. The facial palsy in this case will be peripheral due to damage to the facial nerve nucleus that contains the cells of the second motor neurons.

There is an exception to the rule of brainstem damage leading to crossed cranial nerve and long tract deficits: lesions affecting the corticopontine tract fibers to the face above the nucleus of the facial nerve can induce a contralateral central facial palsy (Fig. 2.10).

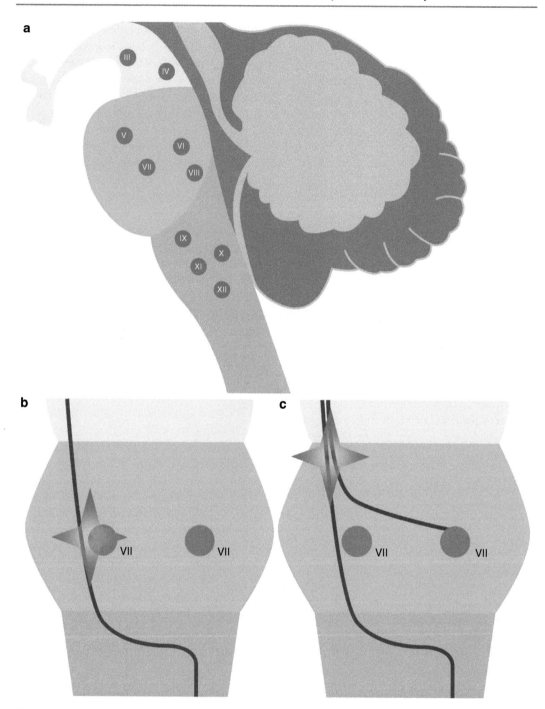

Fig. 2.10 Brainstem. The brainstem consists of the midbrain, the pons, and the medulla oblongata. The CN nuclei are organized numerically from cranial to caudal (**a**). Although the motor nucleus of CN V is in the pons, the sensory CN V nuclei reside within the entire brainstem (not shown). Observe that CN I and CN II do not posses nuclei and are therefore not depicted here. A brainstem lesion typically leads to crossed deficits with ipsilateral CN impairment and contralateral long tract signs, e.g., a right peripheral facial palsy and a left hemiparesis (**b**). However, lesions affecting the corticopontine pathway to the face above the nucleus of CN VII occasionally induce a contralateral central facial palsy (**c**)

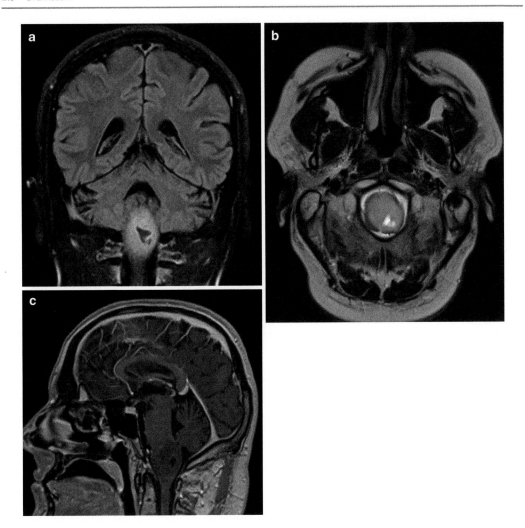

Case 2.6 Brainstem glioma. A 26-year-old male with an unremarkable medical history had noticed subtle difficulties swallowing and slightly slurred speech for the previous 4 months. Recently, he had also noticed visual blurring and subsequently minor double vision during highway driving. (Slowly progressive diplopia is often first noticed during visual tasks at distance, e.g., driving, because small-angle misalignments become symptomatic.) In addition, he had experienced mild sensory symptoms from his left hand for a few days. MR of the brain revealed a large cystic pontine tumor (FLAIR, **a**; T2, **b**) without contrast enhancement (T1-weighted with gadolinium, **c**). The discrepancy between the massive tumor infiltration of the brainstem and the relative paucity of clinical symptoms is typical for a brainstem glioma. Given the classic tumor presentation and the high periprocedural risk, a brainstem biopsy was not performed. The patient was treated with radiation therapy and temozolomide. Two years later, he continued to be independent in his activities of daily living despite moderate dysarthria, a left foot drop, and mild ataxia of gait

Other typical brainstem symptoms are *diplopia*, *dysphagia*, and *dysarthria* (Case 2.6).[13]

Lesions involving the vestibular nuclei (CV VIII) or the cerebellar-pontine tracts may lead to *acute vertigo*.

In conclusion, as a rule of thumb, brainstem lesions lead to ipsilateral CN palsies and contralateral sensory and motor signs in the extremities; CN palsy therefore localizes the lesion in the brainstem both on the cranial-caudal and left-right axes.

---

[13] Please bear in mind that dysphagia, dysarthria, and diplopia are also often due to diseases of the muscle, neuromuscular junction, or cranial nerves. Non-neurological causes are common as well, e.g., dysphagia and dysarthria due to tonsillitis. Also note that distinguishing disturbed speech (dysarthria) from abnormal language (dysphasia) is crucial. The latter is not a brainstem sign; it is a cortical phenomenon.

2.6 Cranial Nerves

2.6.1 Olfactory Nerve

The olfactory nerve (CN I) is not a part of the brainstem, but is discussed here for convenience. The olfactory bulb may be damaged by trauma, an olfactory glioma, or a frontal lobe meningioma. Neurodegenerative disorders such as AD and Parkinson's disease (PD) may affect olfaction before cognitive and motor functions. *Loss of olfaction*, however, is much more frequently due to the common cold and local causes in the nasal cavity.

The patient will normally notice the loss of taste, but not necessarily the olfactory loss. Taste, although mediated by CN VII and IX, is very much a matter of olfaction. (This is why food may seem tasteless when eaten without breathing.) Thus, during the history, ask whether the patient can smell, e.g., coffee or perfume, or whether food no longer tastes as good as it used to do.

Whereas lesions of the primary olfactory cortex in the temporal lobe may lead to epileptic olfactory hallucinations, olfactory bulb tumors can provoke nonepileptic sensations that usually involve rather unpleasant odors. The intimate connection between the piriform cortex, the amygdala, the entorhinal cortex, and the other limbic regions explains why olfaction instantly evokes memories and emotions. (For a complex, poetic, study of this subject, see Marcel Proust's *Remembrance of Things Past*.)

2.6.2 Optic Nerve

Similar to the olfactory nerve, the optic nerve (CN II) is more an outpouching of the central nervous system (CNS) than a true CN and thus lacks a CN nucleus. Its myelin is produced by oligodendrocytes instead of Schwann cells, and it is surrounded by the dura, arachnoidea, and pia mater instead of the epi-, peri-, and endoneurium. Complete loss of optic nerve function leads to *blindness of the affected eye* and may either develop acutely or chronically.

Occlusion of the ophthalmic artery due to an embolus from a carotid artery plaque is a common cause of acute monocular blindness. With the help of an ophthalmoscope, the examiner may sometimes notice a small cholesterol embolus occluding one of the central retinal artery branches, leading to focal ischemic changes distally of the occlusion. More commonly, ischemic retinal infarction does not occur and visual function is restored after a few minutes. This condition is called *amaurosis fugax*. Although atherosclerosis of the internal carotid is by far the most common source of the embolus, cardiac sources of retinal artery emboli are well described. Amaurosis fugax should therefore be dealt with similar to any other transient ischemic attack.

Whereas amaurosis fugax leads to instant monocular blindness, the following conditions develop rather subacutely or chronically and may involve one or both optic nerves.

Patients with *idiopathic intracranial hypertension* (sometimes called pseudotumor cerebri) complain about headache and transient visual obscurations that may progress to blindness. Ophthalmoscopy initially reveals loss of spontaneous venous pulsations (SVP) and later established papilledema. Irreversible loss of vision represents a significant threat, which is why "benign intracranial hypertension" is a somewhat unfortunate term. Visual symptoms and headache may or may not be accentuated by Valsalva-like maneuvers. The vast majority of these patients are obese young females and recent weight gain is often reported. The diagnosis of idiopathic intracranial hypertension requires exclusion of cerebral venous sinus thrombosis, intracranial structural pathology, and extracerebral venous outflow obstruction (e.g., paraganglioma with compression of the jugular veins).

Headache and transient visual obscurations are also common with *secondarily increased intracranial hypertension* due to, as stated previously, a cerebral tumor or cerebral venous sinus thrombosis. Again, ophthalmoscopic examination may reveal papilledema of varying degree. In contrast, if papilledema is absent and spontaneous pulsations of the central retinal veins are visible, intracranial pressure (ICP) is normal—at least at the time of examination.

Orthostatic hypotension commonly leads to transient visual obscurations in the absence of papilledema.

Although bilateral scotomata are much more common, unilateral blindness occasionally occurs during the aura of a *migraine attack*.

Anterior ischemic optic neuropathy (AION) may also present with acute or subacute visual loss of one or both eyes and is divided into *arteritic* and *non-arteritic AION*. AION is much more common in people 50 years of age or older.

- Arteritic AION is almost always due to *temporal arteritis* (or giant cell arteritis). A typical patient is an elderly patient who complains about generalized muscle tenderness (polymyalgia rheumatica), pain in the temples or the jaw while chewing (jaw claudication), and tenderness with palpation of the temporal region. Visual disturbances are an urgent warning that irreversible loss of sight may soon occur. A prominent temporal artery may be seen upon inspection. As a rule, the erythrocyte sedimentation rate should be checked in every patient more than 50 years of age with new-onset headache of unknown origin. Beware that, occasionally, the erythrocyte sedimentation rate is normal and a temporal biopsy negative (if an unaffected part of the artery has been removed). Only rarely is arteritic AION due to *other types of vasculitis*, e.g., polyarteritis nodosa, SLE, or herpes zoster. Takayasu's disease is a large-vessel inflammatory arteriopathy that predominantly affects young females and may lead to transitory neurological symptoms, including amaurosis fugax. The disease is also called "pulseless disease" because stenosis of the brachial arteries can lead to a decrease of pulse and blood pressure in the arms.
- Non-arteritic AION is probably the most common cause of sudden visual loss due to optic nerve damage in the elderly. There are two main risk factors for non-arteritic AION. The first is *congenital small optic discs*, which can be detected on ophthalmoscopic examination

and which may compromise vascular supply of the optic nerve fibers; the second is related to *general cardiovascular risk factors* such as hypertension, smoking, and high cholesterol levels.

Very common, of course, is *optic neuritis*. In the young, this is the most frequent disorder associated with acute or subacute visual disturbance. Pain on movement of the affected eye is a common complaint with acute optic neuritis and may sometimes precede the visual impairment. Complete blindness is very rare and normally only encountered in patients with severe and long-standing MS or NMO. Patients usually complain of blurred or foggy vision. Although the patient may not be aware of a loss or decrease in color vision in the affected eye, this can easily be documented on examination. Ask the patient to close the affected eye and to focus on a red object. (Red perception is usually lost first.) Then ask the patient to close the other (healthy) eye and focus on the object using the affected eye. In the case of optic neuritis, the patient will usually report ipsilateral decrease of color intensity and brightness. An ophthalmoscopy may show papilledema with anterior, but not with retrobulbar, neuritis. In a patient with MS and lack of current visual complaints, optic atrophy and desaturation to red may suggest a former episode of optic neuritis. Some 50–70% of patients presenting with optic neuritis will eventually develop other evidence of MS.

Severe optic neuritis that simultaneously or subsequently involves both eyes combined with myelitis strongly suggests a diagnosis of *NMO*, also called Devic's disease. This is a severe autoimmune neuroinflammatory disorder associated with aquaporin-4 antibodies that may leave the patient blind and paraplegic, if not treated with aggressive immunomodulatory therapy. Consult Chap. 4, the differential diagnosis of demyelinating diseases, for further information.

Leber's hereditary optic neuropathy (LHON) is a mitochondrial disease leading to degeneration of retinal ganglion cells and their axons. It leads to an acute (!) or subacute loss of central vision and affects predominantly, but not exclusively, young adult males. A diagnosis of LHON should be considered in every young patient with sudden visual loss and lack of obvious reasons. Sudden onset of visual loss is usually one-sided in the beginning, but after some weeks or months, the other eye is affected as well. Severe optic atrophy and permanent decrease of visual acuity will eventually result. Examination may reveal an afferent pupillary defect, papilledema in the acute stage, followed by optic atrophy in the chronic stage, decreased visual acuity, loss of color vision, and scotoma.

Toxic optic neuropathy may occur from exposure to carbon monoxide, ethylene glycol, methanol, and toluene or may result from an adverse drug reaction. Many drugs have been associated with optic nerve disease, e.g., amiodarone, ethambutol, linezolid, and phosphodiesterase type 5 (PDE-5) inhibitors (sildenafil, vardenafil, and tadalafil). However, whether or not PDE-5 inhibitors may induce visual loss due to non-arteritic AION is not established beyond doubt. Tobacco-alcohol amblyopia is a toxic-nutritional optic neuropathy encountered in smokers with poor dietary habits and long-standing alcohol abuse. It may be reversible with the replacement of B vitamins and cessation of smoking.

Monocular loss developing over many months or years may occur with an *optic nerve glioma* (typically encountered in patients with neurofibromatosis type I) or a tumor compressing the optic nerve, e.g., a *sphenoid sinus meningioma*. With the latter process, the patient may exhibit the Foster-Kennedy syndrome. This syndrome is revealed by ophthalmoscopy showing ipsilateral optic nerve atrophy due to the tumor compressing the ipsilateral CN II and contralateral papilledema due to increased ICP.

Obviously, the neurologist must remember that many *primary ocular diseases* lead to acute (e.g., glaucoma, retinal detachment) or chronic (e.g., cataract, retinitis pigmentosa) monocular or binocular blindness. Disturbances of the visual system located at or behind the optic chiasm will be discussed together with dysfunction of subcortical white matter pathways and the occipital cortex later in this chapter.

2.6.3 Oculomotor Nerve, Trochlear Nerve, Abducens Nerve

2.6.3.1 Supranuclear, Infranuclear, and Nuclear Dysfunction of Eye Movements

For the sake of convenience, dysfunction of the oculomotor nerve (CN III), trochlear nerve (CN IV), and abducens nerve (CN VI) is reviewed here together with eye movement disturbances due to lesions of the brainstem and cerebrum. But first some words of comfort: Everyone who is not an experienced neuro-ophthalmologist finds that the anatomy of eye movements is difficult, and clinical assessment can be rather frustrating in the beginning. Therefore, most neurologists use an approach based on pattern recognition and try to classify eye movement disturbances into a few easily recognized syndromes. All other cases are termed as unclassifiable, and then an experienced neuro-ophthalmologist is consulted, if available. In many such cases, eye muscle paresis will not be due to defective nervous supply but rather due to disorders of the eye muscles themselves (e.g., external ophthalmoplegia in mitochondrial disorders), the neuromuscular junction (e.g., fluctuating gaze palsies in MG), or the orbit and the eye itself (e.g., exophthalmos and diplopia in Graves' disease).

The following eye movement disturbances due to impaired *supranuclear, nuclear, or peripheral nervous supply* should be recognized by the neurologist at the bedside:

- Lesions of the supranuclear pathways include contralateral and ipsilateral horizontal gaze palsies and supranuclear vertical gaze palsy (Parinaud's syndrome).[14]
- Brainstem syndromes include nuclear CN palsies, internuclear ophthalmoplegia (INO), the one-and-a half syndrome, skew deviation, opsoclonus, and some forms of nystagmus (in addition to ipsilateral horizontal gaze palsy and the Parinaud's syndrome).

---

[14]"Supranuclear" means "above the cranial nerve nuclei," in this case the nuclei of CN III, IV, and VI.

- Lesions of the CNs include external, internal, and complete oculomotor nerve palsy,[15] trochlear nerve palsy, and abducens nerve palsy.

In severe cases, complete ophthalmoplegia may arise with lesions at the supranuclear and nuclear level (e.g., progressive supranuclear palsy (PSP), Wernicke's encephalopathy) or with combined palsies of the oculomotor, trochlear, and abducens nerves (e.g., leptomeningeal carcinomatous infiltration, GBS, basal meningitis due to, i.e., neuroborreliosis, TB) or with impairment of the external eye muscles (e.g., mitochondrial disorders, Graves' disease). For the analysis of eye movements in comatose patients, see Chap. 3.

Supranuclear dysfunction of eye movements can be due to supratentorial and infratentorial lesions. A large ischemic or hemorrhagic stroke in one hemisphere leads to *contralateral horizontal gaze palsy*. For example, a patient with a left hemispheric stroke cannot move his eyes across the midline and look to the right. In the early phase, the eyes typically deviate to the left. Thus, contralateral gaze palsy is associated with ipsilateral gaze deviation. (The patient looks toward the lesion.) With epilepsy, the opposite is the case (*ipsilateral gaze palsy*). A patient with an epileptic seizure due to a left-sided lesion may have gaze deviation toward the right. (The patient looks away from the lesion.) The reason for this, somewhat simplified, is that the hemispheres exert tonic control of the eyes; the right hemisphere "pulls" the eyes to the left and the left hemisphere to the right. With a left-sided stroke, the tonic control of the left hemisphere is weakened, and consequently, the relatively larger tonic control from the right hemisphere induces deviation of the eyes to the left (toward the lesion). With an epileptic seizure, tonic control increases at the site of the epileptic focus; thus, a seizure focus in the left hemisphere will overpower the right hemisphere and "pull" the eyes toward the right (away from the lesion). Because of damage to the pontine gaze center, an infratentorial supranuclear stroke will lead to ipsilateral gaze palsy, and the eyes will deviate toward the contralateral side (away from the lesion); thus, gaze palsies due to a brainstem stroke lead to the exact opposite of what is seen with supratentorial hemispheric stroke.

Supranuclear vertical gaze palsy is usually due to a lesion at the dorsal midbrain at the site of the superior colliculi of the tectum, the third ventricle, or the Sylvian aqueduct. Pineal gland tumors in the young and metastases and thalamic hemorrhages in the elderly are common lesions, but any inflammatory or vascular upper brainstem process may be responsible. Thiamine deficiency due to alcohol abuse is another common cause. Obstructive hydrocephalus due to stenosis of the aqueduct, a pinealoma, or a third ventricle tumor may also lead to a supranuclear vertical palsy; sustained downgaze is called the "setting sun sign." The palsy is supranuclear insofar as vertical gaze is possible with the (vertical) doll's eye maneuver. Thus, both oculomotor nerves and their nuclei (which are part of the vestibulo-ocular reflex pathways) are intact. This is also true for PSP, a neurodegenerative disorder of the parkinsonian spectrum associated with mesencephalic atrophy (see below). Supranuclear vertical gaze palsy is often combined with eyelid retraction (Collier's sign) and pupillary abnormalities (*Parinaud's syndrome*).[16]

Internuclear ophthalmoplegia (INO) is due to a lesion of the medial longitudinal fasciculus (MLF) in the brainstem. The MLF connects the abducens nerve nucleus of one side with the oculomotor nucleus of the other side. This is important for conjugate lateral gaze. If the patient looks to the right, the right eye is abducted (CN VI on the right side) and the left eye adducted (CN III on the left side). This is accomplished with the

---

[15] "External" and "internal" refer to the external eye muscles, respectively, the muscles of the iris. Thus, an external ophthalmoplegia leaves the pupillary function intact, whereas with an internal CN III paresis, there is mydriasis.

[16] Parinaud's syndrome (also known as dorsal midbrain syndrome) includes supranuclear gaze palsy, pupillary dysfunction characterized by poor reaction to light (but normal to accommodation) and convergence-retraction nystagmus.

help of the MLF. With a left-sided lesion of the MFL, adduction of the left eye will no longer be possible. Upon the attempt to look to the right, the left eye will be fixed in the midline, whereas a compensatory nystagmus is seen in the abducted right eye. However, the patient will have no problem looking to the left. As a rule, INO in young patients is due to MS and in the elderly due to a vascular event in the brainstem. INO may also be seen as part of Wernicke's encephalopathy. For all practical purposes, *bilateral* INO is pathognomonic for MS.

Knowing the anatomic substrate of the *one-and-a-half syndrome* does not lead to any clinical benefit, but since the neurologist will encounter the syndrome every now and again, being able to recognize it is a good idea. It is characterized by dysconjugate horizontal gaze palsy in one direction and an INO in the other. Consequently, one eye is completely fixed in the midline, whereas the other eye is turned outward at baseline and fixed in the midline when looking in the opposite direction. The clinical relevance of the one-and-a-half syndrome is comparable to INO.

Skew deviation is a vertical misalignment of the eyes usually seen in the context of brainstem or cerebellar injury from stroke, MS, trauma, or tumors. It can be accompanied by torticollis and a tilt in the subjective visual vertical axis. Skew deviation may be subtle and compensated for by focused gaze. Compensated skew deviation can be detected during the bedside examination. The examiner may prevent compensation by covering one of the patient's eyes (cover test), which makes supranuclear compensation impossible, and the covered eye will deviate vertically from its baseline position. The eye returns to baseline when uncovered again. This vertical movement reveals the compensated skew deviation. Admittedly, it takes some practice until this test provides reliable results, but it is important in the evaluation of the patient presenting with acute vertigo. Skew deviation in such a patient is strongly suggestive of a brainstem or cerebellar lesion, as discussed later. Of course, the cover test may also reveal latent strabismus that is not associated with an acute vascular pathology.

Vertical nystagmus (upbeat, downbeat) also suggests an upper brainstem or cerebellar lesion. Downbeat nystagmus is seen in bilateral disturbance of the cerebellar flocculus and in lesions at the craniocervical junction, such as in Arnold-Chiari malformation. Also, cerebellar degeneration and intoxications (such as with antiepileptic drugs and lithium) can produce downbeat nystagmus. Upbeat nystagmus, when present in the primary position, is usually associated with focal brainstem lesions in the tegmental gray matter, e.g., due to multiple sclerosis, malignancy, ischemic infarction, and cerebellar degeneration. In the young, vertical nystagmus is of course most likely due to MS, and in the elderly, it is usually due to a vascular or neoplastic process. Yet the rule of the three Ws should not be forgotten: Vertical nystagmus may be seen with Wernicke's encephalopathy, Wilson's disease, and Whipple's disease. See-saw nystagmus (one eye rises and intorts, whereas the other falls and extorts, and the other way round) and convergence-retraction nystagmus (repetitive adducting saccades, accompanied by retraction of the eyes into the orbit) are associated with diencephalic or mesencephalic lesions. In contrast, the so-called pendular nystagmus is usually congenital and more frequent in people with albinism. (Chap. 3 discusses *horizontal nystagmus*.)

Opsoclonus is characterized by completely chaotic, fast, multidirectional, and involuntary eye movements that puzzle everyone unfamiliar with this phenomenon. It is typically part of opsoclonus-myoclonus-ataxia syndrome and often of paraneoplastic origin. In adults, it is usually associated with lung, breast, and ovarian cancer; in children, it can be secondary to a neuroblastoma. However, opsoclonus can also be due to a postinfectious autoimmune process, where it has a much better prognosis.

Nuclear and peripheral dysfunctions of eye movements are related to impairment of CN III, CN IV, and CN VI due to damage to their nuclei in the brainstem or along the path of the nerves outside the brainstem. The patient with defective ocular motility due to a CN lesion usually complains of diplopia of recent onset. There are different algorithms for assessing diplopia, all of which are rather complicated, which is why you can also simply ask the patient whether the double images are strictly horizontal or somewhat vertically and diagonally displaced. Sometimes showing the patient a drawing comprised of four circles, two strictly horizontally and two diagonally displaced, is useful. Strictly horizontal double images are likely due to a defect of eye abduction (CN VI) or eye adduction (INO or CN III; however, with a lesion of CN III, there is usually a vertical component as well). Vertically displaced double images make a lesion of CN III or CN IV much more likely. The neurologist should then assess eye movements using the techniques discussed in Chap. 3 and analyze whether the findings are compatible with an INO or a lesion of one of the three CNs as discussed in the following. (Always be sure to rule out monocular diplopia: persisting diplopia when the patient closes the other eye is due to local eye disease and an aberration of the ocular media, e.g., due to a cataract.)

All external eye muscles are innervated by the *oculomotor nerve* (CN III), except the superior oblique muscle, which is innervated by the *trochlear nerve* (CN IV), and the lateral rectus muscle, which is innervated by the *abducens nerve* (CN VI). As a consequence, CN VI mediates horizontal abduction of the eye and CN IV mediates depression and intorsion. If you find the precise movements mediated by CN IV difficult to remember, then recall that the superior oblique muscle allows us to look down and fixate the tip of the nose.[17] All other eye movements are mediated by CN III. This nerve also innervates the levator palpebrae superioris muscle that elevates and retracts the upper eyelid. In addition, CN III has parasympathetic fibers that serve the iris sphincter muscle, the action of which results in pupillary constriction (miosis).

In conclusion, a lesion of CN VI leads to a unilateral deficit of abduction, and damage to CN

IV impairs downward and inward movement of the eye. Injury of CN III may result in complete drooping of the eyelid (ptosis), pupillary dilatation (mydriasis), and displacement of the eye downward and outward. Thus, in a patient with CN III palsy, the affected eye is "down and out" due to the combined action of the preserved CN IV and CN VI.

Along their path outside the brainstem, CN III, IV, and VI may be damaged individually or in combination with:

- Trauma.
- Elevated ICP (leading to CN III or CN VI palsies, so-called false localizing signs).
- Skull base tumors and metastatic infiltration, including lymphoma.
- Aneurysms of the arterial Circle of Willis.
- Cavernous sinus thrombosis.
- Carotid-cavernous fistula (which can be low flow or high flow, traumatic or spontaneous, and direct or indirect via internal carotid artery branches).
- Microvascular infarction as seen with diabetes mellitus.
- Inflammatory diseases (e.g., GBS, vasculitis, SLE).
- Basilar meningitis due to infectious (e.g., tuberculosis, Lyme disease) and noninfectious processes (e.g., sarcoidosis).
- Orbital processes. Lesions within the orbit that produce CN III, IV, and CN VI palsies typically lead to optic neuropathy and proptosis as well.
- Hyperthyroidism (Graves' disease).
- Tolosa-Hunt syndrome, a rare and ill-defined inflammatory disorder of unknown origin that affects the cavernous sinus and superior orbital fissure, characterized by severe unilateral headache and ophthalmoplegia; a granulomatous disorder, it responds to corticosteroids and diagnosis is a matter of exclusion.

2.6.3.2 Oculomotor Nerve

As stated above, CN III palsies can be divided into *internal*, *external*, and *complete oculomotor nerve palsies*. "External" and "internal" refer to the external eye muscles and the internal muscles

---

[17]CN IV is unique in that its axons cross the midline before emerging from the brainstem. Thus, a lesion of the trochlear nucleus affects the *contralateral* eye. Lesions of all other cranial nuclei (CN III, CN V, CN XII) affect the *ipsilateral* side.

of the iris, respectively. CN III palsies can also be divided into those that spare the pupil and those that do not. The nerve fibers supplying the pupil run superficially in the oculomotor nerve. This is why these fibers are damaged early by compression, e.g., due to *cerebral aneurysms* (arising from the internal carotid, posterior communicating, basilar, or SCA) or cerebral herniation due to *elevated ICP*. Thus, the first oculomotor sign that arises during brainstem herniation is anisocoria. A complete CN III only becomes visible later. In contrast, the nerve fibers supplying the external eye muscles run deeply within the oculomotor nerve. This is why they are easily affected by microvascular infarction as seen with *diabetes mellitus*, in which case the superficial fibers and pupil function tend to be spared. In other words:

- It is traditionally thought that CN III palsy is not caused by an aneurysm if pupillary function is preserved; however, this rule should only apply for complete (as opposed to incomplete) CN III palsies. Thus, in an elderly patient presenting with a sudden-onset painless eye muscle palsy of the "down and out" type and sparing of the pupils, blood sugar levels should be checked. Thiamine deficiency because of alcohol abuse and giant cell arteritis are also common causes.
- In contrast, as a rule of thumb, a pupil that suddenly turns mydriatic and is not responding to light (with or without external eye muscle palsies, with or without pain) is a surgical problem until proven otherwise. If consciousness is normal, a non-ruptured aneurysm must be ruled out. If consciousness decreases, cerebral herniation is an imminent threat, especially if other focal signs are present. When a surgical cause has been ruled out, the diagnosis is likely ophthalmological.[18]

Adie's tonic pupil is a benign condition of presumed autoimmune etiology. Injury to the ciliary ganglion or short ciliary nerves results in dener-

vation of the iris sphincter and ciliary muscle. The patient may notice difficulty reading and complain about being easily blinded by light. Examination typically reveals light-near dissociation; i.e., the affected pupil is large and reacts poorly or not at all to light but responds much better (although often delayed) to near stimulation. Subsequent involvement of the other pupil can occur in some patients. Although Adie's tonic pupil occurs most commonly in adult women, it can develop at any age and may affect men as well. The combination of Adie's pupil, loss of deep tendon reflexes, and excessive (or sometimes decreased) sweating is termed *Holmes-Adie syndrome*. This condition is as mysterious as it is harmless.

Another rare syndrome is *hippus*, a prominent, repetitive oscillation of the pupils. Although it can be a physiological variant of pupillary unrest in healthy people, hippus occurring after traumatic or anoxic-ischemic brain injury is associated with increased 30-day mortality (Denny et al. 2008).

2.6.3.3 Trochlear Nerve

Patients with CN IV palsy usually complain of binocular vertical diplopia and the tilting of objects (torsional diplopia). They may have difficulties descending stairs due to *the inability to look down and inward*. They often have a characteristic compensatory head posture with the head tilted to one side and the chin tucked in (Bielschowsky's sign). The compensatory head tilt is usually away from the side of the lesion. A patient with a chronic superior oblique palsy may possess old photographs that clearly show the head tilt. Diabetic microinfarction is not as common as with CN III and CN VI. Due to its long intracranial path, the trochlear nerve is rather susceptible to trauma. Trauma may even provoke bilateral CN IV palsies; less frequent causes include clivus tumors such as lymphoma and metastatic disease.

Superior oblique myokymia is a rare ocular motility disorder with high-frequency, low-amplitude monocular torsional tremor. Superior oblique myokymia is characterized by intermittent oscillopsia (a visual disturbance in which objects in the visual field appear to oscillate) and

---

[18]However, it is not uncommon for neurologists to be asked to evaluate an alert patient after surgery or trauma with a large pupil; these patients often turn out to be friendly and unconcerned people without any other focal signs than habitual anisocoria.

diplopia, which can be particularly troublesome when reading. One hypothesis is that superior oblique myokymia may be due to neurovascular compression at the root exit zone of the trochlear nerve. Thus, the pathogenesis of superior oblique myokymia is analogous to hemifacial spasm and trigeminal neuralgia, which can arise with neurovascular compression of the facial and trigeminal nerve, respectively.

2.6.3.4 Abducens Nerve

Patients with CN VI palsies complain about binocular *horizontal diplopia* being worse in the gaze direction of the paretic lateral rectus muscle. If CN VI palsy develops slowly over time, diplopia typically will not be noticed until fusional capacity becomes inadequate. Failure of fusion and diplopia are then initially intermittent, often influenced by factors such as alcohol and fatigue. In the beginning, blurring and diplopia usually occur when the patient looks at distant objects, e.g., while driving (for many people, the most frequent visual task performed at distance). It is important to note that CN VI palsy, especially if bilateral, can be a *non-localizing sign of increased ICP*. (Also decreased ICP as seen after a lumbar puncture may lead to CN VI palsies.)

Elderly patients with an isolated CN VI palsy and headache, scalp tenderness, jaw claudication, or visual loss should be evaluated for *temporal arteritis*. *Diabetic microinfarction* and *thiamine deficiency* (as part of Wernicke's encephalopathy) are also common causes of abducens nerve palsy.

Due to the close proximity of the CN VI nucleus to the facial nerve, a brainstem lesion affecting the CN VI nucleus will usually lead to additional peripheral facial palsy (see Case 3.6 for illustration).

2.6.3.5 Horner's Syndrome

Horner's syndrome is a dysfunction of the sympathetic nerve fibers in the upper quadrant of the ipsilateral half of the face, leading to the classic triad of *miosis, ptosis, and anhidrosis*. The sympathetic innervation consists of a chain of three neurons:

- First-order neurons. Their cell bodies reside in the hypothalamus, and their axons synapse in the spinal cord with second-order neurons.

- Second-order neurons. Their cell bodies are found in the lateral column of the thoracolumbar spinal cord (T1–L2), and their axons, the so-called preganglionic nerve fibers, synapse with third-order neurons.
- Third-order neurons. Their cell bodies are in the sympathetic paravertebral trunk. The postganglionic nerve fibers that leave the superior cervical ganglion travel along the carotid artery. The sympathetic fibers leading to the face follow the external carotid artery, while other fibers follow the internal carotid artery and join CN III on the way into the orbit.

Lesions leading to Horner's syndrome may therefore be of central or peripheral origin. *Vertebral artery dissection*, for instance, may evoke infarction of the lateral medulla oblongata (Wallenberg syndrome) and damage to the first-order sympathetic neuronal axons, leading to ipsilateral Horner's syndrome. A *tumor of the upper lung apex or lower brachial plexus* (Pancoast tumor) may damage the second-order neurons and provoke Horner's syndrome as well. The third-order neurons may be injured by *carotid artery dissection*; if only the fibers to the orbit are damaged (e.g., due to isolated internal carotid artery dissection), it may lead to Horner's syndrome without anhidrosis. Common non-lesional causes of Horner's syndrome include cluster headache and migraine.

2.6.4 Trigeminal Nerve

The trigeminal nerve (CN V) mediates *sensation in the face* and has motor branches that mainly serve *muscles of mastication*. Facial sensation is mediated by the following branches:

- The ophthalmic nerve (V1) carries sensation from the forehead to the tip of the nose.
- The maxillary nerve (V2) from the tip of the nose to the upper lip.
- The mandibular nerve (V3) from the upper lip to the chin, including the mandibular region.[19]

---

[19]The mnemonic *Standing Room Only* may assist in remembering that V_1 passes through the superior orbital fissure, V_2 through the foramen rotundum, and V_3 through the foramen ovale.

A lesion of one of these sensory branches may therefore lead to hypesthesia in the corresponding facial area. However, also note that lesions of the spinal trigeminal nucleus in the brainstem, representing pain and temperature sensation, lead to a different pattern of facial sensory disturbance.

- The part of the sensory trigeminal nucleus that lies in the upper cervical cord and the part of the lower medulla represents the scalp, ears, and chin.
- The part of the nucleus in the upper medulla represents the nose, cheeks, and lips.
- The most rostral part in the pons represents the mouth, teeth, and pharyngeal cavity.

Thus, a lesion of the lower brainstem may lead to sensory loss according to an onion skin type distribution that is entirely different from the dermatome distribution of the peripheral branches of the fifth nerve. A patient with a *brainstem transitory ischemic attack*, for instance, may complain about paresthesias in an area that covers the entire mouth.

As far as the sensory function of CN V is concerned, simply asking the patient whether sensation in the face is normal is often sufficient. Examination should be restricted to pinprick sensation. Detailed sensory examination in a suggestible patient often leads to unreliable and potentially confusing results.

The pain of *trigeminal neuralgia* is usually highly intense and involves the area served by V3 and less frequently by V2 and V3. The patient describes an electric shock-like sensation lasting from a few seconds to minutes. This may be followed by several hours of monotonous background pain. The involved facial area is exquisitely tender. Light touch, chewing, teeth brushing, or even speaking may trigger a new attack of pain. Patients may be affected to such a degree that they refuse to speak or eat. Suicide was not uncommon in former times when treatment was not available. Often, the patient will reveal a history of frustrating visits to the dentist that resulted in extraction of several teeth on the affected side. Compression of the trigeminal nerve root by the superior cerebellar artery or another blood vessel is a frequent cause for trigeminal neuralgia and can be treated surgically by vascular decompression. In the young, trigeminal neuralgia may also be caused by a demyelinating plaque in the brainstem due to MS.

V1 and V2 are purely sensory nerves, whereas V3 has both sensory and motor functions. The motor branch of V3 innervates primarily muscles of mastication, e.g., the masseter muscle and the temporal muscle. These muscles have bilateral supranuclear innervation, which is why they are not affected by hemispheric brain lesions. In contrast, with nuclear brainstem lesions or lesions that damage the course of the trigeminal nerve outside the brainstem, e.g., *skull base tumors* or *infectious processes*, unilateral atrophy of the masseter muscle may occur. Ask the patient to bite his teeth together and palpate the masseter muscle bulk, which will be atrophic. When the patient is asked to open his mouth, the jaw deviates to the paralyzed side because the healthy contralateral masseter muscle pushes the jaw away from the healthy side.

A *trigeminal schwannoma* arises in the middle or posterior cranial fossa and typically leads to decreased sensation in one or more of the trigeminal dermatomes. The corneal reflex is usually weak or absent, which can be the very first sign recorded during the neurological examination. Pain may or may not be present. Mild weakness of the muscles of mastication is found in one-third of patients. Abnormal function of other CNs is noted in the majority of patients when the tumor reaches a critical mass. The CNs most commonly affected are CN VI, CN VIII, and CN VII, in descending frequency.

2.6.5   Facial Nerve

The purpose of the facial nerve (CN VII) is primarily to *serve the muscles of facial expression*. In addition, CN VII has different functions of less obvious importance, which nevertheless help the clinician in establishing the site of lesion in a facial palsy.

In assessing the patient with facial palsy, the first question to ask is whether or not the patient is able to wrinkle his forehead. This is because the approach to a *central facial palsy* is completely different from that to peripheral nerve palsy. Due to bilateral supranuclear innervation, eye blinking and forehead wrinkling are preserved with central facial palsy, and eye closure may be fairly weak but is always possible. *Signe des cils* ("sign of the eyelashes") denotes that the eyelashes remain more visible on the affected side when attempting to close the eyes completely. Sometimes it may be difficult to decide whether or not there is a facial palsy due to habitual facial asymmetry. In this case, ask the patient to repeatedly show his teeth and purse his lips repeatedly. If one corner of the mouth lags behind, this is likely due to a facial nerve weakness. A similar sign, probably somewhat less reliable, is the fact that the nasolabial groove is less distinct on the paralyzed side.

A central facial palsy may be more pronounced with voluntary or involuntary (i.e., emotional) facial activity. A facial palsy that is more evident when reading aloud from a book or when smiling on command (as compared to when laughing spontaneously) is usually due to a lesion of the main motor cortex. In the opposite case, the lesion is subcortical or affects the caudal cingulate motor cortex, a medial brain region with inputs from the limbic system.

If the neurologist has established that a facial palsy is central, he should ask about symptoms compatible with a UMN lesion affecting the ipsilateral arm and leg and about cortical signs such as aphasia (in patients with right-sided central facial palsy). However, if forehead wrinkling is impossible, if the patient cannot close the eye on the affected side, or if Bell's phenomenon is visible, the *facial palsy* is *peripheral*. A normal protective reflex, Bell's phenomenon denotes the upward movement of the eyes when attempting to close them. If eye closure is impossible, the sclera remains visible. This never occurs with central facial palsy. In less severe cases with preserved eye closure, a decrease in the frequency of spontaneous eye blinking on the affected side as compared to the normal side reveals that the facial palsy is peripheral. Difficulties can arise in cases of very early peripheral facial palsies when the forehead muscles and eye blinking are not yet affected. In these instances, it is important to look for CN VII abnormalities other than facial weakness, in particular loss of taste and hyperacusis. These signs also allow localizing the lesion along the path of the facial nerve, in accordance with the affected nerve branches. During its path through the facial canal, CN VII gives off three clinically relevant branches:

- First, the greater petrosal nerve provides parasympathetic innervation to the lacrimal gland. *Impairment of the lacrimal gland* makes eye dryness because of defective eye closure even worse. Complaints about an ipsilateral dry eye thus point toward a peripheral palsy.
- Second, a nerve branch supplies the stapedius muscle responsible for stabilizing the tympanic membrane, thereby controlling the amplitude of sound waves that reach the inner ear. Loss of stapedius nerve function provokes ipsilateral *hyperacusis* (increased sensitivity to noise). Explicit questioning about this feature is necessary because the patient often fails to mention it spontaneously. Sometimes the patient simply is not aware of hyperacusis but reports increased sensitivity on the affected side when the examiner claps his hands together in front of the patient's ears.
- Third, the chorda tympani consists of nerve fibers that leave the CN VII inside the facial canal, just before the facial nerve exits the skull via the stylomastoid foramen. The chorda tympani carries parasympathetic fibers to the submandibular and sublingual gland and mediates *taste on the first two-thirds of the tongue*. Consequently, a patient with a peripheral palsy often reports that taste is also affected and may complain of a metallic taste.

Bell's palsy, an idiopathic isolated peripheral CN VII dysfunction, is the most common type of peripheral facial palsy. Mild to moderate pain behind the ear on the affected side is highly common with Bell's palsy, often occurring prior to the development of the palsy itself. Lack of awareness of this phenomenon may induce considerable concern in the patient and the respon-

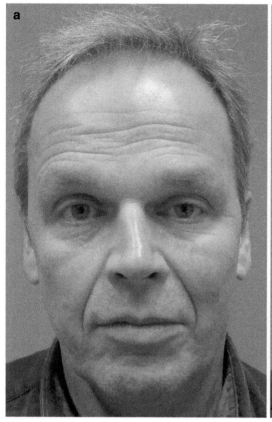
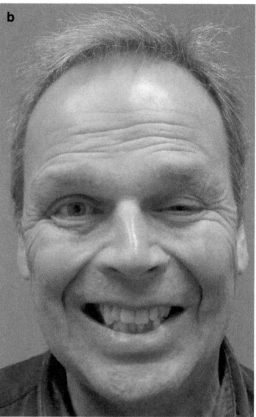

Case 2.7   Facial synkinesis after Bell's palsy. This gentleman demonstrates facial synkinesis 2 years after left-sided peripheral facial palsy. Although his face appears normal at first sight (**a**), smiling leads to involuntary closure of the ipsilateral eye because of aberrant axonal sprouting during recovery from Bell's palsy (**b**). Most cases of synkinesis are acquired following traumatic or inflammatory peripheral nerve injury, but congenital forms exist as well. For instance, the Marcus Gunn phenomenon is a congenital trigemino-oculomotor synkinesis associated with synkinetic movements of the upper lid while drinking or chewing. It is usually unilateral and results from an aberrant connection between trigeminal nerve motor branches controlling masticatory muscles and the superior division of the oculomotor nerve controlling the levator palpebrae superioris muscle ("jaw winking")

sible physician, which often results in unnecessary neuroimaging. Prognosis is usually good, but residual weakness is seen in 10–15% of patients; early steroid treatment can improve the outcome. An unusual long-term consequence of Bell's palsy is Bogorad's syndrome, or the crocodile tears syndrome. Upon recovery of facial weakness, aberrant regeneration of nerve fibers into the lacrimal glands causes the patient to shed tears while eating (gustatolacrimal reflex). This is one form of synkinesis following chronic CN VII injury; other examples are involuntary eye closure with pursing of the lips and forced platysma contraction with smiling (Case 2.7).

Other diseases leading to peripheral facial palsy, often bilaterally, include:

- Infectious basilar meningitis due to tuberculosis (Case 2.8) and neuroborreliosis[20]
- Noninfectious basilar meningitis due to neurosarcoid and meningeal carcinomatosis
- GBS

[20]Lyme disease is a common cause of isolated (unilateral or bilateral) peripheral nerve palsy in children, whereas in adults neuroborreliosis almost always leads to other symptoms as well.

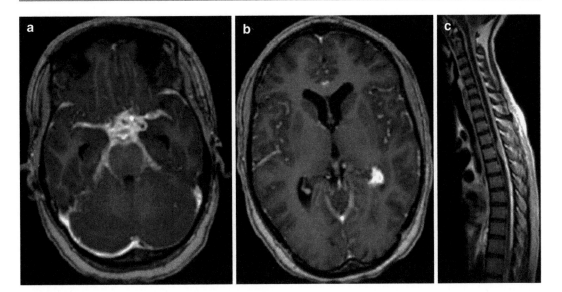

Case 2.8 Tuberculosis of the CNS. A 19-year-old female of Northern African origin developed subacute onset of bilateral facial palsy, hearing loss, dysphagia, and spastic paraparesis. MRI revealed leptomeningeal contrast enhancement in the basal cisterns (**a**) as well as a contrast enhancing lesion in the posterior horn of the left lateral ventricle (**b**) and in the thoracic spine (**c**). CSF PCR identified *Mycobacterium tuberculosis*. The patient was diagnosed as having tuberculosis of the CNS, including basilar meningitis and supratentorial and spinal tuberculoma. The patient was treated with isoniazid, rifampicin, pyrazinamide, and ethambutol for 2 months followed by prolonged therapy with isoniazid and rifampicin. During the course of the disease, she also required a ventriculoperitoneal shunt (note slight dilatation of the temporal horns on axial MRI). Two years later she had a good functional outcome, despite lasting deficits, including bilateral facial weakness and a spastic gait ataxia

Although there are only a few conditions that can lead to bilateral facial palsy, other basal CNs will of course also be involved in many instances.[21]

Ramsay Hunt syndrome is an eponymous term for herpes zoster oticus, an exquisitely painful condition characterized by acute unilateral peripheral facial palsy and erythematous vesicular rash in the ear canal, tongue, and hard palate.

Malignant or infectious processes may also involve CN VII outside the skull base. The first CN VII branch after exit from the stylomastoid foramen is the posterior auricular nerve that controls movements of some of the scalp muscles around the ear. If a patient with a peripheral facial palsy volunteers the information that he still can wiggle his ears (suggesting that the posterior auricular nerve is intact), the lesion affecting CN VII must be distal to the stylomastoid foramen. It should then be assumed that the patient has parotid cancer until proven otherwise, particularly if the patient is an elderly smoker. Restated, patients with a peripheral facial palsy without hyperacusis or impairment of taste should be asked whether they have noticed a lump inside their cheek, and the parotid gland should be palpated in order to search for a tumor.

Hemifacial spasm is a disorder that leads to varying degrees of unilateral facial twitching. Typically, the spasms originate around the eye of the afflicted side and gradually spread to the lower part of the face over the course of months. They can be rather painful and socially stigmatizing. In analogy to trigeminal neuralgia, hemifacial spasm usually is due to compression of the CN VII nerve root by an aberrant vessel. It appears to be much more frequent in the Asian population.

A mysterious syndrome of presumed granulomatous etiology, *Melkersson-Rosenthal syndrome*, usually develops in children and young adults. Patients have a deeply fissured tongue (lingua plicata), episodic unilateral facial palsy,

---

[21] Some myopathies (e.g., FSH) and myasthenia gravis also frequently lead to bilateral orofacial weakness.

and swelling of the face and lips. After recurrent attacks, with intervals absent of attacks ranging from days to years, swelling and facial palsy typically become permanent.

Another rare cause of episodic peripheral facial palsy, occasionally bilateral, is HNPP (see above). Facial palsies typically develop when the patient has slept with his face resting on a hard surface but can also arise without obvious compression.

2.6.6   Vestibulocochlear Nerve

The CN VIII carries auditory information (cochlear nerve) and information about equilibrium (vestibular nerve) from the inner ear to the medulla oblongata, entering the cranial cavity via the internal acoustic meatus.

Damage to the *cochlear nerve* may lead to sudden or chronic progressive *sensorineural deafness* and *tinnitus*. Injury to the *vestibular nerve* may evoke acute *vertigo*, motion sickness, and vomiting, as well as horizontal or torsional (*not* vertical) *nystagmus*. Vestibular nystagmus of peripheral (labyrinthine) origin usually beats away from the side of the lesion and increases as the eyes turn in the direction of the quick phase. (In contrast, nystagmus associated with a brainstem or cerebellar pathology is most obvious when the patient fixates and follows a moving target. The direction of nystagmus changes with the direction of the gaze.)

It is mandatory to verify that the patient actually has vertigo and not dizziness or lightheadedness. Vertigo typically has a kinetic feature, which means that the patient experiences a false sensation of movement. The patient may feel that the world appears to be spinning around him, or he may feel as if something is pushing him to the left or right or pulling him downward or upward. Ask the patient to imagine being on a high-speed merry-go-round and what it feels like to step off the carousel when it suddenly stops.

Then ask if this is the kind of vertigo the patient is experiencing.[22]

Benign paroxysmal positional vertigo (BPPV) is due to sudden and abnormal stimulation of the posterior semicircular canal by otolithes. Occasionally, the patient reports that acute onset vertigo occurs in the morning in bed when turning from one side to the other. Keeping the head motionless improves the vertigo. Movements of the head, often toward one side or the other, trigger another attack of sudden vertigo, typically with a delay of 1–2 s. The patient is nauseous, may vomit heavily, and feels like he is being pushed to the right or the left when walking. Sometimes walking is not possible at all. Gradual improvement usually occurs over several days. There are no auditory symptoms. Chapter 3 discusses the Epley and Dix-Hallpike maneuvers.

Vestibular neuritis is a somewhat ambiguous term that is used for sudden vertigo and unilateral vestibular dysfunction of unknown origin and without the clear association to head movement that characterizes BPPV. Recurrent attacks of sudden vertigo may also be due to a *perilymph fistula* (or labyrinthine fistula) and leakage of inner ear fluid into the air-filled middle ear.

Some disorders of CN VIII impair balance and hearing simultaneously and acutely. *Ménière's disease* is characterized by sudden attacks of vertigo lasting minutes to hours preceded by tinnitus, aural fullness, and fluctuating hearing loss. With recurrent attacks sensorineural deafness occurs. *Trauma, infectious processes* (suppurative labyrinthitis, meningitis, and viral diseases, including mumps and measles), and *ototoxic medications* (aminoglycosides, chemotherapeutics, loop diuretics, salicylates) may lead to acute or subacute vertigo and hearing loss. In addition, *infarction of the anterior inferior cerebellar*

---

[22] In contrast to true vertigo, dizziness is often described as "a lightheaded feeling as if I was about to faint" or as "a spaced out feeling as if I wasn't quite there." The latter description usually points to a functional complaint, whereas the former may also suggest a vasovagal or orthostatic event.

artery (AICA) can present with vertigo and ipsilateral deafness from labyrinthine artery ischemia.

Chronic damage of CN VIII may sometimes evolve without vertigo due to central compensation mechanisms. A *vestibular schwannoma* is a benign intracranial tumor of the myelin-forming cells of the VN that leads to the so-called cerebellopontine syndrome.[23] The earliest symptoms of vestibular schwannoma include ipsilateral sensorineural deafness, gait disturbance, tinnitus, ear fullness, and vertigo with nausea and vomiting. Large tumors may affect other CNs as well, e.g., CN VII involvement leads to ipsilateral peripheral facial palsy, impairment of glandular secretions, and loss of taste sensation in the anterior two-thirds of the tongue, while CN V involvement leads to ipsilateral loss of sensation in the face (including, notably, early impairment of the corneal reflex) and atrophy of the masseter muscle. Nowadays, patients rarely present at an even later stage when compression of the glossopharyngeal and vagus nerves leads to loss of the gag reflex and dysphagia.

Typewriter tinnitus is an intermittent tinnitus with a staccato quality reminiscent of the noise from a typewriter or from popping popcorn. Like hemifacial spasm and trigeminal neuralgia, it may be secondary to vascular compression of the ipsilateral CN (in this case, the auditory nerve) and responds to carbamazepine.

Sudden sensorineural deafness with tinnitus is usually taken care of by an otolaryngologist, or ENT, specialist; however, sensorineural deafness with or without tinnitus may also occur due to *chronic basilar meningitis* (e.g., neuroborreliosis, neurosyphilis), chronic subarachnoidal bleeding (*superficial CNS siderosis*), and other neurological disorders, e.g., *Refsum disease, mitochondrial disorders,* and *Susac's syndrome.*

The leading genetic cause of combined hearing and vision loss (congenital deaf-blindness) is *Usher syndrome*, characterized by sensorineural hearing loss, progressive retinal degeneration, and vestibular dysfunction. It is genetically and clinically very heterogeneous.

2.6.7 Glossopharyngeal Nerve

The glossopharyngeal nerve (CN IX) mediates *taste from the posterior one-third of the tongue* and *sensation from the pharynx, middle ear, and back of the tongue*. In addition, it receives sensory fibers from the carotid bodies.[24] CN IX supplies parasympathetic fibers to the parotid gland and motor fibers to the stylopharyngeus muscle. The afferent limb of the gag reflex is mediated by CN IX, the efferent limb by CN X.

Due to its close proximity with CN X, CN XI, and CN XII and due to the fact that most of its function is shared by other CNs, isolated glossopharyngeal nerve dysfunction is very rare. *Glossopharyngeal neuralgia* has more or less the same etiology and symptomatology as trigeminal neuralgia, with the obvious exception that with glossopharyngeal neuralgia the pain affects the back of the throat and tongue, the tonsils, and part of the ear. Acute pain is typically provoked by swallowing. Episodes of syncope may occur due to involvement of the carotid sinus reflex. Glossopharyngeal neuralgia is somewhat more common in middle-aged men. A differential diagnosis to glossopharyngeal neuralgia is Eagle syndrome, a rare condition where an elongated temporal styloid process is in conflict with the adjacent anatomical structures leading to unilateral neck pain and otalgia.

---

[23] Vestibular schwannoma is also known as "acoustic neurinoma." However, this is a misnomer because, first, the vestibular nerve tends to be affected prior to the cochlear nerve and, second, the tumor is a schwannoma, not a neurinoma.

[24] The carotid bodies are small clusters of chemoreceptors at the carotid bifurcation and are sensitive to changes in the composition of the arterial blood, e.g., alterations of partial pressure of oxygen and carbon dioxide.

CN IX–XII may be affected by:

- Brainstem lesions
  - Ischemic
  - Hemorrhagic
  - Neoplastic (e.g., brainstem glioma)
  - Infectious (e.g., Whipple's disease)
  - Inflammatory (e.g., neurosarcoidosis, neuro-Behçet)
  - Demyelinating (e.g., MS, central pontine myelinolysis)
- Carotid artery dissection (due to compression of the nerves and ischemia in the vasa nervorum because of carotid artery wall hematoma; see Case 2.9)
- Trauma (e.g., surgical injury, basilar skull fracture)
- Motor neuron disease (MND) (ALS)
- Extramedullary neoplasms (e.g., glomus jugulare tumor, meningeal carcinomatosis)
- Syringobulbia
- Basilar meningitis of infectious (tuberculosis, neuroborreliosis, neurosyphilis) and noninfectious origin (sarcoid, lymphoma, carcinomatous meningitis)

2.6.8   Vagus Nerve

The vagus nerve (CN X) exits through the jugular foramen, runs parallel to the internal carotid artery and the internal jugular vein, and continues into the chest and abdomen, where it supplies the *parasympathetic innervation* of most of the viscera, including the proximal half of the colon.

Parasympathetic discharge leads to decreased heart rate and blood pressure and increased GI motility and gland secretion, as well as bronchoconstriction and bronchorrhea. Motor fibers of CN X supply many of the *muscles of the pharynx and larynx, including the vocal cords*. Afferent nerve fibers carry sensory information from the viscera to the brain. In addition, CN X has sensory fibers that innervate the skin of the inner portion of the outer ear. This is why removal of ear wax with a cotton swab may provoke coughing.

The patient with a lesion of the vagus nerve frequently complains of hoarseness, dysphagia, and especially choking with fluid intake. On examination, the gag reflex is lost, the uvula deviates away from the side of lesion, and there is failure of ipsilateral palate elevation. This is the so-called curtain movement (or the rideau phenomenon). Autonomic function can be assessed at the bedside by asking for symptoms of orthostatic hypotension, measuring pulse and blood pressure in supine and upright positions, etc., but referral to a formal physiological assessment can be necessary (Chap. 5).

CN X can be damaged by all of the processes that may affect C IX and that have been listed above. In addition, *thyroid surgery*, *local infections*, and *malignant infiltration* may damage the CN X nerve branch supplying the larynx and the vocal cords (recurrent laryngeal nerve), causing a hoarse voice. The rare syndrome of *superior laryngeal neuralgia* causes shock-like pains radiating from the larynx to the ear, a condition similar to glossopharyngeal neuralgia.

In contrast to CN X lesions, bilateral supranuclear lesions, as seen in *pseudobulbar palsy* (typically due to bihemispheric lacunar strokes), may lead to spastic dysphagia and dysarthria. Laryngeal spasms may occur with PD and other *extrapyramidal disorders*. Autonomic impairment with orthostatic hypotension, obstipation, and sexual dysfunction is common in parkinsonian diseases as well. Rhythmic movement of the palate (*palatal myoclonus*) may occur with *vascular, infectious, demyelinating, and traumatic brainstem lesions* but can also arise without obvious structural pathology (essential palatal myoclonus).

2.6.9   Spinal Accessory Nerve

The spinal accessory nerve (CN XI) is a pure motor nerve that innervates the *sternocleidomastoid muscle* and the *trapezius muscle*. The trapezius muscle elevates the shoulder, whereas the sternocleidomastoid muscle tilts and rotates the head. Patients with CN XI palsy typically have a depression in the shoulder line with downward and lateral displacement of the scapula and moderate scapula winging. Examination reveals muscle atrophy and sometimes fasciculations of the ipsilateral trapezius and sternocleidomastoid muscles, as well as weakness of head rotation and forward elevation of the shoulder.

Injury within the posterior cervical triangle may produce CN XI palsy and occurs during *lymph node biopsy*, *radical neck dissection*, and *carotid endarterectomy* (*CEA*). Hypertrophy of the sternocleidomastoid muscle may be seen with cervical dystonia and torticollis, whereas myotonic dystrophy and other primary muscle diseases lead to significant bilateral atrophy. The remaining differential diagnosis of a CN XI lesion is similar to the differential of other lower CNs.

2.6.10 Hypoglossal Nerve

Also the hypoglossal nerve (CN XII) is a pure motor nerve. Upon leaving the hypoglossal canal, it supplies the muscles of the tongue. Damage of CN XII may occur with the same lesions that can affect CN IX, X, and XI (see above) and leads to *weakness of the ipsilateral half of the tongue*. When protruded, the tongue deviates toward the side of the lesion because the spared contralateral muscle fibers push the tip of tongue away from the healthy side. With bilateral atrophy, such as in MND, the tip of the tongue still points straight forward. Fasciculation and atrophy are best seen when the patient keeps his tongue relaxed and inside his mouth. A patient with *bulbar ALS* shows only limited tongue movements or none at all. The same is true with *pseudobulbar palsy* due to bilateral lesions of the corticobulbar tracts. Pure pseudobulbar palsy, as seen, for instance, with bilateral hemisphere infarction, is per definition a UMN lesion, which is why lower motor signs such as muscle atrophy and fasciculations are lacking. Patients with ALS, however, may have combined bulbar and pseudobulbar palsies.

Since the supranuclear innervation of the tongue is mainly unilateral, one-third of patients with *acute hemispheric ischemic* or *hemorrhagic stroke* may have tongue deviation toward the side of limb weakness. Some patients may also show tongue apraxia and be unable to protrude it on command. Thus, unilateral and bilateral supranuclear lesions may cause dysarthria and dysphagia due to tongue weakness and incoordination. However, tongue deviation associated with an isolated hemispheric stroke is nearly always reversible.

Extrapyramidal disorders can be associated with bradykinetic or hyperkinetic movements of the mouth and the tongue. For instance, choreatic oral movements are seen with tardive *dyskinesia* due to neuroleptic treatment.

In young patients with sudden onset of neck pain and tongue deviation, it is mandatory not to overlook a dissection of the ipsilateral carotid artery (Case 2.9). Damage to lower cranial nerves such as the hypoglossal nerve may arise because of interruption of the nutrient vessels supplying the nerve.

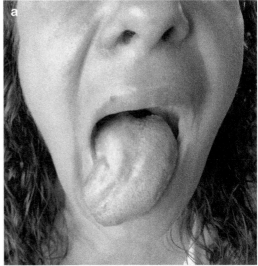

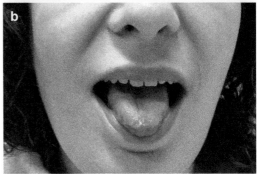

Case 2.9 Hypoglossal nerve palsy due to carotid artery dissection. A 36-year-old previously healthy woman complained of decreased tongue motility resulting in slightly slurred speech and difficulties swallowing. She had experienced an unusual and moderately severe neck pain for a few days prior to consultation. The pain had started suddenly during a roller coaster ride. On examination, tongue deviation to the right was noted compatible with ipsilateral hypoglossal nerve damage (**a**). MR showed a right-sided carotid artery wall hematoma, suggesting a right-sided carotid artery dissection, which was confirmed by CT angiography. A year later, tongue weakness had resolved (**b**)

2.7   Cerebellum

The cerebellum plays a major role in the integration of sensory information, coordination, and movement. It receives afferent information from the cerebral motor cortex, vestibular and inferior olivary nuclei, and spinal cord. It sends efferences to the thalamus, vestibular nuclei, formatio reticularis, and nucleus ruber, and this information is passed further on to the motor cortex and the spinal cord. These feedback loops help to fine-tune motor activity. The anatomy of the cerebellum is much more complicated, but the signs and symptoms of cerebellar lesions are rather simple.

A hemispheric lesion of the cerebellum leads to ipsilateral *cerebellar ataxia* (including dysmetria and dysdiadochokinesia), *intention tremor*, and muscle hypotonia. (The last item is rarely clinically relevant.) All signs are ipsilateral to the lesion because the afferent information to the cerebellum comes from the contralateral side, and the efferent information leaving the cerebellum is again destined for the contralateral cerebral hemisphere. Restated, information processed by the cerebellum crosses the midline twice, which is why a hemispheric cerebellar lesion affects the ipsilateral extremities (Case 2.10).

It is important to note that while lesions of the cerebellar hemispheres cause ipsilateral signs in the extremities, lesions of the midline region lead to ataxia affecting gait and trunk only. Alcohol abuse, for instance, mainly affects the cerebellar vermis, which is why examination often reveals relatively mild ataxia during the finger-nose and knee-heel tests despite obvious gait ataxia.

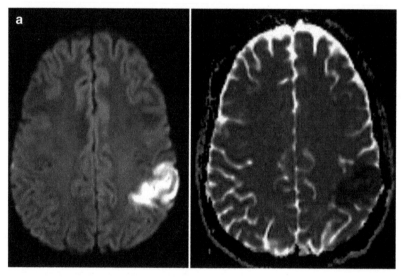

Case 2.10 Crossed cerebellar diaschisis. A 30-year-old previously healthy woman experienced an unusual pain in the neck and around the left eye following a yoga session. The following day, she had a short episode of right-sided facial weakness. She did not seek medical help. On day 3, however, she was admitted with aphasia and a right hemiparesis (NIHSS 18). Following IV thrombolysis, the left MCA (M1) was successfully reopened using stent-retriever thrombectomy. MRI confirmed a partial left-sided MCA infarction (hyperintense signal on DWI (**a**, left) with corresponding hypointensity on ADC (**a**, right), consistent with cytotoxic edema). MR angiography also showed left-sided ICA dissection. Note the absence of the left ICA on time-of-flight sequences (**b**, left) and the carotid artery wall hematoma on fat-suppressed T1-weighted imaging (**b**, right). The next day, the patient had a pronator drift on the right, a subtle right-sided central facial palsy, and minor word-finding difficulties (NIHSS 3). Interestingly, CT perfusion from the day of admission revealed hypoperfusion of the right cerebellar hemisphere (**c**). Crossed cerebellar diaschisis can be detected in roughly one-third of patients with MCA infarctions but may also be seen with other pathologies affecting the contralateral cerebral hemisphere such as trauma or malignancy. It is believed to result from decreased input from the damaged cortex to the contralateral cerebellum via the corticopontocerebellar pathways. Although it is not fully understood and does not have any direct clinical consequences, this phenomenon nicely illustrates the close relationship between the cerebral hemispheres and the contralateral cerebellar cortices with respect to sensory and motor information processing

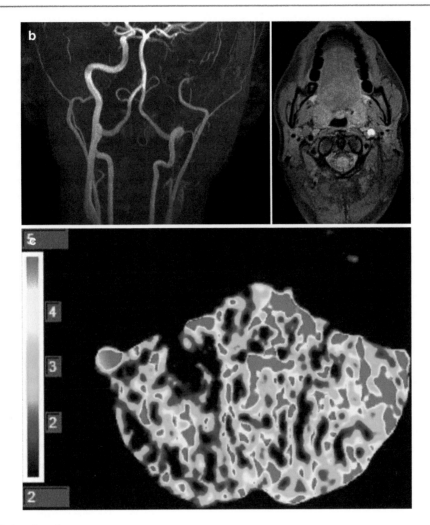

Case 2.10 (continued)

Nystagmus due to a cerebellar or brainstem lesion is usually permanent and direction changing and may occur in the horizontal and vertical plane, in contrast to vestibular nystagmus, which is almost never vertical or direction changing and typically habituates after a while. Usually vascular in origin, acute lesions of the cerebellum are often combined with nausea, vomiting, and vertigo. The patient may complain of occipital headache and neck pain. *Cerebellar hemorrhage* and *ischemic infarction* may lead to acute infratentorial herniation because of mass effect. Therefore, urgent neurosurgical consultation should be obtained. Less acute cerebellar injury can be due to *demyelinating*, *neoplastic*, *infectious*, and *neurodegenerative disorders*. Chapter 4 discusses these and the *hereditary ataxias*, while Chaps. 3 and 4 discuss how to distinguish cerebellar ataxia and tremor from sensory and vestibular ataxia, respectively, from parkinsonian and orthostatic tremor.

Traditionally, the cerebellum was considered to be exclusively involved in the coordination of voluntary movement, gait, posture, balance, and motor speech, but recent neuroanatomical, neuroimaging, and clinical studies provide evidence of cerebellar contribution to linguistic and cognitive function. Evidence is accumulating that cerebellar disorders, both cerebellar degeneration and focal lesions, may lead to certain impairment of working memory and higher language tasks.

2.8 Subcortical Gray Matter

The subcortical gray matter consists mainly of the basal ganglia, thalamus, and hypothalamus.

2.8.1 Basal Ganglia

The basal ganglia include the striatum (caudate nucleus and putamen), pallidum, substantia nigra, and the subthalamic nucleus, but the definition varies somewhat from textbook to textbook. The anatomy of the basal ganglia and its connecting parts is particularly complicated. Fortunately, this is in contrast to the relative simplicity of its clinical signs, which is why no more anatomic considerations will be made here.

Movement disorders associated with disease processes affecting the basal ganglia can be divided into those that lead to *hypodopaminergia* and *parkinsonism* and those causing *hyperdopaminergia* and *hyperkinetic disorders*.

PD should be carefully distinguished from parkinsonism as the first is a disease and the second a syndrome that includes a large variety of neurodegenerative and other disorders.

The cardinal manifestations of PD are *rest tremor*, *bradykinesia*, *rigidity*, and *postural instability*. Of these, bradykinesia tends to have the greatest impact on the patient's life. PD almost always begins with unilateral manifestations. At later stages, both sides are involved more symmetrically, but symptoms still tend to affect one side in particular. PD with an isolated pill-rolling tremor of one hand as the initial symptom has a comparatively better prognosis. A 4–6 Hz tremor sometimes also affects the jaw and the lower limbs. The parkinsonian gait is slow and shuffling with decreased arm swing and a stooped, forward-flexed posture. Extreme cases of forward flexion are termed camptocormia. The patient turns "en bloc" and may exhibit gait freezing (which may be overcome by visual and auditory cueing) and festination (which is the inability to stop once the patient has started walking). Bradykinesia also manifests as impaired handwriting (letters becoming smaller at the end of a sentence, called micrographia), a masklike face (due to hypomimia and pseudo-seborrhea), a monotonous voice, and dysdiadochokinesia. The inability to turn around in bed impairs sleep. Nuchal rigidity (particularly often seen with PSP and rather advanced Parkinson's disease) may lead to the typical posture of a parkinsonian patient lying supine with the neck flexed and the head hanging in the air, several centimeters above the pillow. This sign is sometimes referred to as psychic pillow, an unfortunate and outdated term in light of its organic nature. Dysphagia and drooling occur at rather late stages of Parkinson's disease. Neuropsychiatric symptoms with depression and cognitive defects affect a large part of Parkinson's patients during the course of the disease. Of note, despite obvious gait disturbances, Parkinson's patients remain able to walk until the very late stages of the disease. A useful clinical rule is that a patient referred with a working diagnosis of PD who comes into the office in a wheelchair usually suffers from a different disease (wheelchair sign), typically belonging to the Parkinson plus spectrum (see Chap. 4). Further, it is important to bear in mind that Parkinson's patients also suffer from nonmotor features such as hyposmia, rapid eye movement-sleep behavior disorder, constipation, or depression, which typically start many years prior to motor symptom onset.

Hyperkinetic movements comprise *chorea* (distal, brief, irregular), *athetosis* (distal, slow, writhing, and twisting), *choreathethosis*, *hemiballism* (proximal, large amplitude, violent movements of the left or right extremities), and *dystonia* (focal, segmental, or generalized and sustained muscle contractions causing abnormal postures, which sometimes may be alleviated by a sensory trick, called *geste antagoniste*). The patient may convert choreatic movements into semi-purposeful movements in order to hide his disorder. In cases of mild chorea, the patient can thus mislead the inexperienced observer, who may believe that the patient is simply nervous. Hemiballism is usually of sudden onset and due to a stroke affecting the subthalamic nucleus, but the differential diagnosis of other hyperkinetic disorders and parkinsonism is extensive. Chapter 4 provides a further discussion.

2.8.2 Diencephalon

2.8.2.1 Hypothalamus

The thalamus and hypothalamus are part of the diencephalon. Lesions of the hypothalamus may lead to *vegetative symptoms*, e.g., hypo- and hyperthermia, hypo- and hyperphagia, hypo- and hypertension, brady- and tachycardia, decreased or excessive sweating, polydipsia, alterations of circadian rhythms, and various hormonal disturbances.[25]

Craniopharyngioma and *hypothalamus hamartoma* may lead to precocious puberty. Gelastic seizures are a classical presentation of hypothalamic hamartoma. *Kleine-Levin syndrome*, a very rare disorder affecting adolescent males, consists of striking episodes of hypersomnia only interrupted by short periods of semi-wakefulness with hyperphagia and behavioral changes such as confusion, aggression, and hypersexuality. Between episodes, however, the patient's behavior is rather normal. Although of unknown etiology, the site of pathophysiology clearly involves the diencephalon.

Narcolepsy consists of a the classic tetrad of sleep paralysis, hallucinations on falling asleep or on awaking, imperative sleep attacks during the daytime, and cataplexy, although not all patients have cataplexy. Patients with narcolepsy have a severely reduced number of hypocretin-producing cells in the hypothalamus.

2.8.2.2 Thalamus

The thalamus is the *sensory gating system* of the brain; all sensory information, except for olfaction, is filtered by the thalamus. Only relevant information is allowed to pass through to the cortex, where it may reach consciousness. This is why, for example, someone reading a murder mystery becomes so absorbed in the story that they become completely unaware of their surroundings and do not realize they are hungry until the story gets dull. Another example of the thalamic filter function is evident in exhausted parents who may sleep so deeply as to ignore the loudest noise but who awake the second their baby begins to cry. In addition, the thalamus contributes to arousal and wakefulness, as well as motor and memory function.

For practical purposes, the thalamus can be divided into four areas, each of them having a specific function and a specific vascular supply derived from branches of the posterior cerebral artery (PCA):

- The anterior nuclei are supplied by the polar artery and are important for language and memory function.
- The medial nuclei are supplied by the paramedian artery, contributing to arousal and memory.
- The lateral nuclei are supplied by the thalamogeniculate artery and regulate sensorimotor function.
- The posterior nuclei are supplied by the posterior choroidal artery and are important for visual function.

It follows that injury to the thalamus can lead to a wide spectrum of deficits. Depending on which area is damaged, patients can present with fluctuating levels of arousal and disorientation, dysphasia (left-sided lesions), or hemispatial neglect (right-sided lesions). Other symptoms and signs include disturbed learning and amnesia (anterior and medial nuclei), numbness (hemianesthesia) and a burning sensation in the contralateral half of the body known as thalamic pain (lateral nuclei), and visual field deficits (posterior nuclei). Further deficits associated with thalamic lesions that are well known but poorly understood include gaze palsies and hyperkinetic movement disorders such

---

[25]The hypothalamus produces vasopressin, oxycontin, and growth hormone-inhibiting hormone, as well as release hormones for corticotropin, gonadotropin, thyrotropin, and growth hormone.

as tremor, chorea, and dystonia. In addition, compression of the mesencephalic tectum is a frequent cause of acute supranuclear gaze palsy (Parinaud's syndrome), often seen in the elderly following hemorrhage or a tumor (Case 2.11).

The most common cause of acute thalamic damage is *vascular*, usually affecting one hemisphere at a time. However, bilateral thalamic

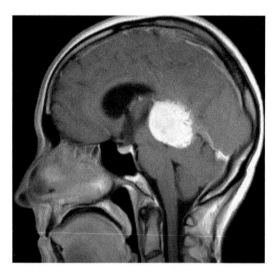

Case 2.11 Parinaud's syndrome. A 50-year-old male complained of new-onset headache and blurred vision, which had started 2 months prior. On examination, there was subtle gait ataxia, as well as conjugate upgaze paralysis, convergence-retraction nystagmus, and light-near dissociation. The latter findings were consistent with Parinaud's syndrome, suggesting a structural lesion at the level of the midbrain. Indeed, MRI showed a contrast-enhancing tumor, leading to compression of the lamina of the mesencephalic tectum and the aqueduct. The patient was treated with surgical tumor removal and a ventriculoperitoneal shunt for obstructive hydrocephalus. Histology revealed a hemangiopericytoma (WHO grade II; a soft tissue sarcoma originating in the pericytes of capillaries), for which he received stereotactic radiation therapy. Three years later, he remained in clinical remission. According to a recent case series of 40 patients with Parinaud's syndrome, the commonest presenting symptoms are diplopia (67.5%), followed by blurred vision (25%), visual field defects (12.5%), gait ataxia (7.5%), and manifest squint (7.5%) (Shields et al. 2016). The complete triad of vertical gaze palsy, convergence-retraction nystagmus, and light-near dissociation is present in only two-thirds of patients. Vertical gaze palsy is the commonest sign (100%), while convergence-retraction nystagmus (87.5%) and light-near dissociation (65.0%) are somewhat less common. The responsible midbrain pathology is typically cerebrovascular or a malignancy

damage is not infrequent and may occur with *deep intracerebral venous thrombosis of the sinus rectus* or *bilateral infarction of the paramedian arteries*, leading to amnesia and akinetic mutism.

The most frequent nonvascular cause of acute diencephalic damage is *Wernicke's encephalopathy* due to severe thiamine deficiency. Wernicke's encephalopathy leads to ataxia, disturbance of consciousness, and oculomotor abnormalities, but bear in mind that the complete clinical triad may be found in as little as 10% of symptomatic patients. Cerebellar ataxia may range from mild incoordination of the extremities and minor problems of balance during tandem gait to severe truncal instability and the inability to stand or walk (astasia-abasia). Disturbed cognition and consciousness can range from minor confusion to coma and oculomotor impairment from slight nystagmus and saccadic pursuit to various oculomotor palsies, including complete ophthalmoplegia in extreme cases. The Wernicke-Korsakoff complex is usually seen in alcoholics but is also encountered in other patients with severe thiamine deficiency (e.g., hyperemesis gravidarum, anorexia). If thiamine deficiency is not rapidly reversed, *Korsakoff's syndrome* may develop with hemorrhages in the mammillary bodies, thus leading to permanent amnesia and confabulation. The latter is the (unconscious) attempt of the patient with severe amnesia to fill in the memory gaps with often bizarre stories that are obviously untrue (Case 2.12).

2.9   Subcortical White Matter

By taking a careful history, the neurologist can distinguish between subcortical white matter damage and cortical lesions by focusing on the absence or presence of visual field defects, cortical symptoms, and epileptic seizures and by elucidating the features of hemisensory and hemimotor symptoms.

Visual field defects strongly suggest subcortical white matter damage, simply because optic radiation involves such a huge part of the subcortical white matter. An isolated lesion of the pri-

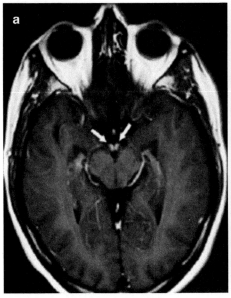
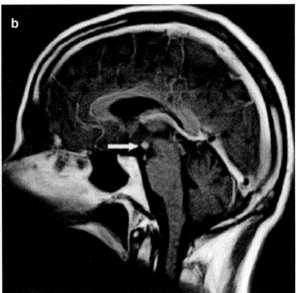

Case 2.12 Wernicke's encephalopathy. A 32-year-old male with alcoholism was admitted because of confusion and gait ataxia. Neurological examination revealed a left CN VI palsy and a course gaze-changing nystagmus. The patient was treated immediately with IV thiamine for Wernicke's encephalopathy. Sagittal and axial T1-weighted MRI showed contrast enhancement of the mammillary bodies (**a, b**; *arrows*), the crucial site of damage in the Wernicke-Korsakoff complex. A few days later, all neurological symptoms had vanished, but the patient was not yet motivated to begin treatment for alcoholism

mary visual cortex is usually far too superficial and small to lead to visual field defects (Fig. 2.11).

Hemiparesis and hemihypesthesia associated with subcortical lesions tend to involve the leg as much as the face and the arm. In contrast, cortical lesions usually spare the leg because the primary motor and sensory cortices representing the legs are localized on the medial aspects of the hemispheres near the falx, where they are well protected. The UMN fibers of the leg join the fibers of the face and arm subcortically in the corticospinal tract (semioval center, internal capsule, cerebral peduncle, brainstem), and here, a lesion is as likely to affect the leg as it is to affect the face and the arm. Restated, subcortical lesions lead to *complete hemiparesis* and *hemihypesthesia*, whereas cortical lesions usually leave the leg rather unaffected (Fig. 2.12).[26] Also, since so much of the cortex from the dominant hemisphere is associated with language function (including reading and writing), a right-sided hemiparesis without dysphasia or other language problems is usually due to a subcortical lesion.[27]

Dense numbness also suggests a subcortical instead of a cortical lesion. This is because the sensory modalities that are represented cortically are rather sophisticated. A patient with an isolated lesion of the sensory cortex has difficulties with recognizing writing on the skin (graphesthesia) or may be unable to perceive the form of an object by using the sense of touch (stereognosis). But he will usually be able to recognize pain, vibration, touch, and position because these primary sensory modalities reach awareness already

---

[26]An exception is falx meningioma compressing bilaterally the areas of the motor cortex that represent the lower extremities, thus leading to paraparesis. This is an important, but rare, differential diagnosis to paraplegia of the UMN type.

[27]Even in two-thirds of left-handed people, language function is localized in the left hemisphere. Thus, when informed that a patient has dysphasia and left-sided hemiparesis, the first question to ask is whether the patient is left-handed. Often it turns out that he is right-handed, which makes dysphasia very unlikely. In most cases, dysarthria or confusion has then been mistaken for dysphasia.

Fig. 2.11 Visual pathways. A visual field defect is a sign of white matter damage, and the configuration of the defect allows conclusions about the localization of the lesion. For instance, a left upper quadrantanopia suggests damage to Meyer's loop in the right temporal lobe

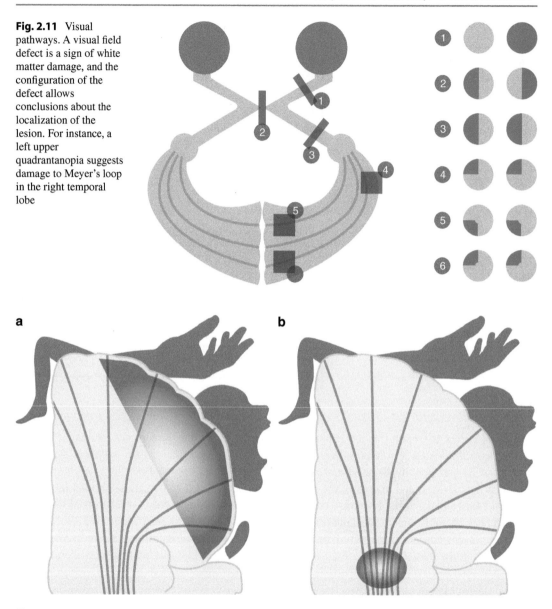

Fig. 2.12 Cortical and subcortical lesions. Cortical lesions usually lead to weakness of the contralateral half of the face and the contralateral arm but tend to spare the leg because its motor and sensory areas are localized on the medial aspects of the hemispheres, where they are well protected (**a**). Subcortical lesions, in contrast, cause hemiparesis and hemihypesthesia that typically involve the leg as much as the face and the arm (**b**)

at the level of the thalamus and its cortical projections. It follows that dense numbness most likely is due to a subcortical lesion.

Bilateral and diffuse white matter damage may evoke decreased psychomotor speed. *Subcortical dementias* (e.g., *hydrocephalus*, *subcortical vascular dementia*, long-standing *MS*) are associated with a striking *decline of psycho-motor speed, executive dysfunction, and a tendency to develop depressive symptoms*, while *higher cognitive functions are less impaired*. In contrast, the archetypical cortical dementia of AD starts with cortical dysfunction such as amnesia, visuospatial problems, aphasia, acalculia, agnosia, and apraxia, and at least in the beginning, psychomotor speed will be preserved. To give a somewhat simplified example, following the question "What year is it?", a patient with established AD may immediately answer with a year long gone, whereas the hydrocephalic patient, after a long latency, provides an answer that differs just slightly from the present date.

Age-related unspecific white matter changes (also called leukoaraiosis) are often seen on brain MRI as small focal or large confluent hyperintense areas on T2-weighted images in older people. Age-related white matter changes may be associated with reduced psychomotor speed, executive dysfunction, depression, difficulties in walking, and urinary incontinence but are also seen in neurologically intact patients. Extensive age-related white matter changes are associated with an increased risk of rapid functional decline.

Adult hydrocephalus can be idiopathic (primary) or symptomatic (secondary to another disease), communicating, or obstructive (with respect to CSF fluid pathway patency), respec-

tively, and chronic or acute. *Normal pressure hydrocephalus* (NPH) is one of the few potentially reversible dementias. NPH can be idiopathic or secondary to, e.g., trauma, meningitis, and intracranial hemorrhage. The classic triad of NPH consists of dementia, urgency incontinence, and frontal gait apraxia. The gait is slow, shuffling, "magnetic," and wide based; the feet are often rotated outward. Postural instability with retropulsion is common. Characteristically, when supine, the patient is often still able to cycle with the legs in the air; this is in striking contrast to the obvious gait disturbance (and probably because of the use of different motor programs). It has therefore been suggested that NPH patients have gait apraxia instead of gait ataxia. Urine incontinence is often quite a late symptom, but slight urgency is very common. Dementia is of the subcortical type and relatively mild; it is characterized by psychomotor retardation rather than cortical dysfunction, as explained earlier (Case 2.13). Notably, not all patients experience the

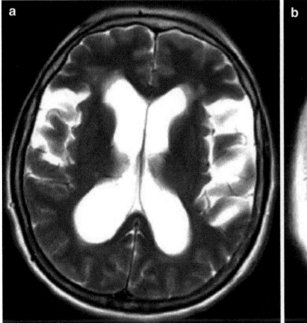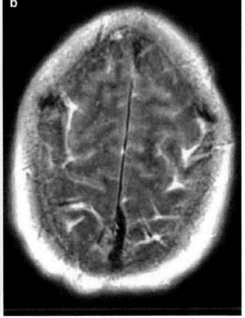

Case 2.13 Normal pressure hydrocephalus. A 68-year-old female with mild gait disturbances and urinary incontinence, but apparently normal cognition, was diagnosed with NPH. An MRI showed ventriculomegaly and characteristic disproportion between dilatation of the Sylvian fissure (**a**) and narrowing of the CSF space at the high convexity (**b**: "mismatch" sign). Following treatment with a ventriculoperitoneal shunt, she realized how unenthusiastic her husband was, got a divorce, and began traveling the world

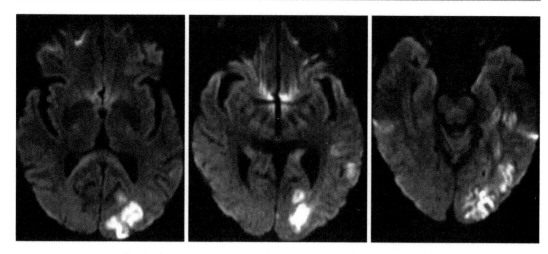

Case 2.14 Alexia without agraphia. A 65-year-old female with atrial fibrillation complained of visual disturbances. Examination revealed a right-sided hemianopia. In addition, although she was able to write, she was unable to read, including what she just had written. MR DWI was consistent with a left cerebral posterior artery stroke, the typical cause of alexia without agraphia

classic triad; some are rather monosymptomatic. See Case 4.40 for an example of a patient with an obstructive hydrocephalus.

There is an important exception to the rule that white matter lesions do not produce cortical symptoms, the so-called disconnection syndrome. White matter lesions that isolate a cortical region due to interruption of the association pathways that connect this region with others can produce symptoms identical or similar to those seen with damage of this particular cortical region. For example, disconnection of the arcuate fasciculus, a deep, white matter tract, disconnects the brain areas responsible for speech comprehension (Wernicke's area) and speech production (Broca's area). The resulting *conduction aphasia* is characterized by relatively preserved speech comprehension and production but poor speech repetition. Another example is *alexia without agraphia* due to a white matter lesion of the left occipital lobe, including the splenium of the corpus callosum. As a consequence, only the right visual cortex can process visual information but is unable to send this information to the left hemisphere, where the language areas reside. Such a patient, who usually has suffered from a left posterior artery stroke, is able to write but unable to read, including what he has just written. Although classic examples of a disconnection

syndrome, both conduction aphasia and alexia without agraphia are relatively often overlooked in clinical practice (Case 2.14).

2.10 Cortex

In contrast to subcortical damage, lesions involving the cortex induce *impairment of higher cognitive function* (e.g., amnesia, aphasia, apraxia, visuospatial deficits, agnosia, neglect, changes in behavior and/or personality, and psychiatric symptoms), *incomplete hemiparesis*, hemihypesthesia, and *epileptic seizures*.

Left-sided vascular cortical lesions often involve disturbance of speech and language processing. *Nonfluent (motor) aphasia* due to left MCA infarction or subdural hemorrhage is typically combined with right-sided hemiparesis that involves the arm and the face but spares the leg. (Broca's area, found in the left inferior frontal gyrus close to the motor area representing the face, is served by the upper MCA branch.) Thus, a history of temporary speech problems is much more likely due to a transient ischemic attack if the patient also reports transitory weakness or numbness of the right half of the face and the right arm. *Fluent (=sensory) aphasia*, in contrast, is usually not associated with motor paresis since Wernicke's area, residing in the posterior section of the left superior temporal gyrus, is served by the lower MCA branch, and is not adjacent to the motor cortex. *Transcortical aphasias* are rare forms of disconnection syndromes due to a stroke that spares the connecting pathways between the motor and sensory language areas; patients typically have a nonfluent or fluent type of aphasia, but strikingly, their ability to repeat the spoken word remains intact. Even more rare is the situation in which a left-sided hemispheric stroke (or rarely, traumatic injury or migraine) affects prosody (rhythm, speech, and intonation), thus leading to the *foreign accent syndrome*. An accent that is vague but distinctly unusual replaces the patient's natural accent, and the listener interprets the new accent as belonging to a foreign language and, hence, may conclude that the patient has turned psychotic, "He suddenly started speaking with a Russian accent!"

Right-sided vascular cortical lesion may cause a left-sided hemiparesis, often in combination with *neglect* and *visuospatial problems*. The latter can affect perception of the patient's body (the patient has difficulties with positioning his arms, trunk, and legs) or of the outer world (the patient has difficulties orienting himself in space).

2.10.1 Frontal Lobes

Lesions of the frontal lobes may lead to *incomplete hemiparesis* and *nonfluent aphasia* if the motor cortex and Broca's area are involved. This and the phenomenon of paraparesis due to bilateral compression of the medial motor cortex by a tumor have been discussed above. Frontal lobe lesions often lead to *personality changes, lack of insight, altered behavior*, and *executive dysfunction*. Even with large frontal tumors or infarction, there can be a complete lack of focal (lateralized) motor deficits during bedside examination (but with large space-occupying lesions, ophthalmoscopy will typically reveal papilledema).

Lesions of the orbital frontal cortex may lead to disinhibition, impulsivity, and confabulation, as well as antisocial behavior, stereotypical behaviors, and overeating. Lesions of the dorsolateral frontal cortex lead to cognitive deficits (poor word generation, reduced attention, working memory deficits, and poor organization and planning). Lesions of the medial frontal circuit are associated with altered energy, motivation, drive, and affect.

Frontal lobe lesions may lead either to a loss of or exaggeration of frontal inhibition. Thus, patients can become lethargic, apathetic, and even mutistic. Lack of empathy and concern for others are particularly distressing symptoms. Patients with apathy present with a lack of goal-oriented behavior and are often disengaged and emotionally unresponsive. Sometimes their drive is decreased to such an extent that they do not complain about extremely painful stimuli, they do not care about their inability to control their bladders and bowels, and they do not take any initiative whatsoever.

Impersistence is the inability to sustain a movement or to stick to a task. When asked to lift their arms and hold them upraised, patients may lift their arms for a second or two but then inevitably lower them again despite understanding what the examiner is requesting. The opposite of impersistence is perseveration. Once in action the patient is unable to stop and may repeat the same sentence again and again or may engage in meaningless repetitive behavior for hours if not interrupted.

Loss of frontal inhibition, in contrast, may lead to reckless, impulsive, and socially inappropriate behavior. Some patients with *frontotemporal dementia*, for instance, show rather well-preserved memory but characteristic frontal disinhibition (Case 2.15). They may drive carelessly in traffic or masturbate in public. They often develop bizarre preferences for certain foods and may eat, e.g., seven or eight bananas at a time. The most famous example of frontal disinhibition is probably the case of Phineas Gage, a 25-year-old railroad construction foreman who survived an accident in 1848 in which a large iron rod was driven through his frontal lobes. Gage became "fitful, irreverent, indulging at times in the grossest profanity […], manifesting but little deference for his fellows, impatient of restraint or advice when it conflicts with his desires, at times pertinaciously obstinate, yet capricious and vacillating, devising many plans of future operations, which are no sooner arranged than they are aban-

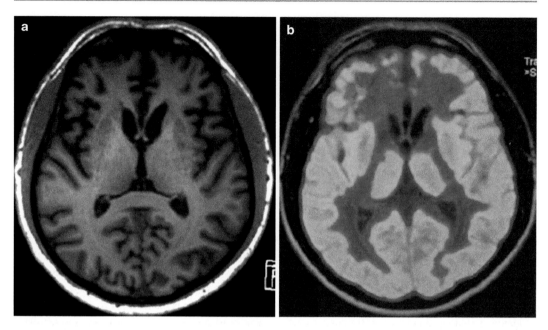

Case 2.15 Behavioral variant frontotemporal dementia (bvFTD) with disinhibition. A 37-year-old male was referred to the memory clinic from a psychiatric ward, where he had been admitted for behavioral symptoms. He had lost his job as a physician 1 year earlier due to inappropriate behavior and attention deficits. Symptoms had progressed, and at the time of referral, he was disinhibited and showed hypersexual behavior, inappropriate social conduct, overeating, motor and verbal perseveration, and mental rigidity. He was unaware of his impairment. CSF analysis and EEG were normal. MRI demonstrated bilateral frontal cortical atrophy, most pronounced in the orbitofrontal region (**a**). FDG PET showed bifrontal hypometabolism (**b**). He was diagnosed with bvFTD (PET images courtesy of Ian Law, Department of Clinical Physiology and Nuclear Medicine, Rigshospitalet, Copenhagen)

doned in turn for others appearing more feasible. [He was] a child in his intellectual capacities, with the general passion of a strong man. [...] Previous to his injury [...] he possessed a well-balanced mind, and was [...] a shrewd, smart businessman, very energetic and persistent in executing all his plans of operation. In this regard his mind was radically changed, so decidedly that his friends and acquaintances said he was 'no longer Gage.'" (Harlow 1868).[28]

Another disorder that deserves mentioning here is Foix-Chavany-Marie syndrome (FCMS), an infrequent neurological condition due to bilateral damage to the anterior frontoparietal operculum. FCMS (or anterior opercular syndrome) affects the voluntary activity of orofacial, masticatory, and pharyngeal muscles, while involuntary and emotional innervation usually remains intact. Although often caused by stroke, there is also a primarily neurodegenerative type.

---

[28]Occasionally, personality changes can be hard to detect for those who have not known the patient prior to the neurological event. A man in his 70s suffered from a right-sided frontal infarction, but on admission to the hospital, he had no focal deficits. Cheerful and with a pleasant manner, he soon became a favorite with the nurses. The real impact of the infarct did not become clear until a few days later when his wife came for a visit and was totally bewildered that this "miserable old man" had turned into such a lovely person.

2.10.2 Temporal Lobes

The temporal lobes include important structures such as the primary and associative auditory cortex and the hippocampal formation. Consequently, the temporal lobes are involved with memory processing and speech comprehension. As stated above, the typical *cortical dementia* of AD starts with cortical dysfunction, primarily of the medial temporal lobes.

A lesion in Wernicke's area causes *fluent aphasia*, as discussed earlier. Lesions involving the geniculocalcarine pathways (Meyer's loop) result in *contralateral upper visual field defects* (colloquially referred to as "pie in the sky"). Hearing is bilaterally represented in the temporal lobes, which is why unilateral destruction of the auditory cortex does not cause deafness (Case 2.16).

Degeneration of left polar and inferolateral temporal structures leads to a striking syndrome called *semantic dementia* (SD), in which patients develop a fundamental loss of semantic memory. Semantic memory is defined as the component of long-term memory that contains the permanent representation of our knowledge about things in the world, concepts, and facts, as well as words and their meaning (Case 2.17). A variant, with degeneration of the right (or bilateral) polar and

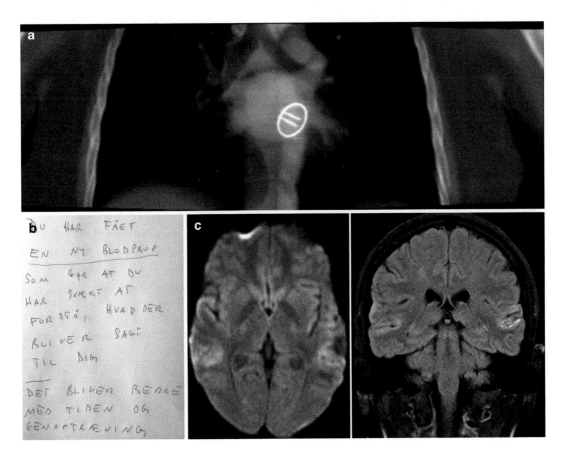

Case 2.16 Pure word deafness due to bitemporal infarctions. A young woman in her thirties with a history of intravenous drug addiction, mechanical mitral valve replacement following endocarditis, (**a**) and poor compliance to anticoagulation therapy was admitted with sudden onset of apparently bizarre cognitive symptoms—although she was able to speak relatively fluently, she did not understand any spoken words. Instead, everything had to be written down (**b** "You have acquired a stroke which makes it difficult for you to understand what is being said. This will get better with time and rehabilitation"). The patient could follow written commands correctly and was able to speak and write but was unable to process spoken language. Hearing thresholds were normal. The remainder of the neurological examination was normal. MRI of the brain (**c**, axial DWI; coronal FLAIR) showed multiple infarctions, including both temporal lobes. Despite the neurologist's optimism ("This will get better with time and rehabilitation"), her deficits remained unchanged on follow-up 6 months later. Pure word deafness with auditory object agnosia may occur with bilateral lesions of the superior temporal sulcus but is exceedingly rare, since auditory processing of language is represented bilaterally (this is probably a form of evolutionary safety mechanism)

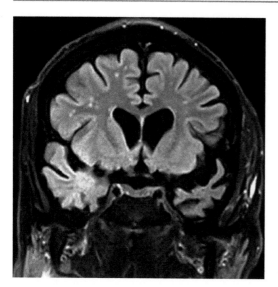

Case 2.17 Semantic dementia. A 65-year-old male was referred for slowly progressive memory loss with word-finding difficulties. His wife reported that the earliest signs had begun more than 5 years earlier. His neurological examination was normal, except for the cognitive deficits. The MMSE score was 28/30. He demonstrated a fundamental loss of semantic memory, which affected naming, comprehension, and object recognition. He frequently used substitute words and phrases and had difficulty reading irregular words. Episodic memory, visuospatial functions, repetition, and psychomotor speed were normal. He also had mild behavioral symptoms. Coronal MRI showed a focal polar and inferolateral temporal lobe atrophy, which was most pronounced on the left side. FDG PET confirmed left anterior temporal and mesial frontal hypometabolism (not shown). He was diagnosed with semantic dementia

inferolateral temporo-occipital structures, including the fusiform gyrus, is associated with *prosopagnosia* (loss of knowledge about faces). Chapter 4 provides more information on both conditions. Of note, prosopagnosia may also occur with bilateral PCA infarctions.

Temporal lobe epilepsy may be divided into mesial (medial) temporal lobe epilepsy and lateral temporal lobe epilepsy. Mesial temporal lobe epilepsy arises in the medial aspect of the temporal lobe where the hippocampus, parahippocampal gyrus, and amygdala are located. It is often due to hippocampal sclerosis. Simple or complex partial seizures, with or without secondary generalization, often occur for the first time in early adolescence but may manifest at any age. A ris-

ing epigastric sensation is the most common aura symptom, fear the second most common. The patient may complain of visual phenomena such as micropsia and macropsia. Another classic feature is memory distortion. *Déjà vu* denotes the experience of peculiar familiarity with an unknown situation, whereas *jamais vu* refers to the illusion that something familiar is strange or new. Hallucinations may also involve gustatory and olfactory qualities. The latter seizures are sometimes called uncinate fits. When observing a patient with mesial temporal lobe seizures, one may notice a motionless stare and automatisms that can be oral (e.g., chewing, lip smacking), gestural, or more complex. Unilateral automatisms are usually ipsilateral to the side of seizure onset, while dystonic posturing is usually contralateral. Head deviation can be both ipsilateral and contralateral to the seizure focus. With seizure origin in the left hemisphere, the patient may have dysphasia ictally and postictally. Dysphasia is probably seen most often with lateral temporal lobe epilepsy that arises in the neocortex on the outer surface of the temporal lobe.[29] Also other signs of neocortical disturbance, such as auditory hallucinations, are more common with lateral than medial temporal lobe epilepsy. Similar to processes of the frontal lobes, neoplasms of the temporal lobe often lead to personality change with psychomotor retardation or agitation, as well as cognitive disturbances (see below) and emotional disturbance, including depression.

Some other conditions affecting primarily the mesial temporal lobes deserve mentioning here.

Transient global amnesia (TGA) is a striking condition in which the patient experiences short-term memory loss and anterograde amnesia for a few hours (rarely longer than 12 h and by definition less than 24 h). The patient appears bewildered and constantly asks the same questions over and over again ("Where are we, what are we doing here?") despite being able to manage fairly complex tasks such as driving or household work (or even conducting a symphony orchestra). Its

---

[29]The neocortex, which represents the vast majority of the cerebral cortex, has six layers and is phylogenetically younger than the archicortex of the three-layered hippocampus.

cause remains unknown but magnetic resonance (MR) diffusion-weighted sequences may reveal hyperintense signaling in the hippocampi and mesial temporal lobes during an attack in keeping with the "focal" deficit of impaired memory processing. TGA more or less exclusively affects people older than 50 years of age. It has a good prognosis, and the relapse rate is low. Importantly, patients can be reassured that there is no association with increased risk for cerebrovascular events (Case 2.18).

Temporary amnesia is occasionally a symptom of focal seizure activity and is then classified as *transient epileptic amnesia*, which may mimic TGA, but the clue to the correct diagnosis is the brevity and frequency of amnesic attacks. Importantly and in contrast to TGA, transient epileptic amnesia carries a risk of persistent memory impairment, and patients might be misdiagnosed as having dementia.

Limbic encephalitis is an autoimmune state that can be of paraneoplastic or non-paraneoplastic origin. Amnesia, personality change, anxiety, and epileptic seizures develop over days to weeks. If left untreated, limbic encephalitis may lead to chronic neuropsychiatric deficits and intractable epilepsy due to lasting damage of the mesial temporal lobes. Chapter 4 provides more information on both TGA and limbic encephalitis.

2.10.3 Parietal Lobes

The parietal lobes comprise the primary sensory cortex as well as the cortex regions associated with integration of visual, auditory, tactile, and proprioceptive information. Damage to the parietal lobe leads to contralateral *hemisensory deficits* and *homonym hemianopsia* (sometimes only inferior quadrantic homonym field defects, "pie on the floor"). With large lesions of the parietal lobe, a contralateral hemiparesis may occur due to compression of the adjacent motor cortex in the frontal lobe. Also, parietal lesions are often associated with striking neuropsychological symptoms, including *visuospatial disturbances*, *apraxia*, and *neglect* for the contralateral half of the body (e.g., the patient may deny ownership of the affected

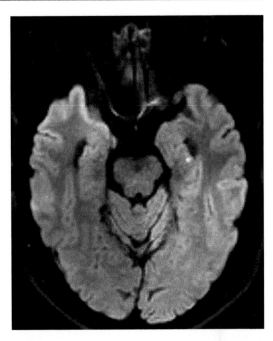

Case 2.18 Transient global amnesia. A 63-year-old male presented with sudden onset of memory loss after an uncomplicated minor medical procedure. He appeared confused and asked the same questions over and over again ("Where are we?"; "What are we going to do?"). On examination, there were no focal deficits. Of note, while recent memory was severely impaired, immediate memory (as tested by digit span), remote and procedural memory, as well as personal identity were intact. The symptoms completely resolved within 24 h. MRI, performed 4 days later, showed a dot-shaped DWI lesion in the left hippocampus; this lesion had vanished on a second MRI 3 months later (not shown). TGA is characterized by the presence of anterograde amnesia (as witnessed by a reliable observer). By definition, there is no clouding of consciousness, no loss of personal identity, no other cognitive impairment than amnesia, no focal neurologic signs or epileptic seizures, no recent history of head trauma, and symptoms resolve within 12–24 h. TGA usually affects people over 50 years, and the prognosis is excellent. Of note, MRI DWI shows punctate lesions in the hippocampus, either unilaterally (and then slightly more often on the left) or bilaterally, in up to 80% of patients. These lesions can no longer be detected on MRI follow-up a few weeks later. Although their exact etiology remains unknown, they precisely localize the site of the functional pathology

limb). Anosognosia is a form of neglect in which a patient denies the existence of an obvious disability or at least seems unaware of it.

Neglect is often somewhat more pronounced with lesions of the right parietal lobe. Thus, the typical patient with a right-sided, MCA occlusion has left hemiparesis, left homonym hemianopsia, and horizontal gaze palsy to the left (resulting in gaze deviation to the right) and ignores everything that happens on his left side. When spoken to from the left side, he will search for the speaker by looking even further to the right. He ignores the left half of his body to such an extent that he may deny being the owner of its extremities. The Eastchester clapping test is a useful test for neglect. When asked to clap, patients with hemispatial neglect repeatedly perform one-handed motions, stopping abruptly at the midline of the visual hemispace, as if pantomiming slapping an invisible board. In contrast, hemiplegic patients without pronounced neglect are able to reach across and clap against their plegic hand. This is an easy, rapid, and unambiguous test for neglect, especially in the setting of acute stroke (Ostrow and Llinás 2009).

Parietal lobe lesions may also lead to gnostic deficits, including impairment of stereognosis, graphesthesia, two-point discrimination, and tactile localization. These deficits are rather subtle and therefore often overlooked during the neurological examination. *Gerstmann's syndrome* is due to damage of the left angular and supramarginal gyri near the junction of the temporal and parietal lobes. It leads to the classic tetrad of agraphia, acalculia, left-right disorientation, and finger agnosia. It is very rare as an isolated syndrome, but it is not uncommon that some of its features coexist with more frequent parietal lobe deficits.

Another rarity, *Balint's syndrome*, is caused by bilateral damage to the posterior parietal cortex, e.g., due to parietal-occipital watershed or embolic posterior circulation infarcts (Case 2.19). Symptoms include:

- Incoordination of hand and eye movement, which is sometimes called optic ataxia. Patients have difficulties grasping for an object despite preserved vision.
- Environmental agnosia (inability to recognize familiar environments).
- Inability to voluntarily guide eye movements; thus, patients move their head instead of their eyes. This phenomenon is incorrectly called oculomotor apraxia (incorrectly because apraxia is the loss of the ability to carry out learned purposeful movements, and oculomotor function is an innate function).

- Simultanagnosia. Patients are unable to analyze a complex picture; instead, they focus on just one object at a time.

Patients with progressive posterior neurodegeneration, *posterior cortical atrophy*, may exhibit symptoms of Gerstmann and Balint's syndrome.

2.10.4　Occipital Lobes

The occipital lobes include the primary and associate visual cortex. Lesions of this region may therefore lead to either negative symptoms (*cortical blindness*) or positive symptoms (*visual hallucinations*).

Acute transitory blindness due to temporary disturbances of occipital cortex function can occur in young children after head trauma. Although it is a frightening experience for everyone, prognosis is excellent. Rarely, acute transitory blindness lasting a few seconds is a sign of a sudden decrease in posterior circulation perfusion due to atherosclerotic basilar artery insufficiency. It is then usually associated with transitory ischemic symptoms of the brainstem. Another cause of temporary cortical visual disturbances is *posterior reversible encephalopathy syndrome* (PRES; see Chapter 4 and Case 4.14 for details).

Cortical blindness is due to bilateral damage of the occipital lobes secondary to hypoxia, vasospasm, or cardiac embolism. Cortical blindness is sometimes associated with *Anton's syndrome*, arguably the most striking form of anosognosia. Patients with this syndrome behave as if they could see despite their obvious loss of sight, and confabulation is frequent (Case 2.20). Anosognosia is usually associated with concomitant dysfunction of the parietal lobe. Both the dominant and the nondominant hemisphere may be affected, although impairment of the latter is perhaps more common. The area of the parietal cortex that integrates visual with other sensory information is separated from inter- and intrahemispheric association pathways (disconnection syndrome, see above).

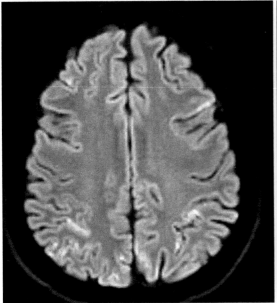 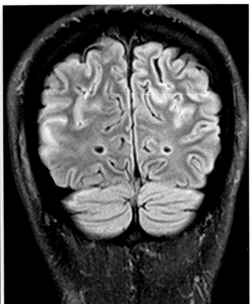

Case 2.19 Balint's syndrome. A 22-year-old man with an unremarkable prior medical history was resuscitated following a cardiac arrest due to a previously unknown cardiomyopathy. He regained consciousness a few days later. On examination, he was able to count fingers and to describe isolated features in his visual fields such as the examiner's eye color, but he was unable to identify more than one visual item at a time (simultagnosia). MRI showed bilateral parietal-occipital cortical ischemia (*left,* axial MR DWI; *right,* coronal FLAIR). Balint's syndrome consists of the triad of optic ataxia, oculomotor apraxia, and simultagnosia, and it is classically associated with bilateral lesions of the borderzone between the parietal and occipital lobes. This may either have a slow onset as in neurodegenerative diseases (see Case 5.5) or arise acutely due to global ischemia as in this case

The opposite of Anton's syndrome is *blindsight*, where patients also have cortical blindness but are fully aware of their loss of sight. Despite destruction of the occipital lobes and the fact that the patient explains he is only guessing, he has a significant ability to perceive and localize visual stimuli presented in a test situation. This is probably due to intact projections from the retina to cortical regions outside the primary visual cortex and to mesencephalic structures, where the visual stimuli do not reach consciousness.

Another striking feature of occipital lobe disease is *palinopsia* ("palin" is Greek for "again" while "opsis" is for "vision") (Case 2.21). Palinopsia is characterized by persistent or recurrent images despite removal of the stimulating object from the visual field and has been associated with lesions of the nondominant occipital lobe. Hallucinations derived from the primary visual cortex (Brodmann's area 17) occur as flashes or light spots. Sensations from the visual association cortex manifest as more detailed objects (area 18) or complex scenic hallucinations (area 19). The differential diagnosis of palinopsia includes, among others, *occipital lobe epilepsy*, *psychedelic drug abuse*, *tumors*, *basilar migraine*, and *visual deprivation hallucinations* (*Charles Bonnet syndrome*).[30]

---

[30] *Charles Bonnet syndrome* is a condition with characteristic hallucinations due to visual deprivation. This syndrome, probably underdiagnosed, usually occurs in the elderly with complete or near-complete blindness due to eye disease such as macular degeneration (or, less often, due to CNS-related visual disturbances). These patients typically have bizarre and complex, dreamlike hallucinations of people and settings. The hallucinations are usually non-frightening and sometimes even pleasurable. The patients are usually aware of the fact that their experiences are hallucinations only (so-called pseudohallucinations). A similar phenomenon is occasionally encountered in elderly hearing-impaired people who develop auditive deprivation hallucinations, usually in the form of repetitive melodies.

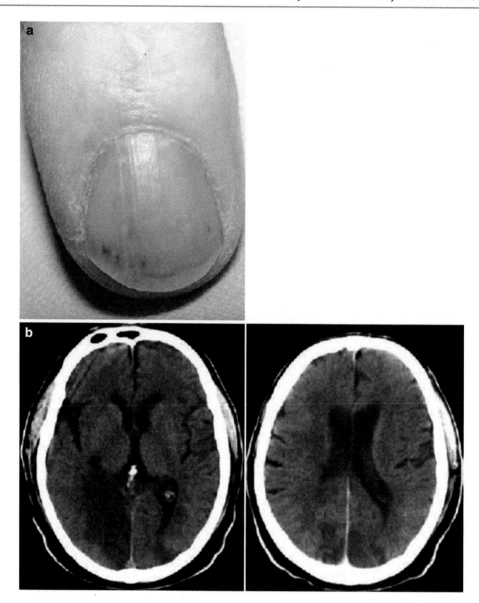

Case 2.20 Anton's syndrome. A 53-year-old female presented with a 2-week history of night sweats and fever. On examination, a systolic cardiac murmur and subungual splinter hemorrhages were noted (**a**). Treatment for infective endocarditis was started, but 2 days later the patient started behaving strangely. She noticed people only when they talked to her and she walked into the furniture. CT of the brain showed ischemic infarction in the territory of both posterior cerebral arteries (**b**). Despite the fact that she obviously was blind, she did not complain and denied any visual disturbance. She had an excuse whenever confronted with her handicap and did not hesitate to describe details in her environment that obviously did not exist

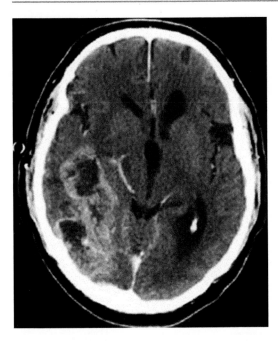

Case 2.21 Palinopsia. A previously healthy 64-year-old male experienced episodes of palinopsia several times a day. At one point, for example, after seeing a picture of a wasp in the morning newspaper, the brightly colored, cartoon-like image of the wasp appeared in his central vision and was projected on every object he looked at for the next 2 h. This occurred despite the fact that he had not looked at the newspaper again. He was aware that the wasp did not exist in reality. Palinopsia as well as episodes of derealization and visuospatial impairment were later preceded by a rising epigastric sensation. Five months after the onset of symptoms, the patient developed headache, vomiting, lethargy, and hemianopsia. A CT revealed a glioblastoma multiforme involving the right temporal-occipital lobe. Derealization, visuospatial impairment, and palinopsia were thus secondary due to partial seizures provoked by the developing glioblastoma multiforme in the occipitoparietal lobe. With the tumor invading the temporal lobe, features of temporal lobe epilepsy such as epigastric sensations occurred (Adapted with permission from Kondziella and Maetzel (2006))

2.11 Cerebrovascular System

The cerebrovascular system is divided into the anterior and the posterior circulation (Fig. 2.13).

The anterior circulation consists of the left and right internal carotid arteries (ICA) that give rise to the anterior cerebral arteries (ACA) and middle cerebral arteries (MCA), as well as the ophthalmic and the anterior choroidal arteries. The anterior communicating artery (AComA) links the left with the right ACA.

The posterior circulation is made up of the two vertebral arteries that give rise to the posterior inferior cerebellar arteries (PICA) before joining into the basilar artery. From the basilar artery arise the anterior inferior cerebellar arteries (AICA), pontine arteries, superior cerebellar arteries, and posterior cerebral arteries (PCA).

The posterior and anterior circulations are connected via the posterior communicating arteries (PCommA), which close the Circle of Willis. Clockwise, the Circle of Willis thus consists of the AComA, the left ACA, the left ICA, the left PCommA, the left PCA, the right PCA, the right PCommA, the right ICA, and the right ACA. Although the MCAs and basilar artery do not contribute to the formation of the Circle of Willis anatomically, they are often considered a part of it functionally.

It is important to note that many anatomical variations of the cerebrovascular system exist. For instance, it is not uncommon that one or both PCAs are supplied mainly by the anterior and not the posterior circulation or that one of the vertebral arteries ends in the ipsilateral PICA and does not contribute to the basilar artery.

Although there are a few notable exceptions, most cerebrovascular events are of course of sudden onset—they happen like a stroke.

2.11.1 Anterior Circulation

Sudden occlusion of the *internal carotid artery* can lead to ischemia of territories belonging to the ACA and the MCA, as well as the ophthalmic and anterior choroidal arteries. Depending on the collateral blood flow through the Circle of Willis, ischemia is transient or permanent. Ischemia in the anterior circulation is usually of acute onset; a fluctuating, crescendo time course is much rarer compared to posterior circulation stroke.

The hallmark of *ophthalmic artery* ischemia is monocular blindness, as discussed earlier.

Occlusion of the *anterior choroidal artery* leads to contralateral hemiplegia, dense hemihypesthesia, and homonym hemianopia due to damage to the posterior limb of the internal capsule and optic tract, a small but critical piece of neuroanatomy. Well-

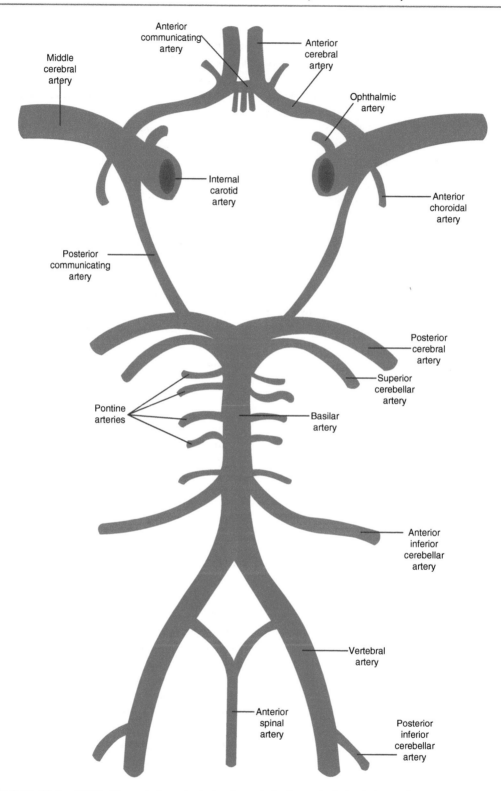

Fig. 2.13 Circle of Willis. The posterior and anterior circulations are connected via the posterior communicating arteries and form the Circle of Willis. This creates collaterals in the cerebral circulation, a "biological reassurance" against intracranial occlusions. Anatomic variants, however, are not uncommon

preserved language and cognition distinguishes this stroke syndrome from MCA infarction.

The *MCA* serves large parts of the medial aspect of the temporal, parietal, and frontal lobes, as well as the insula and most of the basal ganglia and internal capsule (via lenticulostriate branches). In the lateral sulcus (or Sylvian fissure), the MCA splits into two or three branches. As stated above, the upper branch serves Broca's area and the motor cortex situated in the frontal lobe (leading to nonfluent aphasia and contralateral hemiparesis sparing the leg), whereas the lower branch supplies the temporal lobe and Wernicke's area (leading to fluent aphasia). Eye opening apraxia is sometimes encountered early after large hemispheric strokes (especially when MCA and ACA territories are involved simultaneously); this resolves usually within a few days.

The *ACA* supplies the medial parts of the frontal and most of the medial parts of the parietal lobe, as well as the most of the corpus callosum and the anterior portions of the basal ganglia and internal capsule. Occlusion of the ACA may therefore lead to sensorimotor deficits of the contralateral foot and leg and, to a lesser degree, of the upper extremity.[31] Hemorrhage from an *ACOM* aneurysm can lead to sudden onset of paraplegia and urinary incontinence due to injury to the medial aspects of the frontal lobes. Another complication associated with an ACOM aneurysm may arise when the *recurrent artery of Heubner* (an ACA branch that arises distally from the ACOM, supplying part of the head of the caudate nucleus) is sacrificed during surgery. This results in severe cognitive deficits because of damage to connecting pathways between the caudate and the frontal lobe.

2.11.2 Posterior Circulation

Posterior circulation ischemia leads to focal deficits related to the *brainstem, cerebellum, thalamus*, and/or *occipital lobes*.

Vertebral artery dissection and/or *PICA* infarction may cause the *Wallenberg syndrome*, probably the only eponymous brainstem syndrome that is worth knowing because it is the most common. An infarction of the lateral medulla oblongata, it leads to:

- Dysphagia, hoarseness, and ipsilaterally diminished gag reflex (CN IX, CN X)
- Ipsilateral Horner's syndrome (descending sympathetic fibers)
- Ipsilateral ataxia of the extremities (cerebellar peduncle)
- Loss of pain and temperature sensation in the ipsilateral half of the face (spinal CN V nucleus)
- Loss of pain and temperature sensation in the contralateral half of the body (lateral spinothalamic tract)
- Diplopia, nystagmus, and vertigo (vestibular nuclei)
- *AICA* infarction, as discussed earlier, may lead to sudden onset of vertigo and ipsilateral deafness (with or without tinnitus).

Thrombosis of the *basilar artery* often gives rise to early bilateral fluctuating brainstem and cerebellar signs (e.g., left and right fluctuating hemiparesis, CN deficits, dysarthria, vertigo, and ataxia), before brainstem infarction occurs. Indeed, in contrast to anterior circulation ischemia, basilar artery stenosis can lead to symptoms that come and go for many hours and days, and they can take a crescendo course when infarcts in the brainstem and cerebellum accumulate over time. Complete brainstem infarction leads to instant death. Preservation of the mesencephalon and the dorsal pons (and thus the ARAS, which is crucial for arousal) leads to the *locked-in syndrome*. In this tragic situation patients are awake and usually well orientated but tetraplegic and unable to communicate except by using preserved oculomotor function.[32]

Occlusion of the distal portion of the basilar artery, usually embolic in origin, leads to the *top-of-the-basilar syndrome* (Cases 4.22 and 4.23).

---

[31]An anatomical variant, both ACA may also arise from a single stem, and occlusion of this stem then causes bilateral infarction of the anterior and medial aspects of both hemispheres. As a result, patients may develop paraparesis, incontinence, and abulia.

[32]Conditions such GBS, ALS, or myasthenia gravis may occasionally be associated with afferent denervation that is severe enough to mimic the locked-in syndrome.

Infarction of the upper brainstem and occipital hemispheric regions is characterized by dysfunction of oculomotor (external and internal ophthalmoplegia), behavioral (somnolence, dreamlike behavior), and sometimes visual (hallucinations) systems. Characteristically, power in the extremities and face is well preserved. Also, an embolus splitting into two parts when reaching the basilar artery bifurcation may occlude both PCA.

The *PCA* supplies the upper brainstem and the inferomedial parts of the temporal lobe as well as the occipital lobes. Therefore, PCA occlusion produces

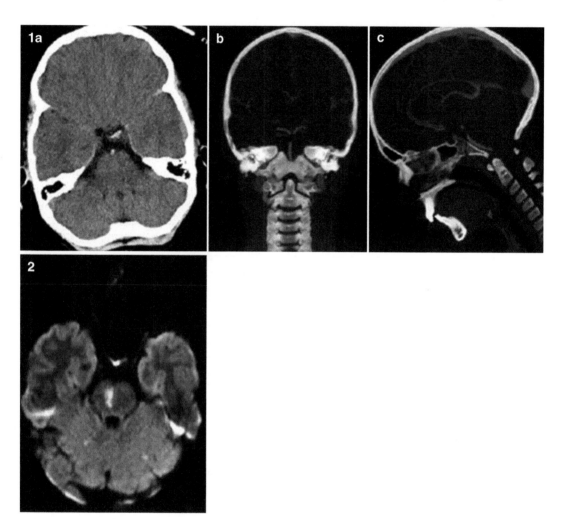

Case 2.22 Pediatric basilar artery thrombosis. A male patient presented with sudden onset of neck pain, double vision, difficulties with articulation, and fluctuating impairment of consciousness. He reacted to loud commands only. On examination, gaze-changing vertical nystagmus, dysarthria, and left Babinski sign were noticed. He was able to move his arms and legs normally. The clinical picture was consistent with a top-of-the-basilar syndrome. CT of the brain showed a dense artery sign, thus suggesting a clot in the basilar artery (**1a**), which was confirmed by CT angiography (**1b**, **1c**). Intravenous thrombolysis with alteplase was initiated, and the patient was immediately referred to the regional stroke center. On arrival, MR DWI revealed acute ischemic infarcts in the pons and the cerebellar hemisphere on the right (**2**). The occluded basilar artery was visualized by digital subtraction angiography (**3a**). Following clot removal using a stent retriever, the basilar artery was fully recanalized 4 h after onset of symptoms (**3b**, **3c**). MR angiogram the next day confirmed persistent basilar artery patency (**3d**). Neurological examination was unremarkable. At 3-month follow-up, the patient had made a complete recovery except for slight dysarthria during periods of physical exhaustion. The most unusual feature of this case is the fact that the patient was a previously healthy 11-year-old boy. An extensive cerebrovascular, cardiologic, and hematologic workup did not reveal the cause of the thrombosis, which is not uncommon in pediatric stroke (Adapted with permission from Fink et al. (2013))

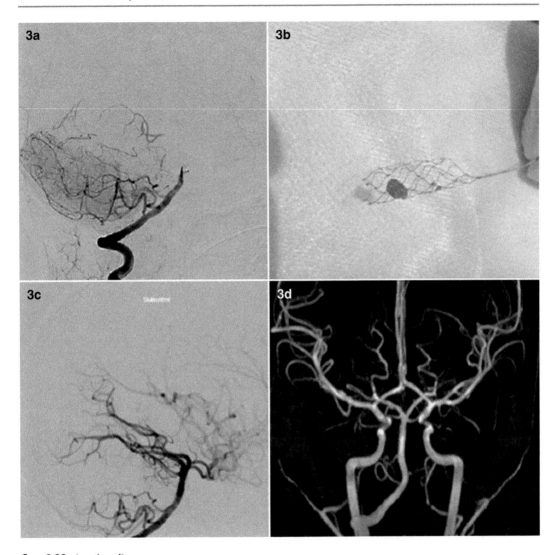

Case 2.22 (continued)

a rather large variety of deficits compared to other intracranial arteries. The *cortical branches* of the PCA supply the occipital lobes, the inferior temporal gyrus, and the uncus. Typical stroke syndromes following occlusion of these branches include homonymous hemianopia (often with macular, or central, sparing because of collateral blood supply of the occipital pole by distal MCA branches), alexia without agraphia (see above), and visual agnosia and memory impairment. Bilateral damage of the occipital lobes leads to partial or complete cortical blindness and, if associated with denial of blindness and confabulation, Anton's syndrome. The *central* (e.g., *thalamoperforating*) *branches* serve large parts of the thalamus and, as explained earlier, may lead to

severe numbness (and possibly thalamic pain) in the contralateral half of the body with or without neglect. Occasionally, infarction of the ventral nuclei and/or the subthalamic nucleus may produce hemiballism or hemichorea, and infarction of the central nuclei may impair consciousness.

Another rare anatomic variant, the *artery of Percheron* is a single arterial trunk arising from the posterior cerebral artery and supplying the thalamus and midbrain bilaterally. Occlusion of the artery of Percheron results in bilateral paramedian thalamus infarction (with or without midbrain involvement) and typically leads to disturbances of consciousness. However, most strokes associated with this infarct pattern are of embolic origin (Case 2.23).

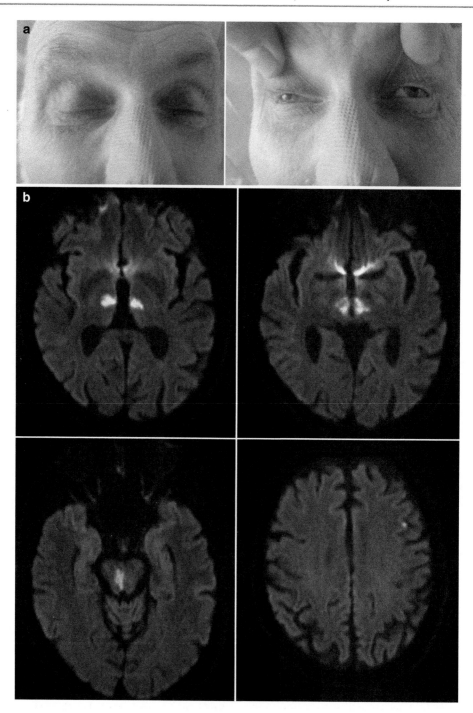

Case 2.23 Top-of-the-basilar stroke. A 72-year-old male with hypertension and previous myocardial infarction was discovered lying on the floor of his home. On admission, he was found to be mute and with bilateral ptosis. Although he tried, eye opening on command was not possible (*upper row*). On passive eye opening, there were divergent eye axes and near-complete external supranuclear ophthalmoplegia. He was unable to swallow (note plaster on his nose to fixate gastrointestinal feeding tube), but power in his arms and legs was relatively spared. MR DWI revealed bilateral infarc-tions in the thalamus and the midbrain, consistent with a top-of-the-basilar stroke (*middle and lower rows*) . Although this is sometimes associated with occlusion of the artery of Percheron (a rare variant of the posterior cerebral circulation characterized by a solitary arterial trunk supplying the para-median thalami and the rostral midbrain on both sides), an embolus to the top of the basilar artery is a much more fre-quent cause. Indeed, as seen in this case, the DWI lesion in the left hemisphere (*lower row, right*) suggests that this patient's stroke was due to an embolic source

2.12   The Healthy Brain

Now that most of the relevant neuroanatomic features have been discussed, let us consider what happens in the normal brain during the acquisition of sensory data, the processing of information, and the resulting vegetative and motor responses. For the sake of discussion, let us assume that I have just heard someone make the statement, "Your new haircut looks rather funny."

What happens initially is that light reflected from the person in question falls onto my *retina* and sound waves traveling through the ear canal hit my tympanic membrane. The light activates retinal photoreceptors (rods and cones) that send signals via bipolar and horizontal cells to retinal ganglia cells, the axons of which make up the *optic nerves*. The tympanic membrane transmits sound from the air to the ossicles inside the middle ear; the sound waves are converted into fluid waves in the inner ear; and the hair cells of the organ of Corti transform the fluid waves into nerve signals that travel along the *cochlear part of CN VIII* into the *brainstem.*

All sensory input (except olfaction) is processed in the *thalamus*, which filters away redundant signals. Important information passes through the thalamic filter and reaches the relevant primary cortex area: the *primary sensory cortex* (gyrus postcentralis), the *primary auditory cortex* (superior temporal gyrus), or the *primary visual cortex* (in and around the calcarine fissure of the occipital lobe). Information is then passed onto the *unimodal (secondary) association cortex* immediately adjacent to the respective primary cortex. The unimodal association cortex analyzes stimuli of the same sensory quality (e.g., recognition of spatial patterns and words). Information is passed further onto the *polymodal (tertiary) association cortex* of the frontal, parietal, and temporal lobes. The prefrontal lobe is the most important one in this regard. In the polymodal association cortex, information from different sensory modalities converges on the same neuron; this is the anatomic basis for the fact that different sensory impressions can be perceived as one (Case 2.24). (Without such cortical computation, major cultural achievements like Mozart's opera *The Marriage of Figaro* would never have been possible.) The information is then processed on an even higher level in the *supramodal association area* in the prefrontal

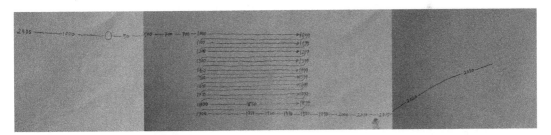

Case 2.24 Time-space synesthesia. A young female physician realized during her residency that she possessed an outstanding ability which she previously had considered normal: She had since childhood experienced units of time, including days, weeks, months, and years, as occupying specific locations in space relative to her own body. Thus, she felt the past was to her left, from around 2500 BC until the present day, while the future was to her right. She would experience the months of the year located on a circle around her. These time-space associations were very specific and experienced consistently. Synesthesia is an unusual brain condition in which people experience merging of sensory modalities, so that activity in one modality automatically, involuntarily, and consistently elicits sensations in another. For instance, grapheme-color synesthesia is a phenomenon in which people may experience that numbers or letters have specific colors (e.g., three may be black, while four yellow). Others may experience that colors have specific tastes (e.g., black tastes bitter, while green tastes sweet; which is termed flavor-color synesthesia), and so on. Time-space synesthesia involves the involuntary association of time events, such as months of the year, with specific spatial locations with two- or three-dimensional forms, such as circles and ellipses. The latter are typically experienced in relation to one's own body. Although the exact mechanisms remain unknown, it has been suggested that synesthesia may be due to extraordinarily rich connectivity between brain regions, e.g., time-space synesthesia may arise with enhanced parietal-occipital network connectivity between regions responsible for temporal sequences and those supporting visuospatial images

and temporal cortices, which is where the information is integrated and associated with previously learned material, e.g., "This statement actually sounded like an insult."

In the end, all information converges on limbic structures, the most important of which are the *hippocampus* and the *amygdala* which serve as an emotional filter. Only emotionally important or otherwise salient information will have an impact on subsequent brain activity; redundant data will be deleted. Emotionally important information ("This is an insult!") will activate the *hypothalamus-septal area*. Electrical stimulation of this region has been shown to induce phylogenetically ancient behaviors such as aggression, flight response, and sexual arousal. The hypothalamus is connected with the brainstem via the *fasciculus longitudinalis dorsalis*. This is the "psychosomatic pathway" and the anatomic substrate for the control of sympathetic and parasympathetic responses by higher cerebral function. Impulses transmitted via this fasciculus activate *parasympathetic dorsal vagus nuclei* and *sympathetic centers in the medulla oblongata*. This results in peripheral vegetative responses, such as flushing of the face, sweating, and tachycardia.

Simultaneously, the *supplementary motor area* and the *premotor cortex* in the frontal lobes come into action as they are the parts of the brain that plan, select, and initiate motor actions. Hopefully, at this stage of the conversation, frontal inhibition will interrupt and prevent me from engaging in a dispute about my new haircut.

References and Suggested Reading

Ahmed RM, Irish M, Piguet O, et al. Amyotrophic lateral sclerosis and frontotemporal dementia: distinct and overlapping changes in eating behaviour and metabolism. Lancet Neurol. 2016;15:332–42.

Al-Chalabi A, Hardiman O, Kiernan MC, et al. Amyotrophic lateral sclerosis: moving towards a new classification system. Lancet Neurol. 2016;15:1182–94.

Blumenfeld H. Neuroanatomy through clinical cases. 2nd ed. Sunderland, MA: Sinauer Associates, Inc.; 2011.

Brazis PW. Localization in clinical neurology. 5th ed. Philadelphia, PA: Lippincott Williams & Wilkins; 2006.

Caplan LR, van Gijn J. Stroke syndromes. 3rd ed. Cambridge: Cambridge University Press; 2012.

Choi BS, Kim JH, Jung C, Kim SY. High-resolution diffusion-weighted imaging increases lesion detectability in patients with transient global amnesia. AJNR Am J Neuroradiol. 2012;33:1771–4.

Denny JC, Arndt FV, Dupont WD, Neilson EG. Increased hospital mortality in patients with bedside hippus. Am J Med. 2008;121:239–45.

Dyck JP, Thomas PK. Peripheral neuropathy. 4th ed. Philadelphia, PA: Saunders; 2005.

Fink J, Sonnenborg L, Lunde Larsen L, et al. Basilar artery thrombosis treated in a child with intravenous tissue plasminogen activator and mechanical thrombectomy. J Child Neurol. 2013;28(11):1521–6.

Gutschalk A, Uppenkamp S, Riedel B, Bartsch A, Brandt T, Vogt-Schaden M. Pure word deafness with auditory object agnosia after bilateral lesion of the superior temporal sulcus. Cortex. 2015;73:24–35.

Harlow JM. Passage of an iron rod through the head. Boston Med Surg J. 1848;39:389–3.

Harlow JM. Recovery from the Passage of an Iron Bar through the Head. Publ Massachusetts Med Soc. 1868;2:327–47.

Hassan A, Mateen FJ, Coon EA, Ahlskog JE. Painful legs and moving toes syndrome: a 76-patient case series. Arch Neurol. 2012;69:1032–8.

Herskovitz S, Scelsa S, Schaumburg H. Peripheral neuropathies in clinical practice. 1st ed. Oxford: Oxford University Press; 2010.

Kiernan MC, Turner MR. Lou Gehrig and the ALS split hand. Neurology. 2015;85:1995.

Kondziella D, Maetzel H. The sting in the tail: syncope and palinopsia. J Neurol. 2006;253:657–8.

Menon P, Kiernan MC, Vucic S. Cortical dysfunction underlies the development of the split-hand in amyotrophic lateral sclerosis. PLoS One. 2014;9:e87124.

Moore AP, Blumhardt LD. A prospective survey of the causes of non-traumatic spastic paraparesis and tetraparesis in 585 patients. Spinal Cord. 1997;35:361–7.

O'Brien M. Aids to the examination of the peripheral nervous system. 5th ed. Philadelphia, PA: Saunders; 2010.

Ostrow LV, Llinás RH. Eastchester clapping sign: a novel test of parietal neglect. Ann Neurol. 2009;66:114–7.

Panayiotopoulos CP. A clinical guide to epileptic syndromes and their treatment. 2nd ed. London: Springer; 2010.

Plum JB, Saber CB, Schiff N, Plum F. Plum and Posner's diagnosis of stupor and coma. 4th ed. Oxford: Oxford University Press; 2007.

Powel R, Hughes T. A chamber of secrets. The neurology of the thalamus: lessons from acute stroke. Pract Neurol. 2014;14:440–5.

Ropper AH, Samuels MA. Adams and Victor's principles of neurology. 10th ed. New York, NY: McGraw-Hill Professional; 2014.

Rubin M, Safdieh JE. Netter's concise neuroanatomy. London: Saunders; 2007.

Shields M, Sinkar S, Chan W, Crompton J. Parinaud syndrome: a 25-year (1991-2016) review of 40 consecutive adult cases. Acta Ophthalmol. 2016; doi: 10.1111/aos.13283.

Sommer WH, Bollwein C, Thierfelder KM, Baumann A, Janssen H, Ertl-Wagner B, Reiser MF, Plate A, Straube A, von Baumgarten L. Crossed cerebellar diaschisis in patients with acute middle cerebral artery infarction: occurrence and perfusion characteristics. J Cereb Blood Flow Metab. 2016;36:743–54.

Waxman S. Clinical neuroanatomy. 27th ed. New York, NY: McGraw-Hill Medical; 2013.

Neurological Bedside Examination: "Can I Confirm My Anatomical Hypothesis?"

3

Abstract

After finishing the history, the neurologist should have a distinct anatomical hypothesis that can be confirmed (or rejected) during the bedside examination. Specifically, the neurologist seeks to elicit the signs compatible with this hypothesis, to confirm the absence of signs irreconcilable with it, and to verify that the rest of the examination is normal. A standard bedside examination includes evaluation of consciousness and cognition, cranial nerves, sensorimotor and cerebellar function, and gait and a general medical assessment. In cooperative patients, this can often be done in less than 10 min. In addition, tactful observation of the patient before, during, and after the consultation can reveal a wealth of information regarding neurological function. In this chapter, the reader will find in-depth information and practice tips concerning the examination of neurological patients, including those with decreased consciousness, epileptic seizures, and functional deficits.

Keywords

Bedside examination • Cerebellar function • Cognition • Consciousness • Cranial nerve examination • Gait • Mental function • Motor function • Sensory function • System overview

The neurological examination has three goals:

- To elicit the signs that confirm the anatomical hypothesis
- To verify the absence of neurological signs incompatible with the anatomical hypothesis
- To assess whether the remainder of the neurological examination is normal based on a complete bedside examination

As the neurologist gains experience, much can be deduced from simply observing the patient during the consultation, and given that time is limited, choosing not to do a complete bedside examination is often an option. Although often acceptable and sometimes inevitable, it is important to be aware of the fact that crucial information may easily be missed. For instance, if the CN examination in a patient presenting with a

© Springer International Publishing AG 2017
D. Kondziella, G. Waldemar, *Neurology at the Bedside*, DOI 10.1007/978-3-319-55991-9_3

symmetric proximal weakness is omitted, the ophthalmoplegia that is essential for the diagnosis of a mitochondrial disorder may be overlooked.

With some experience and unless detailed cognitive testing is necessary, a neurological bedside examination can be performed in less than 10 min. To avoid confusion, arranging the examination according to functional systems and assessing one functional system at a time are advisable (Table 3.1).

Table 3.1 Suggestions for a standard bedside examination in the cooperative patient

Cognitive examination: arousal, consciousness, attention; orientation to personal data, time, place, and situation; episodic memory, praxia, spontaneous language, comprehension, behavior, and mood
Cranial nerve examination:
Ophthalmoscopy
Visual fields and acuity (CN II)
Direct and indirect pupillary reflexes (CN II, III)
Full range of eye movements and smooth pursuit (CN III, IV, VI)
Facial sensation (CN V)
Facial muscle power (CN VIII)
Palatal contraction (CN IX, X)
Head turning and shoulder lifting (CN XI)
Tongue power and diadochokinesia (CN XII)
Motor examination:
Straight arm test
Formal power testing, including:
Elevation and abduction of the arm at 90° (deltoid muscle)
Adduction in the same position (major pectoralis muscle)
Elbow flexion with forearm supinated (biceps muscle)
Elbow extension (triceps muscle)
Extension of the wrist (extensor carpi radialis longus muscle)
Pincer grip (flexor pollicis brevis, flexor digitorum superficialis, and opponens pollicis muscles)
Finger abduction and adduction (interossei muscles)
Hip flexion (iliopsoas muscle)
Knee extension (quadriceps femoris muscle)
Knee flexion (biceps femoris, semitendinosus, and semimembranosus muscles)
Dorsiflexion of foot (tibialis anterior muscle)
Plantar flexion of foot (gastrocnemius, soleus muscles)

Table 3.1 (continued)

Muscle tone in arms and legs
Reflex status, including:
Brachialis (C5/C6)
Brachioradialis (C5–C7)
Finger flexor (C6/C7)
Triceps (C6–C8)
Adductor (L2/L3)
Patellar (L2–L4)
Achilles (S1/S2)
Plantar reflexes
Sensory examination: touch at hands and feet (pin prick only if patient has sensory complaints); vibration and proprioception in the great toe
Cerebellum: finger-(nose)-finger test, knee-heel test; gait (including Romberg's test)
Gait: normal speed, turning around, walking on toes and heels, walking on a line; classification of involuntary movements, if present
System overview: auscultation of heart, carotids, lungs; pulse, blood pressure; temperature

The following neurological examination may be regarded as routine at the bedside:

- Assessment of consciousness, orientation, higher mental functions, behavior, and mood
- CN examination including ophthalmoscopy
- Motor examination including muscle power, tonus, inspection for possible muscular atrophy, deep tendon reflexes, and plantar reflexes
- Sensory examination including assessment of pain, temperature, vibration, and proprioception
- Cerebellar function
- Gait
- System overview, e.g., vital parameters and auscultation of the heart, lungs, and carotid arteries

Assessment of mental function, CN examination, and evaluation of power in the upper extremities are best performed with the patient sitting. Assessment of power in the legs, muscle tone, and reflexes in the upper and lower extremities, sensory function, and cerebellar function (e.g., finger-nose, heel-knee test), as well as system overview, is most conveniently performed with a supine patient. At the end—or at the very beginning of the examination—gait is assessed, which provides an invaluable overview of total performance. (Indeed, informal observation of gait should start when the patient walks down the corridor to the neurologist's office.)

It cannot be overemphasized that neurological assessment of the patient is not restricted to the formal bedside examination. Before, during, and after consultation, careful but discreet observation of the patient may reveal a wealth of information regarding neurological function. To name but a few examples, difficulties with finger movements of one hand while undressing as well as outward rotation of the ipsilateral foot while walking into the office may disclose a mild hemiparesis; gait performance of the patient with a functional disorder tends to be much better outside the office than during the consultation; and a spontaneous smile during conversation may reveal a mild facial palsy. Also, when a patient is in bed, as typically happens during ward rounds, make every attempt to get him out of it. In a patient with a midline cerebellar lesion, for instance, muscle power and coordination in the extremities can be normal, and truncal instability and gait ataxia may only become apparent when the patient is out of bed.

The following section provides an overview of the formal neurological examination. Table 3.1 highlights routine tests, but these and more comprehensive testing of each functional system are reviewed below in greater detail.

3.1 Cognitive and Mental Functions

Bedside examination of the patient with cognitive or mental impairment is challenging, because the abilities used by the patient to construct a history and description of symptoms are also the potentially defective abilities that are under scrutiny. Some patients may not have a clear understanding of the reason for attending the clinic. Memory impairment as well as anosognosia (unawareness of deficits), aphasia, and disturbed mood or behavior may lead to an inadequate or unreliable history when obtained from the patient alone. Therefore,

also obtaining a history from an informant is of the utmost importance. Whenever possible, the informant interview should be conducted in the patient's absence. It is particularly helpful in getting an overview of the impact on activities of daily living of the presenting symptoms and in identifying psychotic and behavioral symptoms. Furthermore, discrepancies in the accounts from the patient and the informant help to assess the level of anosognosia.

3.1.1 The History as Part of the Cognitive Examination

Taking the history from the patient also forms an important part of the cognitive examination and serves to identify areas of particular interest for further formal assessment. During the patient interview, the neurologist will get an impression of memory from the patient's ability to recall events in the autobiographical and medical history and information about language from the patient's spontaneous conversation and ability to comprehend. The examiner will also have the opportunity to get an impression of the patient's insight, mood, behavior, and possible psychotic manifestations. Be sure to inquire into the patients' understanding of the reason for the visit. During the interview, the patient with amnesia or dementia may turn his head back to the spouse or caregiver, as if he is silently looking for some cues directly to the question. This characteristic behavior is called the *head-turning sign*. Many of the following symptoms are delicate—although important—issues and are best enquired about with the informant in the absence of the patient. Explain to the patient why you need to talk with the informant.

3.1.1.1 Cognitive Symptoms
The cognitive history should explore the different cognitive domains:

- Memory:
  - Are there problems with attention, slips, and poor concentration (*working memory*)?
  - Is knowledge about facts and objects impaired and is there loss of memory for words or vocabulary (*semantic memory*)?

- Does the patient have impaired recall of specific events? Does he have difficulties remembering appointments and events, e.g., are there problems recalling details of a recent phone conversation, television program, or a birthday party last Sunday (*episodic memory*)?
- Language and speech:
  - Expression: Are there any problems with naming, with word order, or with word endings?
  - Comprehension: Does the patient have problems with understanding conversations or with "hearing" when many people are gathered in a group?
  - Are there any problems with reading or writing?
- Executive functions:
  - Is the patient easily distracted?
  - Are there problems with organizing, shopping, and other household activities or with using new appliances or electronic devices in the home?
  - Does the patient appear disorganized?
  - Is the patient's ability to plan and set goals impaired?
- Calculation:
  - Does the patient show impaired handling of money, e.g., getting correct change in the supermarket and difficulties handling bills or bank accounts?
- Praxis:
  - Is there disturbed planning of motor functions, e.g., getting dressed and brushing teeth?
- Visuospatial/perceptual abilities:
  - Does the patient have problems in finding his way around?
  - Are there difficulties reaching out for objects? Is there a tendency to miss steps (suggesting biparietal pathology)?
  - Does the patient have trouble recognizing faces (prosopagnosia, suggesting bilateral occipito-temporal pathology)?

3.1.1.2 Mental Functions

Brief assessment scales for depression (e.g., Geriatric Depression Scale, Cornell Scale for Depression in Dementia, or Hamilton Depression Scale) and for neuropsychiatric symptoms (e.g., Neuropsychiatric Inventory) are available for systematic enquiry of mental functions:

- *Personality changes* may arise insidiously many years prior to other impairments in patients with dementia. Disengagement, loss of empathy, apathy, agitation, and/or disinhibition is characteristic for specific dementia disorders.
- *Behavioral changes* may be very disturbing and include aggression, agitation, stereotypical behavior, psychomotor restlessness, and wandering (Case 3.1).
- A person with *Godot's syndrome* is anxious and repeatedly asks questions about an upcoming event—a behavior which may result from decreased cognitive abilities and from the inability to apply remaining thinking capacities productively.
- *Depression* is a common differential diagnosis to dementia, and depressive symptoms occur often in degenerative dementias. Mood disturbances should always be assessed and classified, e.g., anxiety, tiredness, pessimistic ruminations, and suicidal ideation (mania or euphoria is rarer).
- *Hallucinations* in cognitively impaired patients most often occur in the visual modality but may also affect auditory, gustatory, olfactory, and tactile modalities. Hallucinations are a particular feature of dementia with Lewy bodies (DLB) but may also occur in patients with other dementias and delirium.
- *Delusions* are false beliefs, occurring often in patients with neurodegenerative dementias, and sometimes they are associated with misidentifications. The most common delusions are:
  - Abandonment: The belief that the caregiver plans to abandon the patient
  - Theft: The belief that someone has stolen a misplaced object
  - Infidelity of the spouse
  - The delusion that one's home is not one's home
  - Capgras' phenomenon: The belief that the spouse or another relative has been replaced by an imposter who looks exactly like him/her

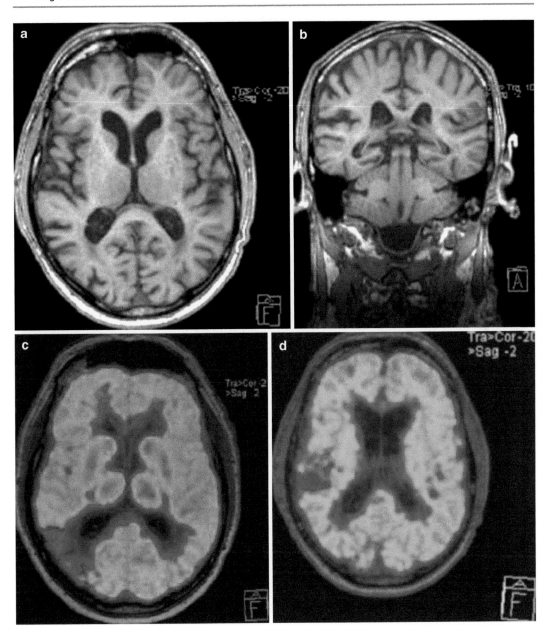

Case 3.1 Alzheimer's disease with atypical onset (behavioral symptoms). A 68-year-old male was referred for diagnostic evaluation of possible frontotemporal dementia. Two years earlier, his wife had noticed gradual onset of personality change with inappropriate (and sometimes disinhibited) social behavior and word-finding difficulties. His symptoms had been progressing rapidly. The neurological and neuropsychological examination revealed a global aphasia with severely impaired comprehension, word finding, and writing, as well as impaired calculation and a mild apraxia. The MMSE score was 11/30. Axial and coronal MRI showed temporoparietal atrophy (more pronounced in the right hemisphere) (**a**, **b**). FDG PET demonstrated classical bitemporoparietal hypometabolism, which was also more pronounced on the right side (**c**, **d**). Amyloid PET (^{11}C-PIB PET) was positive. The diagnosis was AD with atypical onset (PET images courtesy of Ian Law, Department of Clinical Physiology and Nuclear Medicine, Rigshospitalet, Copenhagen)

- Phantom boarder syndrome: The belief that someone uninvited is living in the patient's house
- De Clerambault's syndrome: The belief that someone is in love with the patient
- Misidentification of the patient's own self (the picture sign): The belief that the person in the mirror is not the patient but some other person (self-prosopagnosia)
- Misidentification of events on television (the patient imagines these events are occurring in real three-dimensional space)
- Bizarre delusions may occur in semantic dementia (SD)
- Cotard's syndrome: The belief that the patient is dead, or that parts of his body no longer exist.

Sleep pattern, *eating pattern*, and *sexual behavior* may be altered as a result of neurodegenerative disorders. For instance, preference to certain (sweet) foods or even pica-type syndromes[1] may be characteristic in frontotemporal dementia and can lead to overweight. Common sleep disturbances are REM sleep disorder, fragmented sleep, day-night reversal, nightmares, and nocturnal hallucinations. Changes in sexual behavior include increased or decreased libido.

Other neurological symptoms of particular interest in patients with cognitive impairment are gait difficulty (pointing to involvement of the extrapyramidal system or the cerebellum or to the presence of a hydrocephalus), visual disorientation (suggesting impaired eye movements), parkinsonism, dysarthria, dysphagia, myoclonus, and motor weakness.

3.1.1.3 Onset and Progression

Was the onset sudden or insidious? Was there any event eliciting the onset of symptoms? Even when there was an acute event, carefully ask about any subtle symptoms prior to the event. Is the condition static (e.g., Korsakoff's syndrome), or is there a gradual (neurodegenerative) or step-

wise (multi-infarct) progression? Are the symptoms progressing very rapidly (for rapidly progressive dementias, see Chap. 4)?

3.1.1.4 Past Medical History

Of particular interest is a history of seizures, stroke, encephalitis, traumatic brain injury, and depression. Drug history and establishing the level of alcohol intake are important elements of the history. Non-neurological conditions such as malignancy, metabolic conditions, and infections may also be related to cognitive impairment.

3.1.1.5 Family History

Ask for family history of memory impairment, dementia, psychiatric illness, movement disorder, and ages and causes of death.

3.1.1.6 Activities of Daily Living, Social Consequences, and Driving

Brief assessment scales are available for informant interview on activities of daily living. Ask the informant to describe the patient's typical daily activities at home and at work, if relevant. Ask about the ability to use electronic appliances, personal hygiene, handling finances, as well as shopping, cooking, and other household activities. Interview the caregiver about driving abilities and about accidents while driving.

Further examination is indicated if the history suggests mental changes or cognitive dysfunction.

3.1.2 Bedside Examination of Mental and Cognitive Functions

During the bedside examination of the *mental functions*, pay attention to the following:

- *The appearance of the patient*: The patient's general appearance should be noted, including dressing, grooming, makeup, body odor, overall behavior and attitude (hostile, guarded, cooperative?), and psychomotor features (restlessness, psychomotor retardation?).
- *Mood* (level and stability) and affect: Is the patient depressed, anxious, or euphoric? Is the

---

[1]Pica is an abnormal appetite for substances not suitable as food, e.g., bricks, clay, soil, and laundry starch.

mood fluctuating/labile? Does the patient have an appropriate or blunt affect?

- *Behavior*: Is the patient's behavior in the consultation room appropriate or not (e.g., agitated, disinhibited)?

Bedside examination of *cognitive functions* may seem complex, but it often reveals striking features in patients with cognitive impairment, and a global overview of cognitive functions with a few supplementary tests in specific cognitive domains can be performed in less than 20 min. Be aware that it may not be possible to assess certain specific cognitive domains due to impairment in others. For example, patients with delirium have severely impaired attention, which is why tests for episodic memory are meaningless.

Several brief screening instruments for global cognitive evaluation are available for the clinician, including:

- The Mini-Mental State Examination (MMSE) is a good starting point (Folstein et al. 1975). Sometimes there is a striking difference between the well-preserved facade and a low score on the MMSE. Occasionally, it is helpful to skip the history and start with an MMSE as doing an extensive auto-history is a waste of effort, for example, in a patient with a score of 10. Instead, much time can be saved if a relative or another informant is contacted right away. At the traditional cutoff of 23 points (used in population studies), the MMSE has high sensitivity for cognitive impairment but rather low specificity. Remember that a score of 25 may be perfectly normal for a low-educated worker, but 28 points in an academic may already be pathological. Low scores may also be seen in patients with depression. It is possible (and highly advisable) to learn the MMSE by heart. With practice, it is administered at the bedside in less than 10 min. Note, however, that the MMSE is heavily weighted toward verbal tasks and does not assess executive function. For instance, a patient with frontotemporal dementia (FTD), unable to behave in a socially appropriate manner, and a patient with a severe right hemisphere

dysfunction may score 28/30. Also, well-educated patients with early-phase AD may have very high scores.

- The Rowland Universal Dementia Assessment (RUDAS) (Storey et al. 2004) is a brief cognitive screening instrument specifically designed to minimize the effect of culture, language, and education.
- Addenbrooke's Cognitive Examination (ACE) (Mathuranath et al. 2000) may also be suited for the bedside examination and has a higher sensitivity (traditional cutoff is 83/100).
- The Montreal Cognitive Assessment (MoCA) is another easy-to-use cognitive screening test designed to assist in the detection of mild cognitive impairment and Alzheimer's disease; it is freely available online. The MoCA may be more sensitive than MMSE in detecting mild cognitive impairment.

A full and detailed examination of cognitive function requires referral to a formal neuropsychological examination (see Chap. 5). However, the neurologist may be interested in quickly assessing specific cognitive domains in more detail, as outlined below, putting most emphasis on apparently impaired functions:

- *Orientation and attention*: Orientation to time and place, digit span forward and backward (a normal person should be able to repeat at least six digits forward and a couple less backward), and subtracting backward (e.g., $100 - 7$).
- *Language* (naming, comprehension, reading, and writing): Characterize the patient's spontaneous language (fluency, vocabulary, syntax, grammar, and phonology). Ask the patient to repeat multisyllabic words (impaired in fluent aphasia). Ask the patient to name three objects (e.g., stethoscope, chalk, and toothbrush); then hide each of them in the consultation room in order to assess memory, as outlined below. Ask the patient to name objects on drawings. It is important to use objects of middle-range familiarity and not very familiar objects. Check verbal comprehension by asking the patient to define the

meaning of words and concepts (e.g., retirement, artichoke). Let the patient read a text from a magazine or book and check pronunciation of orthographically irregular words (words not pronounced as spelled, e.g., island). Difficulty with reading irregular words (surface dyslexia) is pronounced in SD. Ask the patient to write a sentence.

- *Memory*:
  - Episodic memory: Let the patient learn and recall (after 5–10 min of delay) a name and address; ask the patient to recall the name and location of the three hidden objects mentioned above. The patient with AD or amnesic syndrome will be able to learn and repeat an address or word list—but will have difficulty recalling all items after a delay.
  - Semantic memory: Ask the patient to name the three most recent prime ministers or presidents and three major capital cities, to name objects, and to define the meaning of words.
- *Visuoperceptual and visuospatial abilities*:
  - Bilateral posterior pathology may lead to difficulty describing a complex picture, and the patient may only be able to describe individual details (*simultanagnosia*). There are validated drawings available for this test, but a suitably complex picture in a magazine will also suffice.
  - Visuospatial skills are tested by letting the patient draw a cube, overlapping pentagons, or a clock face. The *clock drawing test* checks neglect as well as general visuospatial skills and executive functions. Give the patient a sheet of paper and ask him or her to draw a circle on it. Instruct the patient to draw numbers in the circle to make it look like the face of a clock and then to draw the hands of the clock to read "20 min past 10." The patient with neglect tends to ignore the objects on one side, usually the left. Tests of line bisection or letter cancellation serve similar purposes.
- *Praxia*: Apraxia is usually bilateral but may be unilateral or asymmetric in corticobasal degeneration (CBD). Check for *apraxia* using

verbal instructions ("Show me how to brush teeth, how to comb your hair."); if this fails, use visual instructions ("You brush teeth like this—now can you imitate me?"). Also, the patient can be asked to imitate a few complex hand movements. A patient with normal praxia should be able to follow these instructions completely. Minor deviations, e.g., using the finger as a virtual toothbrush instead of showing how to actually hold the toothbrush, may already be pathological. Oral (buccofacial) apraxia (e.g., difficulties licking the lips, blowing out matches) is common in nonfluent aphasia.

- *Stereognosis*: Ask the patient to close his eyes and to identify an object, e.g., a coin or a key, using tactile sensation of one hand only.
- *Executive functions*:
  - In category fluency, the patient is asked to produce as many examples as possible in 1 min from a given category (e.g., animals) and in letter fluency, to generate as many words as possible starting with a given letter (e.g., "S"). Normal subjects can name more than 15 words for letter fluency and a few more on category fluency. The tests are differentially impaired in frontal-subcortical dementias (the normal difference between category and word fluency is exaggerated) and AD and SD (worse on category fluency).
  - Abstraction may be tested by asking the patient to explain the meaning of sayings like "too many cooks spoil the soup" or by asking the patient to explain differences and similarities, e.g., "How are a table and a chair similar?" or "What is the difference between a canal and a river?" Judgment may be tested by asking the patient to estimate the size of objects unknown to them, e.g., "How tall is the Eiffel tower?" or "How many people fit into a London sightseeing bus?"
  - Disinhibition may be revealed by the go/no-go test in which the patient with frontal pathology is unable to stop. Ask the patient to tap the desk once if the examiner does so, but if the examiner taps twice, the patient should not tap at all. Further, the so-called applause test is useful in a patient

with suspicion of a neurodegenerative disorder. When asked to clap three, and only three, times as quickly as possible after seeing a demonstration by the examiner, prolonged clapping is suggestive of a neurodegenerative disease. Reports have suggested that the specificity of the applause sign is 100% in distinguishing parkinsonian patients from normal subjects with the highest sensitivity in patients with CBD and PSP, although the applause sign can also be seen in other neurodegenerative disorders, including AD.

3.1.3 General Neurological Examination in the Cognitively Impaired Patient

The following aspects of the general neurological examination require particular attention in the cognitively impaired patient:

- Primitive reflexes are those that are present in early life but suppressed during adolescent brain maturation. They commonly reemerge during advanced stages of dementia and are then called frontal release signs (e.g., snout, rooting, palmomental, and grasp reflexes). It is important to note, however, that some of them such as the palmomental reflex may be elicited in perfectly healthy individuals, and they all lack localizing value.
- Utilization behavior may be pronounced in FTD: The patient will begin to use any object placed in his hand, even if instructed not to. Give the patient several pairs of glasses, one at a time, and the patient will attempt to put them all on, one after the other. Imitation behavior may also be a striking feature in FTD, e.g., the patient will imitate the examiner's movements automatically.
- Speech: Dysarthria raises the suspicion of MND and parkinsonian syndromes/parkinsonism. Echolalia (repeating the examiner's words), palilalia (repeating sounds), and palilogia (repeated utterance of words) may be observed in patients with frontal pathology.

- Dysphagia suggests MND or atypical parkinsonian syndromes.
- Eye movements and the eyes themselves are important to examine (e.g., supranuclear palsy or slowing of saccades suggests PSP; Kayser-Fleischer ring suggests Wilson's disease).
- Motor function: Look for extrapyramidal features suggesting Parkinson's disease or other parkinsonian syndromes, weakness and fasciculations (seen in FTD-MND), myoclonus (Huntington's disease (HD), Creutzfeldt-Jakob disease (CJD), CBD and advanced AD), chorea (HD), limb dystonia (CBD or Wilson's disease), and asterixis (metabolic encephalopathy). The patient with the alien limb phenomenon, typically seen in CBD, complains that one arm is becoming increasingly useless and performs movements and actions "on its own."
- Gait: Gait ataxia may suggest cerebellar involvement (neurodegenerative disorders, alcohol-related cerebellar degeneration, MS, leukodystrophy, or CJD), a slow and unsteady ataxic gait may suggest NPH, and a shuffling gait with small steps suggests PD.

3.2 Cranial Nerves

With practice, a complete CN examination in a cooperative patient can be assessed in less than 90 s.

CN I is rarely tested; usually it is enough to simply ask if the patient can smell his partner's perfume or the coffee in the morning. Otherwise, the patient can be examined using a selection of odors, testing one nostril at a time. Remember that ammonia and other irritants activate trigeminal fibers, not CN I.

Examination of *CN II* may begin with an *ophthalmoscopy.*[2] The presence of spontaneous

---

[2]It is advisable to buy an ophthalmoscope and to use it routinely during the neurological examination. Ophthalmoscopy is undoubtedly the most difficult of all neurological bedside techniques. Considerable practice is needed to master this technique – it has been said that no other bedside examination is associated with as many lies as ophthalmoscopy.

venous pulsations (SVPs) as revealed by ophthalmoscopy is a useful finding in a patient with headache and should be documented in the charts. SVPs occur at the optic disc where the retinal veins leave the orbit (the retinal veins are the darker, broader vessels; the arteries are lighter and thinner). With some practice, SVPs can be detected in nine of ten people. Video demonstrations of SVP can be found on youtoube.com. Venous engorgement and the lack of spontaneous pulsations are the earliest signs of raised intracranial pressure. Full papilledema usually takes a few days to develop and leads to blurring of optic margins, elevation of the optic disc, hemorrhages from congested retinal veins, and nerve fiber damage (cotton wool spots) (Case 3.2). Thus, the presence of SVP suggests that ICP is normal, at least at the time of examination. Although SVPs do not fully exclude an intracranial cause for the patient's headache, their presence nevertheless allows the conclusion that headache is not due to raised ICP (e.g., as seen with sinus venous thrombosis, a cerebral tumor, or idiopathic intracranial hypertension). This is highly useful when evaluating a patient with headache.

Ophthalmoscopy may also reveal chronic optic neuropathy (small, pale, and atrophic optic disc), drusen (optic disc elevation due to mucoproteins and mucopolysaccharides without other signs of papilledema—usually a normal variant without any pathological value), diabetic and hypertensive changes (retinal hemorrhages, cotton wool spots, and atherosclerotic vascular changes), and optic neuritis (although with retrobulbar neuritis, inspection can be normal). Occasionally, one may see retinitis pigmentosa, cholesterol emboli and retinal infarction, retinal melanoma, and retinal toxoplasmosis.

If the history suggests loss of *visual acuity*, assess this using the classic Snellen chart. Optic correction (if needed) is important since the function of nervous tissue and not the lens apparatus should be assessed. If a Snellen chart is not available, a simple test of visual acuity is to let the patient read a newspaper using one eye at a time. Is he able to read the small text or only the big letters in the headings? If neither, can he count fingers from 20 in. away?

Testing the *visual field* is part of a standard neurological examination. For finger perimetry, the examiner uses his visual fields as a reference. If the patient's history does not suggest any visual field loss, asking the patient if he can see finger movements in each quadrant of the eyes is usually sufficient. Each eye should be assessed independently by covering the other eye. Another more sensitive examination technique is to slowly move a finger or another object from each corner of the periphery toward the center of the patient's visual field and to ask when the patient can see the object. *Visual attention*, however, is best tested using double confrontation. Show the patient both hands and ask him to point at the hand where the fingers are moving. Also, move both hands simultaneously at some time during the examination to assess for possible extinction. With complete visual neglect, there is extinction of visual stimuli of one side at all times; with visual hemineglect there is extinction only with double confrontation. Examination of visual fields and visual attention assesses not only CN II but the entire visual system and its cortical projections.

Color vision is normally only assessed when suspecting (chronic) optic atrophy, e.g., due to optic neuritis in MS. Since the color red is most significantly affected, the patient is shown a red object and asked to look at it first with one, then with the other eye. Is there desaturation of red with one of the eyes?

Optic atrophy leads also to an *afferent pupillary defect*, which can be tested for by applying the *swinging-flashlight test*. If the optic and oculomotor nerves and their parasympathetic connection (Edinger-Westphal nucleus) are intact, both pupils constrict and stay miotic when moving a flashlight quickly from one eye to the other. This is because of the consensual light response. With unilateral optic dysfunction, however, both pupils will constrict as light falls into the healthy eye, but they will dilate as light falls into the affected eye. The *direct and indirect (consensual) pupillary reflexes* can also be tested in a well-lit room by first covering one eye and then the other. This is especially useful in small children, who often do not like the glare of a pocket lamp.

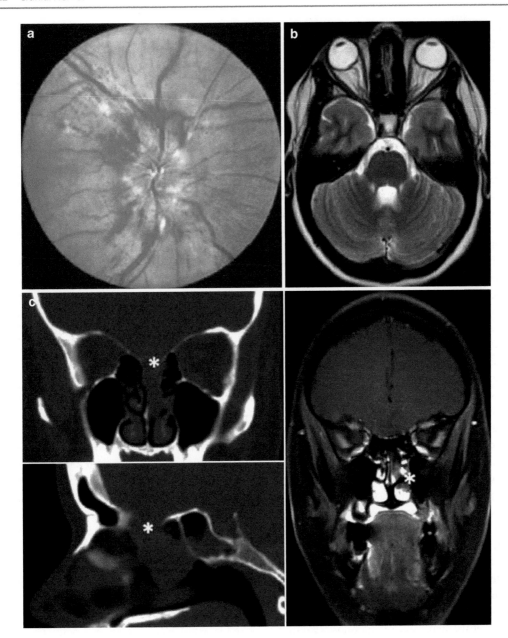

Case 3.2 Idiopathic intracranial hypertension and spontaneous CSF fistula. A 29-year-old female was diagnosed with IIH based on a history of headache, obesity, papilledema (**a**), increased CSF opening pressure, and lack of a mass lesion or CVST on an MRI of her brain. Although the MRI initially was reported as normal, it showed signs of increased intracranial pressure, such as vertical kinking of the optic nerves and flattening of the posterior sclera (**b**). She was treated with diuretics and acetazolamide, as well as given dietary advice. At a 2-year follow-up, her headaches had disappeared, and the fundus examination was normal. Treatment was discontinued. In the following years, she experienced continuous watery nasal discharge, consistent with CSF rhinorrhea, and two episodes of bacterial meningitis. CT and MRI revealed a left-sided nasal cavity meningocele (**c**, *asterisk*). Spontaneous CSF leaks have epidemiological and clinical features very similar to IIH. In one case series of spontaneous CSF leaks, 85% of patients were obese, 77% were women, and the CSF lumbar opening pressure increased following closure of CSF leaks. Increased ICP and constant pulsatile pressure lead to bone erosion. Spontaneous CSF leaks probably represent a variant of IIH, which is why after operative closure of a spontaneous CSF leak, patients must be carefully followed for signs of increased ICP to prevent recurrence of the leak (Adapted with permission from Kurtzhals et al. (2011))

Accommodation can be tested by asking the patient to fixate on a point on the wall and then to fixate on the examiner's finger moving into the visual field just in front of the patient's nose. Accommodation leads to constriction of the pupils and convergence of the eyes.

In contrast to afferent pupillary defects, *efferent pupillary defects* are due to *CN III* palsy, e.g., due to increased ICP, autoimmune mechanisms (Adie pupil), or infections such as neurosyphilis (Argyll-Robertson pupil). Drug intoxication is another cause, with atropine and sympathetic drugs leading to mydriasis and opioids to miosis.

It is important to actively look for *Horner's syndrome*, because it is easily missed otherwise. Horner's syndrome consists of miosis, ptosis, and anhidrosis. See Chap. 2 for a discussion of the relevant neuroanatomy. *Anhidrosis* is loss of sweating in the upper quadrant of the ipsilateral half of the face. It is tested with the back of the hand or—even better—with a plastic card moving over the forehead. With anhidrosis, the skin is smooth and dry, and the plastic card will not stick to the skin as much as on the unaffected side. When physical activity provokes facial flushing, the affected skin area remains pale. However, anhidrosis can be lacking when the sympathetic fibers traveling along the external carotid artery are spared. *Miosis* and pupillary efferent dysfunction are most easily assessed in a semi-dark room as miosis is most visible because the contralateral pupil dilates. When the light is turned on, the healthy pupil will constrict as well. (In contrast, mydriasis is most visible in a well-lit room.) *Ptosis* can be evaluated by comparing the border of the upper eyelids with the level of the pupils when the patient looks straight forward and upward.

Oculomotor function, mediated by *CN III, IV, and VI*, is assessed by evaluating gaze axis, range of eye movements, smooth pursuit, saccades, and, if present, nystagmus. The examiner moves a finger slowly to both sides and up and down in an H-like movement and asks the patient to follow it. The examiner's finger should not be held too close to the patient's eyes. Many patients will instinctively move their head slightly, which the examiner can avoid by fixating the patient's head with the other hand. Oculomotor function is analyzed according to whether *gaze is conjugated or divergent*, whether *pursuit is smooth or saccadic*, and whether the *range of movements is full or restricted* (Case 3.3). If nystagmus other than end-gaze nystagmus is present, determine whether it is conjugate or unilateral, unidirectional or gaze changing, and horizontal or vertical, whether it occurs after a latent phase of a few seconds or immediately, whether it is positional or independent, and whether it is transient or constant. (The first adjective of each pair is consistent with *vestibular nystagmus*; the second suggests *nystagmus of central origin*.) For assessment of saccades, ask the patient to fixate on the examiner's face. The examiner then holds up his hands and moves them suddenly and in a random manner. The patient has to look at the moving hand and then immediately at the examiner again. Are eye saccades precise, or does the patient need to perform corrections due to either overshoot or hypometric saccades?

Skew deviation may be revealed by asking the patient to fixate on the examiner's face, while the examiner covers one of the patient's eyes with his hand. Skew deviation, as well as *latent strabismus*, is revealed by a corrective movement of the affected eye when the hand is removed (Chap. 2).

The VOR or oculovestibular reflex is a reflex eye movement that stabilizes the image on the retina during head movement by producing an immediate eye movement opposite to the movement of the head. Thereby, the image remains fixed in the center of the visual field. The head impulse test can be used for assessment of the VOR. Again, ask the patient to fixate on your face. Take the patient's head in both hands and turn the head quickly 10–20° to one side. With vestibular failure, the eyes will follow the head movement for a fraction of a second until a compensatory saccade in the opposite direction allows the patient to fixate on you again. Take care not to miss this compensatory saccade as it

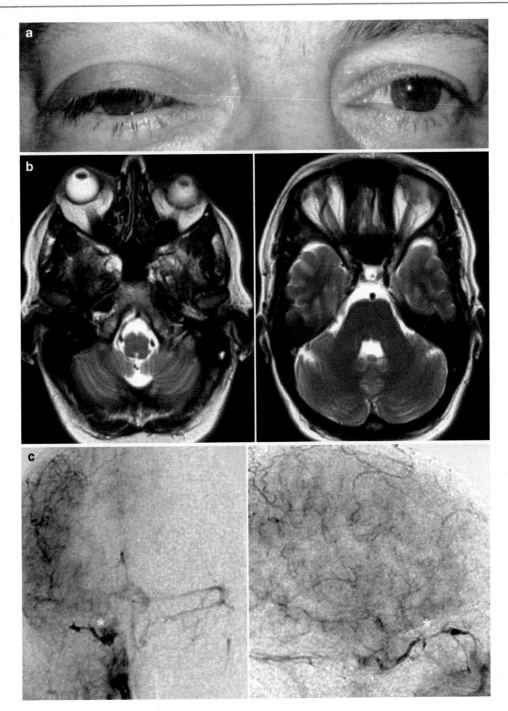

Case 3.3 Carotid-cavernous fistula. A 53-year-old previously healthy male presented with a 6-month history of watering of the right eye, double vision, and pulse-synchronous tinnitus. Examination revealed ptosis, ciliary injection, and restricted movements of the right eye (**a**). MRI showed exophthalmos, orbital edema, and a dilated orbital vein on the right side (**b**). A digital subtraction angiography was consistent with a low-flow carotid-cavernous fistula (*asterisk*) (**c**). The fistula was successfully embolized, and the symptoms disappeared (Digital subtraction angiography images courtesy of Markus Holtmannspötter, Department of Neuroradiology, Rigshospitalet, Copenhagen)

is minute.[3] With smooth pursuit, in contrast, VOR must be suppressed in order to allow a stable image on the retina. Ask the patient to extend both arms, to put his thumbs together, and to fixate them while you turn the patient en bloc. With correct VOR suppression, the gaze is fixed on the thumbs; with deficient VOR suppression (e.g., in a patient with MS), the patient's gaze constantly lags behind, and compensatory saccades are necessary to catch up with the moving thumbs.

Oculomotor function is often impaired in *neuromuscular junction disorders* such as MG. For assessment of fatigability and ptosis, ask the patient to look upward for 60 s and look for occurrence of ptosis (Jolly's test). When ptosis is subtle, it may be difficult to establish whether or not the Jolly's test is positive. Ptosis is best detected when focusing on the decreasing gap between the upper eyelid and the upper border of the pupil. For other relevant bedside tests (tensilon test, ice-on-eyes test), consult the differential diagnosis of neuromuscular junction disorders in Chap. 4.

Facial sensation, mediated by *CN V*, is assessed by touching both halves of the face gently. There is usually no need to test the different qualities of facial sensation. Most sensory disturbances are obvious. One exception is sensory disturbance due to vestibular schwannoma, which initially is subtle and may sometimes only manifest as impaired corneal sensation leading to a decreased corneal reflex. Also, it is crucial not to miss complaints of circumoral sensory symptoms as these may point toward a brainstem lesion, as discussed in Chap. 2. The skin area innervated by V3 ends at the lower mandible; thus, sensory disturbances including areas below the mandible may suggest that these complaints are nonorganic in nature. Also, keep in mind that minor differences in pain and temperature sense between the right and left facial halves are often described by suggestible patients; again, such complaints are seldom due to an underlying organic disorder if the patient has not mentioned them spontaneously during history taking.

To test CN V *motor function*, have the patient bite his teeth together and palpate the masseter muscle bulks; one-sided atrophy suggests chronic damage to the motor nucleus or the peripheral axons, e.g., secondary to an ipsilateral skull base tumor.

CN V motor fibers constitute the efferent pathway of the *jaw jerk*. A hyperactive jaw jerk points toward bilateral UMN lesions such as in pseudobulbar palsy.

Frontal headache may be due to congestion of nasal sinuses and may increase with percussion of the bony area above the relevant sinus as well as with bending of the head forward. In the elderly, with new-onset headache and complaints of generalized muscle ache, weight loss, and/or pains in the jaw while chewing (jaw claudication), it is important to look for a prominent painful temporal artery suggestive of giant cell arteritis.

The most important question in a patient presenting with a facial palsy (*CN VII*) is, "Can you wrinkle your forehead?" This *distinguishes central from peripheral facial palsy*. In a patient with a subtle facial palsy, examine all three CN VII branches. Ask the patient to whistle, to show his teeth, and to repeat this maneuver rapidly, while you look for a slight palsy as revealed by one corner of the mouth lagging behind the other. Sometimes a mild facial palsy (whether central or peripheral in origin) is best detected during observation of spontaneous facial activity. An asymmetry of the nasolabial fissure may also occasionally reveal a facial palsy better than voluntary muscular activity. *Facial reflexes* are hyperactive with bilateral UMN impairment, e.g., due to multiple vascular lacunes (pseudobulbar palsy) and other neurodegenerative disorders. One of these reflexes is the so-called snout reflex (a frontal release sign), which leads to pouting or pursing of the lips elicited by a slight and constant pressure on the philtrum (essentially a variation of the tactile rooting response). Another example of a frontal release sign is the palmomental reflex, which consists of a twitch of the chin muscle elicited by stroking the thenar eminence and the palm. However, although it is held dear by many neurologists, the palmomental

---

[3]When testing for compensatory saccades, it is advisable to strictly focus on one eye at a time as the compensatory saccades are much easier to observe this way. Alternatively, focusing on the patient's nose permits the examiner to see the compensatory saccades in his own peripheral vision.

reflex lacks sensitivity, specificity, and localizing value; and therefore it should be considered obsolete (Schott and Rossor, 2016).

In a patient with a peripheral CN VII palsy (e.g., Bell's palsy), ask about a *loss of taste* or an unusual metallic taste in the mouth. A useful but uncomfortable examination is the salt test. Ask the patient to protrude his tongue, fixate its tip with your hand (using gloves), and rub salt on the left and right side of the tongue. The patient with a peripheral CN VII palsy that also affects the chorda tympani will report loss of salt taste perception on the ipsilateral side of the tongue. Also test for *hyperacusis* by clapping your hands together in front of the patient's ears. Consult Chap. 2 regarding localizing the lesion in peripheral facial palsy.

Lesions of the *vestibular part* of *CN VIII* may lead to vestibular ataxia and nystagmus, as discussed earlier. In vestibular damage, horizontal or torsional nystagmus occurs with a latency of a few seconds after position change and is habituating.

The *Dix-Hallpike maneuver* is used to diagnose the symptomatic side of the vestibular lesion. Youtube.com provides excellent demonstrations of the Dix-Hallpike maneuver. Have the patient sit upright and stand behind him, holding his head with both hands. Then rotate the patient's head approximately 45° to one side. Afterward, help the patient to lie on his back with his head hanging over the edge of the examination table at roughly a 30° angle. When the Dix-Hallpike maneuver is positive, rotatory nystagmus occurs after a latency of 2–10 s, and the fast phase is toward the affected ear. If no nystagmus occurs, the maneuver is repeated with the head rotated to the other side.

The *Epley maneuver*, also demonstrated on youtube.com, can be used to cure benign paroxysmal positional vertigo. The first steps are identical to the Dix-Hallpike maneuver, but the patient remains in the position that provokes nystagmus for 1–2 min, after which the patients rotates his head 90° to the other side, remaining in this position for another 1–2 min while maintaining his head at a 30° angle. Then, have the patient roll over onto his side in the direction he is facing while keeping the head and neck in a

fixed position relative to the body. Now the patient's face should be pointing downward (toward the floor). Let the patient remain in this position for 1–2 min before slowly returning to an upright sitting position, where he should remain for up to 30 s. The entire procedure can be repeated once or twice.

The *Unterberger stepping test* can be useful in assessment of vestibular pathology. Ask the patient to walk in place for 60 s with his eyes closed. If the patient turns more than 45° to one side, this is pathological and suggests a labyrinthine lesion on that side. A similar test is the finger-pointing test, in which the patient lifts both arms up and down a few times, again with eyes closed, while trying to keep his fingers pointed in the same direction. Deviation suggests an ipsilateral vestibular lesion.

Sensorineural deafness (due to injury of the *cochlear part* of CN VIII) is usually obvious during normal speech. If not, rub your index finger and thumb together in front of the patient's ears to reveal slight hearing impairment. The Weber and Rinne tests allow distinguishing sensorineural from conductive hearing impairment. During the *Weber test*, a vibrating tuning fork is placed in the middle of the patient's head. If available, a 512 Hz tuning fork is preferable; otherwise, a common 256 Hz fork will do as well. With conductive hearing loss, the patient will hear the sound lateralized toward the affected ear, whereas the opposite is true with sensorineural hearing loss. Then, perform the *Rinne test* by placing the vibrating tuning fork on the patient's mastoid. When the patient no longer hears the sound, hold the fork in front of the ipsilateral ear. Since air conduction is normally better than bone conduction, the patient should hear the sound again and at least twice as long as with bone conduction. For instance, with conductive hearing loss of the left ear, the Weber test will be lateralized to the left, and, since bone conduction is better than air conduction in this case, the Rinne test will be negative on the left side. In contrast, with left sensorineural hearing loss, the Weber test will be lateralized to the right, while the Rinne test will remain positive (showing that air conduction is still better than bone conduction).

CN IX and *CN X* are assessed together. In most cases, simply asking the patient to stick out his tongue and say "aaah" and watching whether or not the soft palate and uvula are lifted symmetrically are sufficient. If the patient is able to clear his throat, this suggests preserved diaphragmatic function and sufficient closure of the epiglottis. Chapter 2 discusses the gag reflex and the curtain phenomenon due to ipsilateral uvula paresis. Dysphagia can be assessed at the bedside by having the patient (carefully) drink a glass of water. Dysarthria is usually obvious when taking the history but can be formally tested for by having the patient say "p-p-p" (CN VII), "t-t-t" (CN XII), and "k-k-k" (CN IX/X). The examiner needs to decide whether dysarthria is spastic (high-pitched sounds, e.g., due to supranuclear pseudobulbar palsy), atactic ("eve-ry syl-la-ble-tends-to-be-pro-nounced-by-it-self," encountered in cerebellar disease or MS), or of the LMN type (flabby and nasal speech, e.g., due to neuromuscular disorders such as ALS and MG).

CN XI is tested by asking the patient to press his head against the examiner's hand (sternocleidomastoid muscle function) and by providing resistance as the patient lifts his shoulders (trapezius muscle function).

Chronic injury to *CN XII* leads to tongue atrophy and fasciculations. The latter are best seen when the patient relaxes his tongue in his mouth. Also ask the patient to stick out his tongue in order to look for possible deviation (to the paralyzed side). Assess tongue power and mobility by having the patient move his tongue quickly from one side to the other. Dysdiadochokinesia of the tongue is occasionally seen in extrapyramidal diseases and may occur early in the course of PD disease. General tongue weakness due to pseudobulbar or bulbar palsy is revealed by slow side-to-side movements or the patient may not be able to move his tongue at all.

3.3 Motor Function

The examination of motor function includes:

- Formal power testing of defined muscle groups. Here the examiner systemically quan-

tifies weakness by offering resistance to the patient's movements
- Observation of spontaneous and unrestrained motor movements. This is usually more sensitive for detection of slight central palsies

For *formal power testing* of defined muscle groups, the examiner needs to stabilize the proximal and distal limbs of the joint in question to make sure to test well-defined muscle groups, e.g., when testing power of elbow flexion and extension, hold the upper arm with the left hand and the forearm with the right (if the examiner is right-handed). Be sure to use the principle of leverage to your advantage. The more distally on the patient's extremity force is applied, the better the chances to quantify power in even muscular patients. When testing for shoulder abduction, for example, press the forearm down instead of the upper arm.

Muscle power can be graded according to the British Medical Research Council (MRC) scale:

- MRC 0: Lack of any muscle contraction
- MRC 1: Visible muscle contraction without movement
- MRC 2: Movement with elimination of gravity
- MRC 3: Movement against gravity
- MRC 4−: Movement against resistance, 25% of normal strength
- MRC 4: Movement against resistance, 50% of normal strength
- MRC 4+: Movement against resistance, 75% of normal strength
- MRC 5: Normal strength

The MRC scale was established for quantification of peripheral palsies secondary to military injuries, but it can also be used, albeit somewhat less reliably, for quantification of other neuromuscular and central palsies.

The abovementioned formal power testing is often inferior to other techniques when it comes to detection of slight central palsies. *Observation of asymmetries* of unrestrained motor movements may reveal such palsies even in cases when formal power testing does not. *Isotonic movements* include hand and foot tapping, playing the piano, screwing in light bulbs, alternating fast supination and pronation of the hands, and hopping on one foot. Unilateral decrease of fine motor movement suggests a central palsy. Examine each extremity independently, because simultaneous examination tends to lead to synchronization, which may obscure asymmetric motor performance. *Isometric techniques* include the straight arm test and the flexed leg test.[4] To perform a straight arm test, ask the patient to close his eyes, lift both arms over his head, and extend the elbow and finger joints with the hands supinated. Finger flexion, pronation of the wrist, elbow flexion, or lowering of the arm occurring on one side suggests a contralateral central lesion. Sometimes the patient may only complain that one arm feels heavier than the other, and if consistent with the history, this is the mildest sign of a central palsy. In contrast to the straight arm test, which is easily performed, the flexed leg test demands greater effort on the patient's part and should therefore be reserved for cases in which the history suggests a mild central paresis of the lower extremity. The supine patient is asked to lift both legs by flexing 90° at the hips, the knees, and the ankles. Asymmetric weakness suggests a central palsy of the affected leg.

If MG or another neuromuscular junction syndrome is suspected, it is advisable to assess *fatigability* by counting the number of repetitive movements (e.g., knee bending, neck flexion) the patient is able to perform or by counting the seconds the patient is able to maintain certain postures (e.g., lifting his head off the pillow when lying in bed). These are also excellent ways to clinically monitor the effect of medical treat-

ment. Furthermore, the Cogan lid twitch is a relatively specific sign for MG. It occurs due to transient improvement in eyelid strength after rest of the levator in downgaze, followed by droop in the primary position as the levator fatigues. Patients with ptosis and possible MG are asked to look straight ahead, down, and straight ahead again. The eyes are carefully assessed immediately after this movement for the presence of a brief upward twitch of the upper eyelid, indicating a positive test. Other bedside tests for MG include the tensilon and the ice-on-eyes tests, which will be explained in Chap. 4.

After these general considerations, let us review the *practical part* of the motor examination. Ideally, the examination should begin with the patient undressed and sitting at the bedside in a well-lit room. If the history suggests LMN impairment, check for possible *atrophy* and *fasciculations*. The latter may be very difficult to detect unless enough time is reserved to examine each extremity carefully. Fasciculations can sometimes be elicited by slightly tapping the muscle. Then, proceed with a *straight arm test* to gain an immediate impression of power in the upper extremities.

Subsequently, formal power testing in the *upper extremities* should be performed. The following movements may be tested routinely ("UMN" denotes movements especially affected by UMN lesions; key myotomes shown in italics):

- Elevation and abduction of the upper arm at 90° (UMN, *C5/C6*, axillary nerve, deltoid muscle)
- Adduction of the upper arm (C6/*C7*/C8, lateral and medial pectoral nerves, major pectoralis muscle)
- Outward rotation of the upper arm at the shoulder (*C5/C6*, suprascapular nerve, infraspinatus muscle)
- Elbow flexion with forearm supinated (*C5/C6*, musculocutaneous nerve, biceps muscle)
- Elbow extension (UMN, C6/*C7*/C8, radial nerve, triceps muscle)
- Extension of the wrist, radial side (UMN, *C6*, radial nerve, extensor carpi radialis longus muscle)
- Pincer grip (*C8/T1*, median nerve, flexor pollicis brevis and opponens pollicis muscles)

---

[4]A patient with a complete spastic hemiparesis has the arm adducted and the elbow, wrist, and finger joints maximally flexed, whereas the joints of the leg (hip, knee, ankle, and phalangeal joints) are fully extended. This leads to the characteristic "short arm, long leg posturing" and is due to increased activity of the antigravity muscles that arise with central spasticity. The result is the typical gait disorder in which the hemiparetic patient has to circumduct the foot in order to clear it from the ground (Wernicke-Mann gait). A mild central palsy will therefore be best detected by testing the anti-antigravity muscles, or, in other words, by long arm, short leg posturing (extension of the arm and flexion of the ipsilateral leg).

- Finger abduction and adduction (UMN, C8/*T1*, ulnar nerve, interossei muscles)

Note that radial palsy may falsely simulate additional ulnar palsy if not examined correctly. This is because finger abduction is impaired (for simple mechanical reasons) when the hand is flexed at the wrist. In order to properly assess ulnar nerve function in a patient with radial nerve palsy, the hands need to be examined with the wrist dorsiflexed. This is best achieved by asking the patient to stand up and put the affected, dorsiflexed hand on a table. Now abduction and adduction of the fingers can be examined. In a patient with isolated radial nerve palsy, power will be normal.

To proceed with formal power testing of the motor examination in the *lower extremities*, test the following movements with the patient in a supine position:

- Hip flexion (UMN, *L1*/*L2*/L3, femoral nerve, iliopsoas muscle)
- Hip extension (*L5*/*S1*/S2, inferior gluteal nerve, gluteus maximus muscle)
- Hip abduction (*L4*/*L5*/S1, superior gluteal nerve, gluteus medius and tensor fasciae latae muscles)
- Hip adduction (*L2*/*L3*/L4, obturator nerve, adductor muscles)
- Knee extension (L2/*L3*/L4, femoral nerve, quadriceps femoris muscle)
- Knee flexion (UMN, L5/*S1*/S2, sciatic nerve, hamstring muscles)
- Dorsiflexion of the foot (UMS, *L4*/L5, deep peroneal nerve, anterior tibial muscle)
- Dorsiflexion of the great toe (*L5*/S1, deep peroneal nerve, extensor hallucis longus muscles)
- Ankle inversion (L4/*L5*, tibial nerve, tibialis posterior muscle)
- Ankle eversion (*L5*/S1, superficial peroneal nerve, peroneus longus and brevis muscles)
- Plantar flexion of the foot (*S1*/S2, tibial nerve, gastrocnemius, soleus muscles)
- Plantar flexion of the toes (*S1*/S2, tibial nerve, flexor digitorum longus et brevis, flexor hallucis longus et brevis muscles)

An excellent test of proximal power in the lower extremities is to ask the patient to rise from a chair without the help of his arms or to perform knee bends. Also, if the patient can stand and walk on his toes and heels, power for dorsiflexion and plantar flexion over the ankles is normal. Assessment of muscle power in a patient with a functional disorder is discussed below.

If the history suggests a conus medullaris or cauda equina syndrome, tonus and power of the anal sphincter should be assessed (S2–S4, pudendal nerve, perineal muscles). For medicolegal reasons, having another person in the room when examining a patient of the opposite gender is advisable.

Now *muscle tone* is assessed. In both the arms and legs, slight *spasticity* due to corticospinal tract dysfunction may lead to the catch phenomenon. When you take the patient's hand, as with a normal handshake, and quickly supinate the forearm, you will feel the catch as instant but very slight resistance that vanishes immediately. To test for spasticity in the legs, lift the supine patient's knee abruptly. In the spastic limb, the foot will be lifted from the ground as well. Alternatively, rotate the thigh back and forth and watch the foot—does the foot dangle or is it stiff? Clonus is another sign of spasticity and appears most commonly in the ankles. Quickly dorsiflex the patient's foot and hold it in this position, at which point spasticity leads to a series of involuntary muscular contractions due to sudden stretching of disinhibited muscle spindles. If the contractions only stop when the limb is immobilized, this is true clonus; if they stop spontaneously, it is called subclonus. One or two contractions, however, can be normal in patients with physiologically lively reflexes, e.g., young females. In severely spastic patients, patellar clonus can sometimes be triggered by quickly pushing the patellar downward, but this can be rather unpleasant for the patient and does not reveal any additional information, which is why this test is considered obsolete.

A mild form of increased muscle tone is *paratonia*. It indicates functional disconnection between the basal ganglia and higher cortical centers. Paratonia is characterized by the patient's inability to relax the extremities despite repeated requests from the examiner. The patient appears to actively resist when the limbs are passively stretched or flexed, although he may claim to be fully relaxed. Hence, the German term *gegenhalten* roughly translates as oppositional resistance. Conscious relaxation requires concentration. Paratonia may appear if concentration is difficult due to dementia, confusional states, frontal lobe pathology, leukoencephalopathy, or NPH.

Paratonia is not the same as *rigidity*, which is a sign of a basal ganglia disorder. Rigidity and the cogwheel phenomenon (a circular, jerking rigidity with superimposed tremor) are best tested for using slow passive movements over the wrist. Rigidity is enforced by emotional stress and cognitive tasks (e.g., when the patient has to count backward) and simultaneous movements of the contralateral extremity (e.g., when the patient is asked to repeatedly raise and lower the opposite hand).

Another, rarer form of increased muscle tone is *tetany*, usually due to low calcium levels leading to muscle cell membrane instability and increased membrane depolarization. The most common cause of tetany is hyperventilation during panic attacks, which may cause characteristic posturing of the hands termed Trousseau sign (spasm of the muscles of the hand and forearm with flexion of the wrist and metacarpophalangeal joints, extension and adduction of the fingers). Chapter 4 discusses tetanus due to clostridium tetani.

Examination of the *deep tendon reflexes* is preferentially performed with the patient in a supine position. Testing reflexes requires a great deal of experience with examining healthy patients in order to develop a feeling for what is normal and what is not. The Queen Square and Trömner reflex hammers offer the best power and precision. Contrary to what many non-neurologists believe, evaluation of reflexes often only confirms what the neurologist already knows; the experienced neurologist will rarely discover unexpected findings when testing reflexes. For instance, in a patient with a history suggestive of polyneuropathy, it is unusual to find that the reflexes are not hypoactive. In a patient with a myopathy, reflexes

are normal or, with severe weakness, slightly hypoactive. A central hemiparesis, in contrast, is typically accompanied by ipsilateral hyperreflexia, but the neurologist is usually already well aware of the hemiparesis after having observed the patient enter the consultation room and having obtained a history.

Sometimes, however, the examination of deep tendon reflexes offers crucial information. Examples include patients with subacute tetraparesis (areflexia would suggest GBS, hyperreflexia cervical myelopathy), with asymmetric limb weakness, atrophy, and fasciculations (hyperreflexia would indicate ALS), and with pes cavus deformity and gait ataxia (hyporeflexia combined with a Babinski sign might point toward a diagnosis of Friedreich's ataxia).

Baseline reflex activity can vary considerably from patient to patient—old men with diabetes and alcoholism have sluggish reflexes, whereas young and female patients tend to have lively reflexes. If the patient has lively reflexes, adapt the blow of the hammer to elicit a slight reflex response only. Are there extended reflexogenic zones or crossed reflexes (e.g., crossed pectoralis or adductor reflexes), thus suggesting true hyperreflexia? Enhanced physiological reflexes can occur, however, with an increase in voluntary muscle tone (which is why nervous people tend to have lively reflexes), a phenomenon called facilitation. Facilitation is used to reinforce difficult-to-elicit reflexes. Ask the patient either to bite his teeth together or to hook the flexed fingers of his two hands together and forcibly try to pull them apart, which is a distraction tactic known as the Jendrassik maneuver.

Testing the following *monosynaptic reflexes* is useful:

- Pectoralis (C5–C8, TH1)
- Brachialis (C5/C6)
- Brachioradialis (C5–C7)
- Finger flexor (C6/C7)
- Triceps (C6–C8)
- Adductor (L2/L3)
- Patellar (L2–L4)
- Achilles (S1/S2)

If a spinal cord lesion is suspected, looking for weakness of the abdominal musculature is helpful. The *Beevor sign* is the upward movement of the navel when the patient is lying supine and bends his neck. (The normal response is that the navel is fixed in its position on the abdomen due to simultaneous contraction of the upper and lower abdominal muscles.) The Beevor sign is caused by weakness of the lower abdominal muscles and typically occurs with spinal cord injury between levels T6 and T10, but it is sometimes also encountered in patients with a generalized myopathy such as myotonic dystrophy. *Abdominal reflexes*, which are polysynaptic, may be tested by briefly and lightly striking the skin of each abdominal quadrant using a sharp device. Note that only unilateral loss of abdominal muscle contraction is a pathological sign, because abdominal reflexes are hard to elicit in many people.

Somewhat simplified, there are two schools of thought when it comes to testing the *plantar responses* and the *Babinski sign*. Some argue that this is a polysynaptic reflex, the afferent pathway of which is mediated via skin receptors and the reason why only light pressure with a rather sharp object should be applied to elicit it. Others believe that considerable pressure and a blunt instrument are needed. As is so often the case, both points of view are right. The necessary degree of pressure and sharpness is usually proportional to the degree of hyperkeratosis of the foot sole. Thus, the examiner should stroke the lateral side of the sole of the foot with a blunt or sharp device from the heel in a curve to the toes, with more or less force, but without causing pain or injury to the skin. The normal plantar response is flexor. The Babinski sign refers to extension (=dorsiflexion) of the great toe as well as abduction of the other toes. There are many eponymous techniques for eliciting a similar plantar response (e.g., Oppenheim, Gordon). Of these, the *Chaddock maneuver* is particularly useful because hyperkeratosis of the foot sole is not a problem. A short, light stroke with a sharp object on the lateral side of the foot just above the site of usual skin thickening is a very efficient way of eliciting the plantar response. Consequently, apply the Chaddock maneuver if the Babinski maneuver is negative. With severe spasticity, elicitation of the plantar reflex may lead to simultaneous flexion of the hip and knee, as well as dorsiflexion of the foot and the big toe. This is the so-called triple flexion response and should not be confused with voluntary withdrawal of the leg. Occasionally, in a patient with a structural myelopathy, e.g., due to a thoracic meningioma or cervical spinal canal stenosis, the Babinski sign and foot clonus are more pronounced when sitting as compared to the supine position because of increased traction of the spinal cord.

As stated in Chap. 2, the patient with radiculopathy usually complains of chronic neck or lumbar pain with exacerbation in the form of acute shooting pain radiating into the extremity. Patients with radiculopathic pain typically have *paraspinal and neck muscle spasms* as well as decreased spinal mobility. In patients with lower back pain, the *straight leg test* may be positive (*Lasègue's sign*). This test has low specificity but high sensitivity, and a negative straight leg test makes a symptomatic lower lumbar disc herniation very unlikely. To diagnose cervical radiculopathy, the foraminal *compression test of Spurling* may be useful. For this test, ask the patient to extend his neck and rotate his head; then apply slight downward pressure on the head. The test is considered positive if pain radiates into the arm ipsilateral to the side of head rotation. In comparison with the straight leg test, Spurling's test has less sensitivity but higher specificity.

3.4   Sensory Function

The bedside examination of sensory function is entirely subjective; the patient can tell the examiner whatever he feels like. Thus, as a general rule, the examiner is well advised not to spend too much time on the examination of the somatosensory system. If the patient denies sensory disturbance in the history, only a few seconds should be reserved for the sensory examination; otherwise, there is risk for considerable confusion, particularly if the patient is suggestible and the examiner inexperienced. However, if the patient complains of sensory disturbances, let him *point out the area of disturbed sensation* and focus on the anatomic hypothesis as suggested by the history. As a result:

- Ask for left-right difference if the history suggests hemihypesthesia due to a hemispheric lesion.
- Look for a truncal sensory level in a patient with a possible myelopathy.
- Evaluate any differences between distal versus proximal sensation in the arms and legs if a diagnosis of polyneuropathy is likely.
- Assess without delay the extremity in question if finding hypesthesia associated with a specific dermatome or peripheral nerve distribution is a possibility.
- Examine the perianal area in the event of conus or cauda equina syndrome.

According to convention, spinothalamic qualities (pain, temperature) are assessed first, followed by examination of the dorsal column qualities (vibration, proprioception).

For *pain evaluation*, use a sterile needle or break a wooden spatula into two pieces; for assessment of *temperature*, one side of a tuning fork can be heated using warm tap water and the other side cooled with cold tap water.

Vibration is best tested at the great toes. If vibration is normal there, testing at other sites of the body is usually unnecessary. Ask the patient to indicate when the *vibration* stops, which is important to make sure that the patient has truly understood that the examiner wants to assess vibration (and not, as many patients believe, just the touch of the fork). It also allows a more precise quantification of possible impairment of the vibration sense. If the patient is not able to perceive vibration at the great toes, vibration is then tested at the ankles, tibias, knees, and hips. In order to test *proprioception*, move the patient's great toe up or down in a random fashion (making sure not to touch anything but the sides of the great toe) and ask the patient to close his eyes and indicate which direction the toe is moving. Again, if proprioception cannot be felt by the patient at the level of the great toes, the examiner should test it at the ankle and then at the knees. Note that

for each trial the patient has a 50:50 chance of guessing right (up or down), which is why proprioception should be tested at both extremities a few times, in addition to a zero sample.

As previously discussed in Chap. 2, the patient with *sensory ataxia* has a gait unsteadiness of the so-called stamp and stick type. Additional signs of large fiber involvement include *absent or hypoactive reflexes* and (in severe cases) *pseudo-athetoid finger movements*, when the patient elevates the arms and closes the eyes. (The last sign mentioned is comparable to Romberg's sign for the legs.)

If the patient is very suggestible or not able to cooperate in a detailed sensory examination, the best option is usually to ask the patient to close his eyes and simply say "Now!" or give a thumbs-up whenever he feels the fine touch of a few cotton wool strands (posterior column-medial lemniscus pathway) or the prick of a needle (spinothalamic pathways). This is a relatively "objective" sensory bedside examination.

For evaluation of stereognosis, see the discussion of testing of higher cortical function earlier in this chapter.

3.5 Cerebellar Function

Midline cerebellar damage leads to *truncal and gait ataxia*, whereas *ataxia of the extremities* is secondary to lesions of the ipsilateral cerebellar hemisphere. The *finger-nose test* may reveal both intention tremor and cerebellar ataxia. The normal way of performing the finger-nose test, however, has disadvantages. The patient is usually asked to extend his arms and to point repeatedly to his nose tip with his left and right index fingers, but simply flexing the elbow joint means the index finger will more or less automatically find its way to the tip of the nose. This can be overcome by asking the patient to execute a large curve and to approach the nose tip from the front instead from the side. Alternatively, a finger-nose-finger test can be performed. Another disadvantage is that patients with severe cerebellar ataxia have been known to inflict eye injuries on themselves. The *finger-finger test* (the patient points to the examiner's finger) is much safer in this regard.

The equivalent of the finger-nose test in the lower extremities is the *knee-heel test*. Ask the patient to lift the leg in question high up into the air. Many instances of ataxia already become apparent when the patient is unable to precisely place the foot on the knee. The knee-heel test should be tested with open eyes first and then closed. As with Romberg's test, sensory ataxia can be compensated for by vision, whereas this is not the case for cerebellar ataxia. A variant of the knee-heel test is the *great toe-finger test*, which is analogous to the finger-finger test.

Other features of cerebellar injury include *atactic dysarthria* (arrhythmic pronunciation of every syllable; seen with demyelinating or neurodegenerative diseases) and *decreased muscle tone* of the ipsilateral extremities.[5] *Occipital headache and neck pain* can occur with sudden expansion of a cerebellar process, e.g., hemorrhage or ischemic stroke, and is an ominous sign of beginning brainstem herniation.

Differentiation of cerebellar from sensory ataxia can be done using *Romberg's test*. Sensory ataxia, usually due to impaired dorsal column function or large fiber polyneuropathy, can be compensated for by visual fixation. Cerebellar ataxia, in contrast, is largely unaffected by vision. The differential diagnosis of vestibular and cerebellar ataxia has been discussed above (see CN examination).

Cerebellar impairment is often associated with disturbed eye movements. A *three-step oculomotor bedside examination* can differentiate acute cerebellar dysfunction due to stroke from benign vestibular impairment. When evaluating a patient with vertigo and ataxia of sudden onset, look for:

- Skew deviation
- Gaze-changing nystagmus
- A lack of compensatory saccades during VOR testing using the head impulse test

The presence of one or more of these findings is even more sensitive for the diagnosis of posterior circulation stroke than early diffusion-weighted MRI (DWI) (Case 3.4) (Kattah et al. 2009). The presence of completely normal eye movements, in contrast, including smooth pursuit and normal saccades, makes any form of cerebellar disorder unlikely.

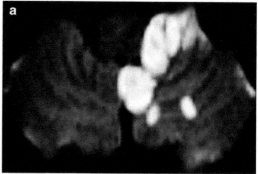
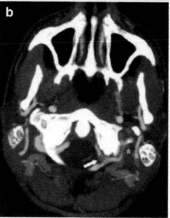

Case 3.4 Vertebral artery dissection. (**a**) A 23-year-old male consulted a chiropractor for chronic neck pain. During neck manipulation he experienced a sudden worsening of the pain in the neck. Three days later he presented with complaints of vertigo and nausea. Examination revealed subtle ataxia and intention tremor of the left extremities as well as a course gaze-changing nystagmus and skew deviation. (**b**) MR DWI showed hyperintense signal changes in the territory of the PICA and AICA on the left. Although an MR angiography of the intracranial vasculature was read as normal, CT angiography including the neck vessels showed dissection of the left VA at the C1 level (*asterisk*) and fresh thrombus material attached to the vessel wall (*arrow*). The patient was managed with anticoagulation and recovered completely. A control CT angiography (not shown) following a 3-month course of warfarin revealed complete recanalization of the left VA and dissolution of the wall thrombus

---

[5]Decreased muscle tone can be revealed by larger amplitude of arm pendulating on passive shoulder shrug or the Stewart-Holmes test. However, this rarely offers additional significant information.

3.6   Gait

Gait should be assessed *informally* when the patient enters the room and *formally* during the bedside examination. Allow for enough space when examining the gait; if the consultation room is too small, make the patient walk down the hallway. Let the patient go back and forth with *normal speed* and let him turn around. Then ask him to walk on his *heal and toes* (this is actually a test of distal motor function in the lower extremities) and to walk on a *line*, maybe even with his eyes closed (this serves the same purpose as Romberg's test). Ataxia of any kind is excluded if the patient is able to walk backward on a line with his eyes closed. Even healthy young people need excellent balance to manage this; try it yourself.

Having observed the patient walk, the neurologist must first decide whether the gait is normal or abnormal. Remember that the gait of an 80-year-old is very different from that of a 20-year-old. If the gait is abnormal, is it a neurological, an orthopedic, a vascular (intermittent claudication), or a psychological problem? If it is a neurological gait disorder, is it of central or peripheral origin?

Gait disorders of *central origin* include:

- Hydrocephalic (magnetic gait, outwardly rotated feet, retropulsion).
- Bizarre (as in paroxysmal dyskinesias, chorea, dystonia, and functional disorders).
- Spastic hemiparetic (circumduction and "short arm, long leg" posturing with cerebral hemiparesis).
- Diplegic spastic (scissor gait of cerebral palsy).
- Cerebellar (broad based, staggering).
- Myelopathic (the patient may require bilateral crutches for ambulation and drag the legs behind).
- Parkinsonian (bradykinetic, flexed posturing, shuffling gait, decrease of spontaneous arm pendulating, turning en bloc with the need for many additional steps, possibly gaze freezing and festination). Interestingly, a recent study suggests that the simple question "Are you still able to ride a bike?" has excellent discriminative power to differentiate between atypical parkinsonism and Parkinson's disease. Whereas patients with PD can maintain their ability to ride a bike for many years, those with atypical parkinsonism typically lose this skill very early (Aerts et al. 2011).
- Camptocormia is encountered in parkinsonism and dystonia and occasionally in MND. It is characterized by a near-90° forward flexion of the trunk. Typically, truncal forward bending disappears when the patient is lying down.[6]

In contrast, gait disorders of *peripheral origin* include:

- LMN type gait (unilateral—drop foot, e.g., due to peroneal palsy or L5 hernia; bilateral—stepper gait, e.g., due to polyneuropathy or the post-polio syndrome)
- Sensory atactic gait (stamping gait, clapping feet on ground with hyperextended knees)

3.7   System Overview

The *first impression* may reveal important diagnostic clues. General hygiene and care, for instance, may be deteriorating in a patient with beginning dementia. Hypomimia, monotonous voice, and mournful body language may point toward a major depression. Registration of the body mass index is crucial in patients prone to cerebrovascular and cardiovascular disease, as well as in young women with suspected idiopathic intracranial hypertension.

Formal medical evaluation is performed with special attention to the *heart* and the carotids. Findings such as atrial fibrillation and systolic murmur suggest cardiac embolism, and arterial hypertension is the most important modifiable risk factor for ischemic cerebral stroke and vascular dementia. For auscultation of the *carotids*, let the patient breath in, then out; then let him stop breathing and listen for noises suspicious of an

---

[6]In very long-standing camptocormia, secondary hip and trunk contractures may prevent disappearance of trunk flexion in the supine position.

underlying stenosis. The examiner should hold his own breath at the same time in order not to exhaust the patient. If the patient complains about pulse-synchronous tinnitus (e.g., due to dural sinus fistula), then listen for sounds over the neck and the temples. As a rule, if the examiner cannot hear a pulse-synchronous noise, there is little likelihood that angiography will reveal a fistula.

In every patient with respiratory problems or with neuromuscular disorders associated with *respiratory failure* (e.g., GBS, ALS, MG), check the *vital capacity*. It is grave malpractice to believe that normal arterial blood gases in a patient with GBS indicate sufficient respiratory function. Hypoxia and hypercapnia only develop late in the course of respiratory muscle fatigue, and then the opportunity for early intubation has been missed. Therefore, the crucial physiological parameter to monitor is the vital capacity. As a rule, a vital capacity of <1.5 L suggests imminent respiratory failure, and arrangements should be undertaken to guarantee ICU support, intubation, and ventilation. Another useful bedside test is to ask the patient to take a deep breath and count aloud as long as possible. Healthy young adults can count to at least until 60. If the patient cannot count further than 30, this suggests severe respiratory impairment and roughly corresponds to a vital capacity of 2 L. Being able to count to 10–15 usually indicates imminent danger of respiratory collapse. Also keep in mind that the diaphragm is innervated by C3–C5[7]; thus, weakness of neck flexion and shoulder abduction in a patient with GBS is a red flag for threatening respiratory failure.

Gastrointestinal symptoms such as abdominal pain, weight loss, and diarrhea are seen with Whipple's disease, celiac disease, and malabsorption syndromes leading to B12 or copper deficiency myelopathy.

With suspected meningitis (fever, headache, confusion, and impairment of consciousness), assess neck rigidity—is the patient able to flex his neck and put his chin on his chest? Remember that *meningism* can be lacking in the very young, the elderly, and the comatose. Other signs of meningism are involuntary lifting of the legs when the patient's head is flexed forward (Brudzinski's sign) and knee flexion during the straight leg test (Kernig's sign).

Inspect the *skin* for stigmata of alcoholism (spider nevi, palmar erythema, caput medusa), diabetes (painless foot ulcers, necrobiosis lipoidica, warm dry feet), atherosclerosis (painful foot ulcers, cold cyanotic pulseless feet), and intravenous drug abuse. Various skin rashes are associated with acute infections, e.g., meningococcal sepsis. Basal cell carcinoma and other skin cancers may lead to retrograde perineural cancer spread toward the cranial cavity. A butterfly rash in the face suggests SLE. Malignant melanoma is the third most common cause for intracranial metastases after lung and breast cancer. The classic erythema migrans often, but not always, occurs during the first 30 days after a tick bite and is sufficiently distinctive to allow a clinical diagnosis of Lyme disease in the absence of laboratory confirmation.

Hallmarks of neurocutaneous disorders include:

- Axillary freckling, café au lait spots, iris hamartoma, and cutaneous fibromata in *neurofibromatosis type I* (Morbus Recklinghausen).
- Nasolabial angiofibroma, subungual fibroma, hypomelanic macules, and areas of thick leathery skin dimpled like an orange peel in *tuberous sclerosis.*
- Telangiectasias of the eyes and skin in ataxia-telangiectasia.
- Facial port-wine stains in *Sturge-Weber syndrome* (Case 3.5).
- Angiomatosis and café au lait spots in *von Hippel-Lindau disease.*
- Vascular anomalies that involve the skin as well as the brain and other internal organs include telangiectasias in *Osler-Rendu disease* and bluish, painless, rubbery venous anomalies in the *blue rubber bleb nevus syndrome* (BRBNS) (Case 3.6).

Lymphadenopathy and *splenomegaly* should be looked for if viral exposure (e.g., HIV or Epstein-Barr infection) is suspected. Splenomegaly may also indicate a metabolic dis-

---

[7]"C3, 4, 5 keeps the diaphragm alive."

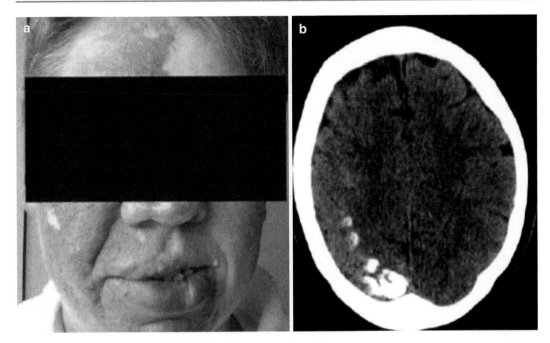

Case 3.5 Focal epilepsy due to Sturge-Weber syndrome. This 35-year-old female with a facial port-wine stain had suffered from focal epilepsy since childhood (**a**). Seizures typically start in the left extremities and may generalize. Unlike other patients with Sturge-Weber syndrome, there was no history of glaucoma or psychomotor retardation. CT of the brain showed ipsilateral gyral calcifications (**b**)

ease, e.g., Niemann-Pick disease type C. The abdomen, breasts, rectum, and testes should also be examined for *mass lesions* if a systemic malignancy is suspected. *Gynecomastia* may signify the presence of pituitary adenoma or a diagnosis of Kennedy's disease.

Several phenomena may point toward a *rheumatologic disease*, including facial rash such as in dermatomyositis and SLE, Raynaud's phenomenon, finger ulcers, tobacco pouch mouth in scleroderma, and joint deformities such as in rheumatoid arthritis and psoriasis arthritis. (Beware of atlantooccipital subluxation in rheumatoid arthritis.) Vitiligo, alopecia, and signs of hypo- and hyperthyroidism may reveal a general disposition for autoimmune disorders.

Spinal congenital malformations, including spina bifida occulta, dermal sinus, or a tethered cord, may be revealed by abnormalities over the lumbar area, such as fistula and dermal sinus, tufts of hair, lipoma, birthmarks, and dimples in the skin. *Foot deformities* with high arch and hammer toes are often encountered in hereditary polyneuropathies such as CMT and in Friedreich's ataxia.

Somatic stigmata of *hereditary and nonhereditary congenital diseases with cognitive dysfunction* include:

- Oblique eye fissures with epicanthic skin folds on the inner corner of the eyes (previously known as mongoloid folds), flat nasal bridge, protruding tongue, small chin, single palmar fold, short neck, and excessive joint laxity including atlantoaxial instability belong to the phenotype of Down syndrome.
- Large testes and a Marfan-like body shape, including an elongated face, a high palate, hyperextensible finger joints, and flat feet, are typical for fragile X syndrome, the most common genetic cognitive disorder in boys.
- Skin folds at the corner of the eyes and a short nose with a low nasal bridge are facial features of fetal alcohol syndrome; other facial

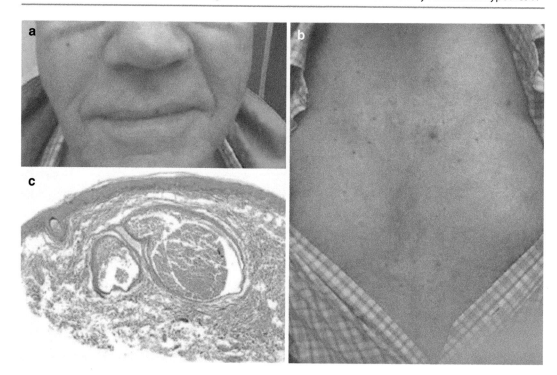

Case 3.6 Blue rubber bleb nevus syndrome. A 75-year-old male presented with sudden onset of diplopia due to palsy of the right abducens nerve and a right-sided peripheral facial palsy (**1a**). During the last 10 years, he had developed a large number of small bluish, compressible, rubbery, and painless nodules, primarily on his face and trunk (**1a, b**). Nodules were also found affecting the oral mucosa. MR imaging of the brain 4 years earlier, ordered during the evaluation of a minor stroke, had revealed multiple vascular anomalies in both the cerebrum and cerebellum. A skin biopsy from nodules of the chest had shown irregular dilated and congested vascular spaces, consistent with a venous malformation (**1c**). A new MRI of the brain revealed a lesion in the dorsal pons at the level of the abducens nucleus and the facial colliculus (**2a–c**; the lesion, marked by an "X" in **2c**, affects both the nucleus abducens and the facial nerve). A strongly hypointense signal on T_2*-weighted MRI was consistent with venous blood and hemosiderin deposits (**2b**). Review of the first MRI revealed that this venous malformation had not been present before and thus had developed de novo (**2d**). Based on the histopathology and appearance of the bluish nodules on the skin, gastrointestinal mucosa, and brain, the patient was diagnosed as having BRBNS with isolated cranial neuropathy due to a pontine venous malformation (Adapted with permission from Kondziella et al. (2010))

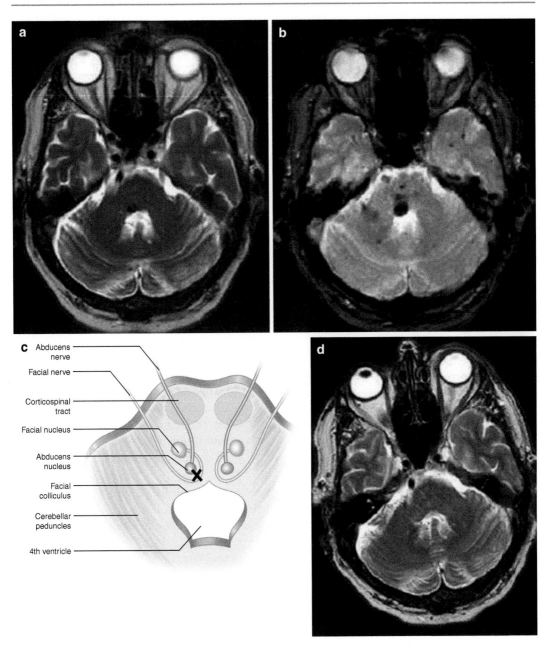

Case 3.6 (continued)

stigmata include an indistinct philtrum, a thin upper lip, a small midface, and a short head circumference.

- Cataracts, temporalis muscle atrophy, ptosis occur in myotonic dystrophy.
- Repetitive wringing hand movements are typically seen with Rett syndrome, the most common genetic cognitive disorder in girls.

3.8 Examination of the Comatose Patient

Coma can be defined as a *state of unresponsiveness and non-arousal in which the patient is aware neither of his surroundings nor of himself.* Coma must be differentiated from:

- Locked-in syndrome
- Psychogenic non-arousal
- Other impairment of consciousness ranging from mild drowsiness to the minimal conscious and vegetative states (see Sect. 4.2)

Prior to examination of the comatose patient, make sure that all *vital functions are secured* according to the ABC approach. Then start with an external inspection and look for trauma (e.g., revealed by retroauricular and periorbital subcutaneous hemorrhages (Case 3.7)) and signs of intoxication (e.g., cherry-red skin coloration such as in carbon monoxide poisoning; mydriasis with sympathicomimetics, e.g., cocaine; or parasym-

patholytics, e.g., atropine; miosis with opioids) or drug abuse (e.g., injection sites). Perform a short medical system overview and note possible fever, neck stiffness, and skin rash (e.g., as in meningococcal meningitis), abnormalities of the breathing pattern (e.g., Kussmaul breathing in diabetic ketoacidosis and other metabolic derangements), hypertension and vomiting (suggesting increased ICP), and so on. Do not forget to contact paramedics, family, friends, and other witnesses to ensure that crucial information has not been overlooked; if necessary, ask for phone numbers and make a phone call. Then proceed with the neurological assessment.

The neurological examination in the comatose patient has four objectives:

- To verify and quantify the level of unconsciousness
- To assess brainstem function
- To search for focal neurological deficits
- To search for neurological causes for coma

3.8.1 Verification and Quantification of Unconsciousness

Unconsciousness should always be verified and graded. (Consult Chap. 2 for discussion of the locked-in syndrome; see below for assessment of psychogenic coma; see Sect. 4.2 for the minimal conscious and vegetative states.) Several grading scales are

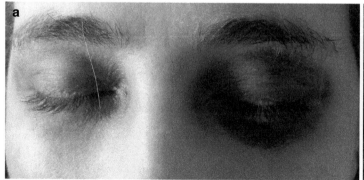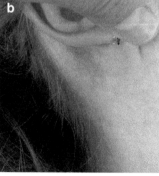

Case 3.7 Raccoon eyes and Battle's sign. Following a traumatic brain injury, this young female developed periorbital (**a**, raccoon eyes) and mastoid (**b**, Battle's sign) ecchymosis, consistent with fractures of the anterior, respectively, posterior cranial fossa

available, but none comes even close to the *Glasgow Coma Scale* (GCS) in terms of popularity.

The GCS has three categories (eye opening, verbal response, motor response; Table 3.2). Always note the total GCS score as well as all three subscores in the charts. According to the GCS, brain injury is classified as severe (GCS ≤ 8), moderate (GCS 9–12), and minor (GCS ≥ 13). GSC ≤ 8 usually indicates impairment of airway protection reflexes and the need for intubation. GCS was designed for trauma victims, and it is less well suited for grading and following coma of metabolic or ischemic origin. Besides, failure to assess the verbal score in intubated patients and the inability to test brainstem reflexes are shortcomings of the GCS.

Alternative grading scales include, among others, *Full Outline of UnResponsiveness* (FOUR, Wijdicks et al. 2005) and *Reaction Level Scale 85* (RLS85; Starmark and Lindgren 1986). FOUR provides greater neurological detail than GSC, has excellent inter-rater reliability, recognizes a locked-in syndrome, and is superior to the GCS due to the availability of brainstem reflexes, breathing patterns, and the ability to recognize different stages of herniation; hence, neurologists should use it more often (Table 3.2) (Case 3.8). The main principle of RLS85 is that it focuses completely on wakefulness and motor response, in contrast to GSC and FOUR, which makes it especially easy to use (Table 3.2). RLS85 has better interobserver agreement than GCS, and in one study it was superior to the GCS in predicting intracranial pathology. Its main disadvantage is that it is virtually unknown outside Scandinavia (Table 3.2).

3.8.2 Assessment of Neurological Deficits, in Particular Signs of Brainstem Injury

For a review of brainstem function and anatomy, refer to Chap. 2. *Brainstem reflexes* can be used to define the site of lesion on a *vertical axis*:

Table 3.2 Scales for grading unconsciousness

Glasgow Coma Scale (*GCS*; Teasdale and Jennett 1974)
Eye opening (*4/4*): spontaneous (4), to speech (3), to pain (2), none (1)
Best motor response (*6/6*): obeys commands (6), localizes pain (5), withdraws from painful stimuli (4), flexion posturing with painful stimuli (3), extensor posturing with painful stimuli (2), none (1)
Best verbal response (*5/5*): orientated (5), confused speech (4), inappropriate words (3), incomprehensible sounds (2), none (1)
Full Outline of UnResponsiveness (*FOUR*; Wijdicks et al. 2005)
Eye response (*4/4*): eyelids open or opened, tracking, or blinking to command (4), eyelids open but not tracking (3), eyelids closed but open to loud voice (2), eyelids closed but open to pain (1), eyelids remain closed with pain (0)
Motor response (*4/4*): thumbs-up, fist, or peace sign (4), localizing to pain (3), flexion response to pain (2), extension response to pain (1), no response to pain or generalized myoclonus status (0)
Brainstem reflexes (*4/4*): pupil and corneal reflexes present (4), one pupil wide and fixed (3), pupil or corneal reflexes absent (2), pupil and corneal reflexes absent (1), absent pupil, corneal, and cough reflex (0)
Respiration (*4/4*): not intubated, regular breathing pattern (4), not intubated, Cheyne-Stokes breathing pattern (3), not intubated, irregular breathing (2), breathes above ventilator rate (1), breathes at ventilator rate or apnea (0)
Reaction Level Scale 85 (*RLS85*; Starmark and Lindgren 1986)
1. Alert, no delay in response
2. Drowsy or confused, responsive to mild stimulation
3. Very drowsy or confused, responsive to strong stimulation
4. Unconscious, localizes but does not ward off pain
5. Unconscious, withdrawing movements to pain stimulation
6. Unconscious, stereotype flexion movements to pain stimulation
7. Unconscious, stereotype extension movements to pain stimulation
8. Unconscious, no response to pain stimulation

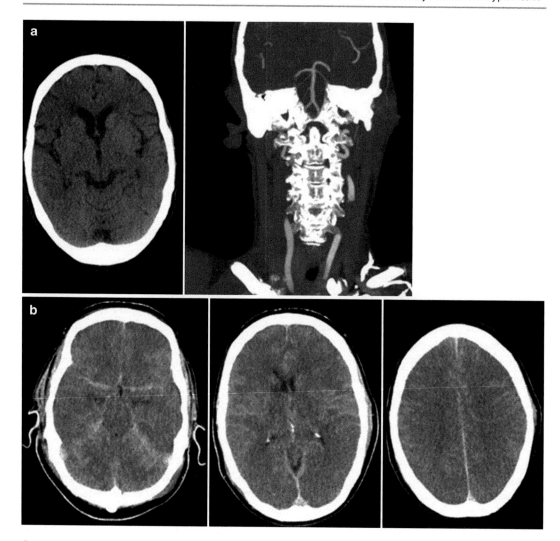

Case 3.8 Cerebral fat embolism. A 72-year-old woman with a history of diabetes mellitus, hypertension, and a fracture of the left femur 6 years previously was scheduled for a total hip replacement. After the operation, she was awake and responsive, but 3 h later, she became obtunded. CT of the brain, including CT angiography, was unremarkable (**a**). However, her level of consciousness further declined, and she was transferred to the intensive care unit. On examination, she was comatose but had preserved pupillary and corneal reflexes. Her FOUR score was 12 (eye response 1, motor response 3, brainstem reflexes 4, intubation 4). A few hours later, she developed respiratory failure, anuria, and hypoxemia. Blood tests were compatible with disseminated intravascular coagulation. Petechial hemorrhages were noted on the skin of the face and abdomen. Her pupils became fixed and dilated. Sternal rub induced decerebrate posturing. The FOUR score was 5 (eye response 0, motor response 2, brainstem reflexes 2, intubation 1). Repeated CT of the brain showed fulminant cerebral edema with loss of white and gray mat-

ter discrimination due to increased intracranial pressure; the resulting brain hypoattenuation and relative hyperintense signal related to engorgement of superficial venous structures were compatible with "pseudo-subarachnoid hemorrhage," suggesting imminent brain death (**b**). Autopsy confirmed cerebral fat embolism. This condition arises within a few hours (usually <48 h) following fractures related to long bones or orthopedic surgery. Tiny fat bubbles accumulate in the arterioles which may lead to multiorgan failure and death, although the prognosis is better in less severe cases, especially in the young. MRI is more sensitive than CT and consistently shows multiple small, scattered, non-confluent intracerebral hyperintensities on T_2-weighted and DWI scans ("starfield pattern"). Focal neurological deficits do typically not occur because major cerebral arteries are not occluded. Instead, the neurological course is characterized by subacute and progressive decline of consciousness (followed in fatal cases by a classical pattern of central brain herniation) because of widespread buildup of fat emboli in brain arterioles

- Pupillary reflex, in, CN II; out, CN III
- Corneal and eyelash reflexes, in, CN V; out, CN VII
- Vestibulo-cephalic reflex and VOR, in, CN VIII; out, CN III, CN VI
- Gag reflex in, CN IX; out, CN X

Asymmetrical brainstem signs can be used to define the site of a lesion on a *horizontal axis*. Thus, nuclear signs are ipsilateral, long tract signs contralateral to the lesion. With metabolic derangements and intoxication, the reflexes and the size of the pupils are usually normal except with atropine, tricyclic antidepressants (TCAs), cocaine, and other sympathicomimetics (mydriasis) and opioids (miosis). Apart from pupillary reflexes, the shape and size of the pupils offer important information. With mesencephalic damage, the pupils tend to be mydriatic, and with pontine lesions miotic. Traumatic compression of CN III leads to a mydriatic unilateral pupil with irregular shape. For evaluation of eye axis deviation and spontaneous conjugate or disconjugate eye movements, see Chap. 2.

The *VOR* stabilizes images on the retina during head movement by producing an eye movement in the direction opposite to the movement of the head. The reflex is driven by vestibular signals from the inner ear (vestibulocochlear nerve) and leads to activation of the contralateral abducens nerve (lateral rectus muscle) and (via the MLF) the ipsilateral oculomotor nerve (medial rectus muscle). An intact VOR suggests two things. First, the oculomotor CNs and central eye movement structures in the mesencephalon and tegmental pons are intact. Second, there is loss of cortical suppression of VOR. Spontaneously "rowing" eye movements indicate loss of supranuclear conjugate eye control, but intact eye movement centers in the brainstem, a good prognostic sign. Thus, the coma is not due to structural mesencephalic damage but rather widespread cortical dysfunction, e.g., due to metabolic-toxic impairment of cortical activity. The VOR is tested by rotating the head of the patient from one side to the other and observing for reflex eye movements in the opposite direction. Allow enough time (a few seconds) for the reflex eye movements to occur. Caloric testing of the VOR in the ICU is usually performed as part of a brain death diagnostic procedure.[8]

The best way to examine the *gag reflex* is to assess cough response to bronchial suctioning; simply moving the endotracheal tube to and fro is usually not a sufficient stimulus. Lack of the gag reflex, however, is rather common in ICU patients and, if isolated, is not necessarily associated with a bad outcome.

The *ciliospinal reflex* produces mydriasis after painful stimuli, e.g., squeezing the side of the neck or inner parts of the arms or supraorbital or sternal pressure. (This is a rather redundant examination technique.) Painful stimuli also lead to an increase of blood pressure and heart rate observable on the monitor.

The *apnea test* is a fairly advanced test only used during brain death evaluation; its main purpose is to assess whether carbon dioxide (CO_2) retention still elicits spontaneous ventilation (see below).

Several breathing patterns are associated with coma. Cheyne-Stokes respiration as an isolated phenomenon is not necessarily a grave sign. Yet, it is an ominous sign if breathing becomes more irregular (e.g., central neurogenic hypoventilation, atactic breathing, apneustic breathing).

Abnormal posturing, spontaneously or after painful stimuli, occurs in patients with severe brain injury and during transtentorial cerebral herniation. Posturing with flexion of the arms and extension of the legs is compatible with the decorticate state, suggesting damage or functional impairment at or above the level of the diencephalon (e.g., cerebral hemispheres, internal capsule, and thalamus). Patients in the decerebrate state show posturing with extension of

---

[8]When flushing the ear canal in a conscious patient, the fast phase of the nystagmus will be to the opposite side with cold water and to the same side with warm water. The acronym COWS (Cold Opposite, Warm Same) has been taught for generations as a mnemonic. However, as stated above, this denotes the fast phase of the nystagmus, which is seen typically in conscious patients. In unconscious patients who lack supranuclear gaze control but who have an intact brainstem, there may only be gaze deviation in the other direction (CSWO (Cold Same, Warm Opposite)).

arms and legs, suggesting damage at or below the level of the midbrain (and thus, often a more advanced stage of brain herniation).

For assessment of *hemiplegia*, begin by observing possible asymmetry of spontaneous movements and postures. Restless but rather symmetric movements of the arms and legs suggest intact corticospinal tracts. If this is not the case, then proceed by applying painful stimuli distally at every extremity. Be sure not to injure the patient. Look for an asymmetric motor response; also look for an asymmetric facial response, e.g., facial winking with pain on one side but not the other suggests *hemisensory loss* or a facial palsy. In addition, in acute hemiplegia, muscle tone is decreased. When lifting and releasing the plegic extremities, they will fall much more heavily than the non-plegic ones.

When *epileptic seizures* occur, rhythmic motor activity can occasionally be limited to the extremities controlled by the unaffected hemisphere. In these cases, the hemiplegia simply prevents epileptic motor manifestations on the paretic side. Beware of the fact that in long-standing status epilepticus visible seizure activity may be reduced to nystagmoid eye movements and flickering of the eyelids. Careful inspection is needed to detect these subtle signs of status epilepticus. The clinical implications of myo-clonic status epilepticus following hypoxic-anoxic encephalopathy are explained below.

3.8.3 Neurological Causes for Coma

Acute hemiparesis associated with coma suggests a *cerebrovascular accident* in the contralateral hemisphere.[9] Alternating hemiparesis, vertigo, and brainstem signs (that sometimes may go on for days) are typical for a *basilar artery occlusion*. For discussion of the top-of-the-basilar syndrome and other brainstem ischemic

syndromes, see Chap. 2. Dissection of the ascending aorta may lead to sudden loss of consciousness and focal neurological signs (Case 3.9).

Decreased consciousness and a unilateral dilated pupil suggest a *subarachnoidal hemorrhage* or *acute uncal brain herniation* due to another cause of sudden increase of ICP (Case 3.10).

Fever and meningism suggest *bacterial meningitis*. Beware that meningism can be lacking in the very young, in the very old, and in the deeply comatose.

A short history of headache, neck pain, and ataxia followed by decreased consciousness and brainstem signs is characteristic for acute brainstem compression from a *cerebellar stroke*.

Acute hydrocephalus is associated with deteriorating consciousness, headache, Cushing response (hypertension, bradycardia, and respira-

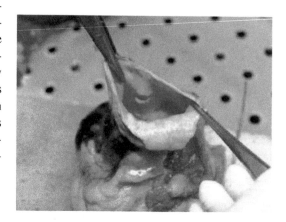

Case 3.9 Type A aortic dissection. A 65-year-old female with arterial hypertension, but otherwise in good general condition, suddenly collapsed. Pulseless electrical activity was noted and resuscitation started. Twenty minutes later the patient was breathing and had a normal blood pressure. ECG showed sinus rhythm. Laboratory results including cardiac enzymes, blood glucose, and blood gases were noncontributory. The patient was unconscious and had gaze deviation to the right. On painful stimuli, she reacted with decerebrate posturing (GCS 5: eye 1, verbal 1, motor 3). There was bilateral Babinski sign. CT of the brain was normal, including CT angiography (limited to the intracranial circulation; CTA including the neck vessels and the aortic arch would have revealed the dissection). Four hours later the patient suffered cardiac arrest and died. Autopsy showed a tear originating in the ascending aorta, confirming a diagnosis of type A aortic dissection

---

[9]Occasionally, hemiparesis and Babinski sign are ipsilateral to the hemispherical lesion. This is the so-called Kernohan's notch phenomenon and occurs when the mass lesion leads to lateral brain displacement pressing the opposite cerebral peduncle, and thus the opposite corticospinal tract, against the tentorium.

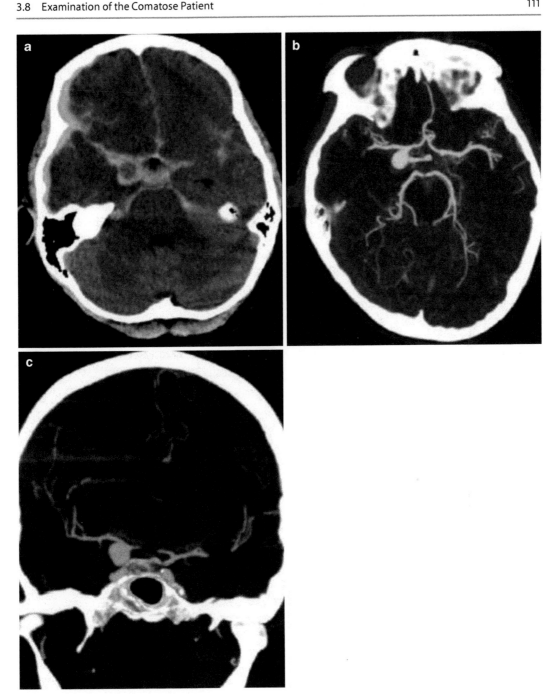

Case 3.10 Subdural hemorrhage due to ruptured intra-cranial aneurysm. A 46-year-old male experienced a sudden excruciating headache before losing consciousness. On arrival of the ambulance, he was comatose and had bilaterally dilated pupils. Following intubation and IV administration of hypertonic saline, both pupils constricted. However, in the emergency room, the right pupil was dilated again. CT of the brain (**a**) and CTA (**b, c**) showed extensive subarachnoidal hemorrhage due to a right-sided ICA aneurysm. As in this case, an aneurysm at the level below the division of the carotid artery into the MCA and ACA (the "carotid T") may occasionally lead to additional subdural hematoma because of bleeding through an arachnoid tear (CT images courtesy of Vagn Eskesen, Department of Neurosurgery, Rigshospitalet, Copenhagen)

tory depression), small pupils, eye movement disturbances (e.g., sustained downgaze, the sunsetting sign), increased tone in the legs, and bilateral Babinski signs.

Metabolic derangements and various forms of *intoxication* may also lead to decreased consciousness combined with (usually reversible) focal neurological signs, e.g., bilateral Babinski sign in a comatose patient with *hypoglycemia*.

Consult Chap. 4 for an in-depth differential diagnosis of coma.

3.8.4 Coma, Vegetative, and Minimal Conscious States

Searching for consciousness in noncommunicating brain-injured patients by clinical examination is essential, yet challenging. The origin of many clinical signs is not entirely clear, and their significance as to whether or not the patient is conscious

is even less certain. In addition, consciousness may wax and wane within seconds to hours and days to months (Fig. 3.1). Indeed, as many as 40% of patients with disorders of consciousness (DoC) are misclassified as being in a vegetative state (VS) (Schnakers et al. 2009). Although these patients may not show any signs of consciousness during clinical examination because of lost motor output, some are able to willfully modulate their brain activity on command, as shown by fMRI and EEG studies, occasionally even answering yes or no questions by performing mental imagery tasks. For patients with acute brain injury and their caregivers, this has significant ethical and practical implications, not least for prognostication, treatment decisions, resource allocation, and end-of-life considerations.

The term DoC includes patients in coma, VS/unresponsive wakefulness syndrome (UWS), and MCS, as well as those who have emerged—but not completely—from MCS (eMCS).

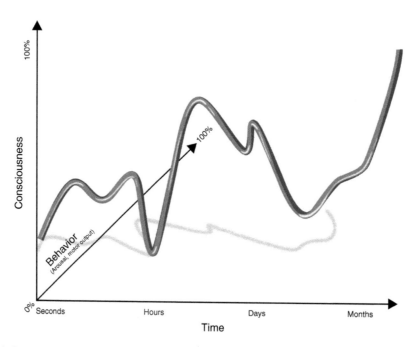

Fig. 3.1 This figure depicts a 3D-model of consciousness in non-communicating patients, including those with a diagnosis of vegetative or minimal conscious states. The degree of consciousness typically fluctuates with time (*x*-axis) both in the short term (seconds to hours) and long term (days to months). The correct evaluation of con-

sciousness (*y*-axis) depends on the patient's behavior (*z*-axis), which can be conceptualized as a product of arousal and motor output. Clinical evaluation at the bedside is critically reliant on measurable motor activity and a sufficient degree of arousal. (Adapted with permission from Kondziella et al. 2016)

- Coma, as stated earlier, may be defined as a state of profound unawareness from which patients cannot be aroused. A normal sleep-wake cycle is absent, and eyes are closed. Coma lasts usually only a few days or weeks following acute brain injury because patients either die or their brainstem function recovers; thus, if patients survive long enough, they will wake up—with or without regaining awareness.

- In contrast to coma, *VS/UWS* is a condition of wakefulness without awareness. Although patients in this condition have alternating periods with eyes open and eyes closed, they exhibit only reflex behaviors and are therefore considered unaware of themselves and their surroundings. While patients are bladder and bowel incontinent, their autonomic hypothalamic and brainstem function is preserved to such a degree that it permits survival (usually with medical or nursing assistance).

- In comparison, patients in *MCS* show unequivocal signs of nonreflex behaviors occurring inconsistently, yet reproducibly, in response to environmental stimuli. Thus, they may show visual pursuit or prolonged fixation of objects or people; they may show emotional responses that are congruent with the situation (e.g., smiling or crying when being visited by a relative); they may reach out for, hold, or touch an object in a manner which is adapted to its shape or size; and when being spoken to they may react to the linguistic content by making sounds or gestures. By definition, although some may follow commands to a certain degree, accurate communication is impossible. Patients may be classified into MCS plus (i.e., if they are able to obey commands) or minus (i.e., if they only localize pain, exhibit visual pursuit, or show appropriate emotional expressions). When patients regain the ability to communicate, albeit rudimentarily and inconsistently, they are classified as *eMCS* (*emerged from MCS*). Of note, one of the earliest clinical signs that distinguishes the MCS from VS/UWS is the presence of eye tracking occurring in direct response to a moving stimulus. It is important to be aware of the fact that autoreferential stimuli are the most salient (this is arguably true for people with normal consciousness as well); hence, when assessing patients for visual pursuit, it is important to use a mirror because MCS patients tend to track their own reflection best (Vanhaudenhuyse et al. 2008). Also, when evaluating patients with DoC, beware of confusing the grip reflex with a sign of voluntary action; thus, instead of asking the patient to "squeeze my fingers," you may ask her to "open your fist."

VS/UWS and MCS most likely exist on a spectrum rather than being categorically distinct. Traditionally, VS/UWS has been considered permanent 3 months after non-traumatic injuries and 12 months following TBI, although late recovery is increasingly recognized. Patients may evolve from VS/UWS into MCS (or better) and they may or may not relapse.

3.8.5 Prognostication of Neurological Outcome Following Cardiac Arrest

All brain function ceases after a few minutes of cardiac arrest. If circulation is restored in time, the brain recovers successively. Brainstem reflexes return first, followed by stereotyped reaction to pain, and, finally, cortical activity and consciousness. The likelihood of a good outcome decreases the longer the patient remains unconscious, and brainstem reflexes and reactivity to pain are lacking. American guidelines published in 2006 for the prediction of outcome in comatose survivors following cardiopulmonary resuscitation (Wijdicks et al. 2006) have been widely implemented and should be basic knowledge for neurologists seeing patients in intensive care units (ICUs). The guidelines' main message was that, following 72 h of observation, "pupillary light response, corneal reflexes, motor responses to pain, myoclonus status epilepticus, serum neuron-specific enolase, and somatosensory evoked potential studies can reliably assist in accurately predicting poor outcome in comatose patients after cardiopulmonary resuscitation for cardiac arrest." In the meantime, however, therapeutic hypothermia (typically for 24 h at 32–34 °C) has become standard of care in many countries for survivors of out-of-hospital ventricular fibrillation cardiac arrest, and prognostication of these patients is not included in the aforementioned guidelines. It follows that the neurologist must be especially careful when evaluating unconscious patients treated with hypothermia, and it is recommended to postpone prognostic evaluation for 72 h following return to normothermia.

The most important tool for evaluation of brain injury following cardiac arrest is the daily clinical examination, which should focus on the presence or absence of brainstem reflexes, reactivity to pain, and clinical seizures. Bilateral loss of the pupillary light response 72 h after cardiac arrest is a reliable clinical sign for an unfavorable outcome even in patients after therapeutic hypothermia. Although lack of bilateral corneal reflexes and reactivity to pain (or abnormal posturing) 72 h after cardiac arrest is traditionally regarded as indicating a bad prognosis, there have been a few reports of recovery in patients following hypothermia. By the time they are evaluated in the ICU, only a minority of patients following cardiac arrest will have lost all brainstem reflexes, suggesting brain death (see below). As always, it is of utmost importance to exclude possible remaining effects from anesthesia and sedation, as well as metabolic derangements. Generalized myoclonic seizures during the first day after cardiac arrest indicate a poor prognosis in the vast majority of patients. (In contrast, action myoclonus developing a few days or weeks after the event, termed Lance-Adams syndrome, is not incompatible with good mental recovery.)

As stated above, unless brain death is suspected or the patient has generalized myoclonic seizures, prognostic evaluation should be postponed for 72 h after cardiac arrest in patients without hypothermia and for 72 h following normothermia in patients who have been subject to therapeutic hypothermia. The clinical evaluation should always be supplemented by laboratory investigations. Bilateral absence of the so-called N20 potential in comatose patients examined by somatosensory evoked potentials (SSEP) (Chap. 5) is associated with a specificity of almost 100%

for death or the vegetative state if performed 24 h after cardiac arrest. Even in patients after therapeutic hypothermia, the specificity is still very high, assuming that the examination has been performed after return to normothermia. However, presence of the N20 potentials does not by itself signify a good prognosis. Other laboratory results that are helpful for prognostication after brain death, suggesting a poor prognosis, include an unfavorable EEG pattern (burst suppression, status epilepticus, nonreactive background activity, and electrical silence), loss of discrimination of white and gray matter on a computed tomography (CT) of the brain, widespread hyperintense signal change on MR DWI, and increased levels of certain biomarkers (S100B, neuron-specific enolase).

3.8.6   Diagnosis of Brain Death

In the past, death was determined by cessation of cardiorespiratory function. With better intensive care medicine and the rise of transplantation medicine, brain death criteria were defined in the early 1980s. Brain death is the irreversible loss of all brain and brainstem function (Wijdicks 2012). In adult organ donors, the most common causes of brain death are *trauma* and *subarachnoidal hemorrhage*. In contrast, the time it takes for patients with *hypoxic-ischemic brain injury* or other neurological disorders to enter the stage of brain death is usually much longer, and by then the body organs are typically no longer in a sufficiently healthy condition to be harvested. Therefore, neurosurgical patients are much more often potential organ donors than neurologic patients, and neurologists only rarely perform a brain death diagnostic procedure (Case 3.11). The precise regulations of how to perform brain death testing vary from country to country and sometimes even from hospital to hospital. The neurologist should therefore be familiar with the instructions at his workplace. The principles of brain death diagnostics are covered in the following[10]:

---

[10] Please observe that the diagnostic procedures in children are significantly different due to the immaturity of the brain; these procedures will not be reviewed here.

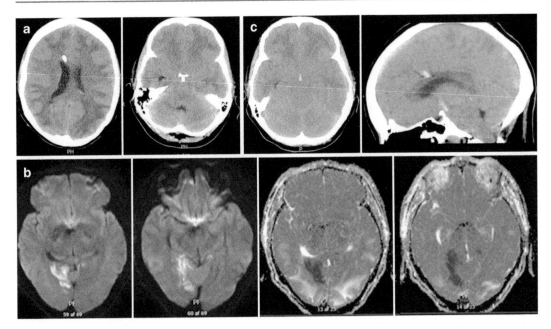

Case 3.11 Dialysis disequilibrium syndrome. A 32-year-old woman had received a kidney transplant because of renal failure and glomerulonephritis 6 years prior to presentation. Due to major depression, the patient had stopped taking all medication for 2 months prior, leading to acute uremia and failure of the renal transplant. Following onset of hemodialysis, the patient became comatose (GCS 3, FOUR 2 (e0, m0, brainstem 1, respiration 1)). CT showed generalized cerebral edema and enlargement of the temporal horns of the lateral ventricles (**a**, also note the external ventricular drain). A diagnosis of PRES associated with the dialysis disequilibrium syndrome was made. MRI DWI and ADC showed vital brain tissue except for a minor right-sided PCA stroke (**b**). In order to prevent further brain swelling due to osmotic shift, intermittent hemodialysis was stopped, and continu-ous renal replacement therapy was started instead. Decompressive occipital craniotomy was contemplated but not performed. The same evening, ICP increased to >70 cm H_2O. CT showed worsening brain edema leading to incarceration (**c**). Dialysis disequilibrium syndrome is a rare but potentially serious complication of hemodialysis. Signs and symptoms vary from mild headache to coma and death. White matter lesions are thought to represent interstitial edema derived from osmotic shift, but the exact mechanisms remain poorly understood. Other neurological syndromes associated with hemodialysis include subdural hematoma, Wernicke's encephalopathy, carpal tunnel syndrome, and dialysis dementia. Fortunately, the latter is rare nowadays due to the use of aluminum-free dialysate

1. Confirm that the patient has a known structural and irreversible cause that fully explains brain death; e.g., following a traumatic brain injury, an MRI may show fulminant transtentorial brain herniation.
2. Exclude medical conditions that may mimic brain death, including:
   (a) Hypothermia. Body temperature should be at least above 32 °C (89.6 °F). Hypothermic patients after a drowning accident should be warmed to at least 35 °C (95 °F).
   (b) Hypoglycemia and hyperglycemia. Blood glucose should be between 3.3 and 22 mmol/L (60 and 400 mg/dL).
   (c) Hypotension. Blood pressure should as a minimum be above 90/40 mmHg
   (d) Other metabolic disorders, e.g., electrolyte, acid-base, and endocrinological disturbances.
   (e) Drug intoxications.
   (f) Anesthetic agents. Ensure that the patient has been taken off all sedatives, anesthetics, and neuromuscular blocking agents and that enough time has been allowed for these substances to be metabolized or secreted. The anesthetist usually knows when enough time has been passed.
3. Confirm unresponsiveness and absence of brainstem reflexes, including:

(a) Absence of pupillary reflexes.

(b) Absence of corneal reflexes. (Be sure not to damage the cornea; it may be harvested during organ donation. A drop of sterile saline can be used for assessment of the corneal reflexes instead of a cotton swab.)

(c) Absence of gag reflex.

(d) Absence of vestibulo-ocular and oculocephalic reflexes.

(e) Absence of motor response in the face or the extremities following facial (e.g., supraorbital pressure) and distal (e.g., pressure on the nail beds in all extremities) painful stimulation. Observe that flexor and extensor posturing are brainstem reflexes, and, if present, they are not consistent with brain death. In contrast, certain spontaneous limb movements (Lazarus movements), deep tendon reflexes, and the triple flexion response (see above, Sect. 3.3) are spinal reflexes, and their presence therefore does not exclude brain death.

(f) Absence of autonomic responses following painful stimulation, e.g., absence of pupillary dilation and tachycardia.

(g) When a lack of the brainstem reflexes listed above has been confirmed, an apnea test may be performed to demonstrate the inability of the brainstem to trigger spontaneous breathing in the presence of hypercapnia. (An apnea test is not routinely carried out at every center.) Confirm that the patient has normal body temperature, sufficient blood pressure, and blood volume as well as a normal $PaCO_2$ and PaO_2. Prevent hypoxemia by preoxygenating the patient with 100% oxygen for 10 min while on the ventilator and by delivering oxygen at 6 L/min through a catheter in the tracheal tube after disconnection from mechanical ventilation. When the patient is removed from the ventilator, observe for (the lack of) spontaneous respiratory movements for at least 10 min and then demonstrate hypercapnia by arterial blood gas measurement. During the test, the $PaCO_2$ should reach >8 kPa in order to be consistent with brain death.

4. As a rule, confirmatory paraclinical investigations are only needed if the situation remains unclear, e.g., with severe facial trauma rendering brainstem reflex assessment impossible. Testing is performed to demonstrate:

(a) Absence of intracerebral circulation. Four-vessel cerebral angiography, transcranial Doppler sonography, and radionuclide cerebral blood flow (CBF)

Case 3.12 Fatal cerebral edema due to inborn error of metabolism. Following a period of gastroenteritis, a 15-year-old boy developed rapidly progressive, ascending tetraplegia with acute respiratory failure and severe lactic acidosis over 2 days. He was admitted with a working diagnosis of GBS. However, MRI showed hyperintense signal changes with decreased diffusion centrally in the brainstem, mesencephalon (**a**, sagittal T_2), basal nuclei including the thalami, mesial temporal lobes, and cerebral cortex (**b**, axial DWI), as well as in the spinal cord (**c**, sagittal T_2). His medical history was notable for slightly delayed motor milestones, a several weeks long period of severe encephalopathy and generalized weakness following a gastrointestinal infection at the age of 4, as well as aversion for meat and other high-protein foods. Metabolic screening revealed diagnostic levels of increased leucine, isoleucine, and valine, consistent with the intermittent form of maple syrup urine disease (MSUD). Despite immediate treatment with low-protein diet (to reduce catabolic metabolism), dialysis (to decrease toxic branched-chain amino acid levels), and parenteral thiamine substitution, the patient developed fatal brain edema within a few hours (**d**, unenhanced CT).

Clinical examination was consistent with brain death, and digital subtraction angiography confirmed this by showing absent intracranial circulation (**e**). MSUD is an autosomal recessively inherited enzyme defect that leads to massive accumulation of leucine in the body. In the intermittent form of MSUD, patients may do well during most of their lives, but acute metabolic stressors such as gastrointestinal infections put them at risk. Cerebral edema is a typical terminal manifestation. MSUD belongs to the so-called inborn errors of metabolism (IBM) which are caused by deficiencies in enzymes or other proteins involved in cell metabolism. They can present at any age from infancy to late adulthood. Late-onset presentations are often triggered by seemingly unspecific factors such as benign fever episodes, surgery, or prolonged periods of exercise or fasting. IBM presenting acutely in adults or adolescents can roughly be divided into intoxication syndromes such as hyperammonemias, hyperhomocysteinemias, aminoacidopathies, and organic acidurias and disorders of energy metabolism such as fatty acid β-oxidation defects and cerebral glucose transporter (GLUT1) deficiency. MSUD belongs to the first category

studies can be used. In some countries cerebral angiography is mandatory to confirm non-traumatic brain death (Case 3.12).

(b) Absence of electrical activity. Thirty minutes of silent EEG registration together with bilateral absence of N20/P22 response on SSEP examination are consistent with

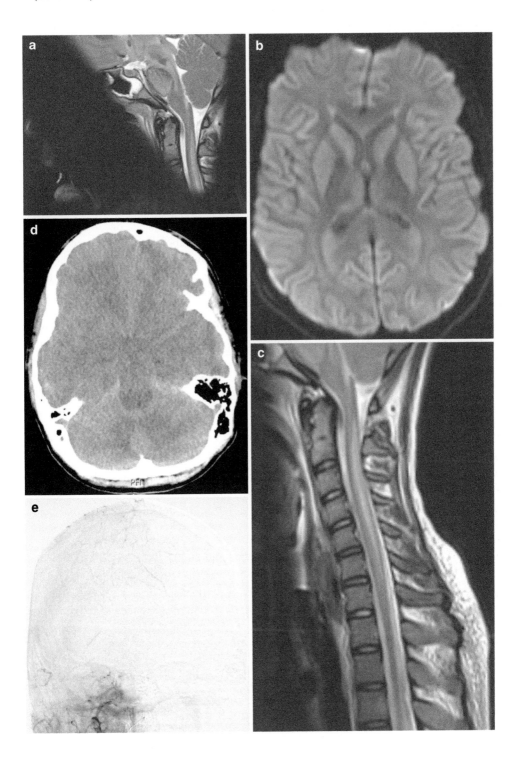

brain death if the minimum technical standards suggested by the American Clinical Neurophysiology Society are met.[11]

3.9 Examination of the Patient with an Acute Ischemic Stroke

The National Institutes of Health Stroke Scale (NIHSS) was created in the late 1980s (and updated in the 1990s) to detect treatment-related differences in clinical trials and to measure right- and left-sided cerebral hemispheric function. However, with the advent of acute treatment options for ischemic stroke (intravenous thrombolysis, mechanical thrombectomy), the NIHSS has become the standard scale to evaluate and monitor stroke patients in emergency settings because it is fast and valid, requires little practice, and has an acceptable inter-rater reliability. It is provided free of charge by the National Institutes of Health (ninds.nih.gov/doctors/NIH_Stroke_Scale.pdf), including online user certification. There are, however, a few pitfalls that should be recognized:

1. The NIHSS tends to underestimate patients with right hemispheric stroke. Of the 42 possible points on the NIHSS score, 7 points are related to language function (assessment of orientation, command following, and aphasia) but only 2 to neglect. Since the left hemisphere is the language-dominant hemisphere in right-handed persons ($\geq 90\%$ of the population) and in 60% of left-handed persons, the NIHSS measures the severity and size of strokes in the right hemisphere differently than strokes in the left hemisphere. For instance, in one study the median infarct volume was 48 mL for patients with a left hemisphere stroke and 133 mL for patients with a right hemisphere stroke, although they all had an NIHSS score of 16–20 (Woo et al. 1999). In another study, 6 h after symptom debut, the

minimum baseline NIHSS score for fatal brain swelling in left hemisphere strokes was 20 as compared with a score of 15 for right hemisphere strokes (Krieger et al. 1999).

2. The NIHSS is not designed for patients with posterior circulation stroke. In contrast to anterior circulation stroke, posterior circulation stroke has a fluctuating course much more often. Patients with basilar artery thrombosis may have minor symptoms for many hours, days, or even weeks, and despite a low NIHSS, they are in danger of suffering fulminant brainstem infarction.

3. Some items (e.g., ataxia, consciousness) have a low inter-rater reliability. Frequent issues of uncertainty include, for instance, how to assess the level of consciousness if the patient is intubated, how to rate orientation if the patient is aphasic, how to rate ataxia in a patient with a paretic limb, and how to rate dysarthria if the patient is aphasic. Fortunately, the original instructions by the National Institutes of Health offer guidance here:

(a) When assessing the level of consciousness, "the investigator must choose a response if a full evaluation is prevented by such obstacles as an endotracheal tube, language barrier, orotracheal trauma/bandages. A 3 is scored only if the patient makes no movement (other than reflexive posturing) in response to noxious stimulation."

(b) When rating the level of orientation, it is important to note that the "answer must be correct—there is no partial credit for being close. Aphasic and stuporous patients who do not comprehend the questions will score 2. Patients unable to speak because of endotracheal intubation, orotracheal trauma, severe dysarthria from any cause, language barrier, or any other problem not secondary to aphasia are given a 1. It is important that only the initial answer be graded and that the examiner not 'help' the patient with verbal or non-verbal cues."

(c) When examining for ataxia, one must remember that this "item is aimed at find-

---

[11] For discussion of SSEP and other evoked potentials, see Chap. 5.

ing evidence of a unilateral cerebellar lesion. Test with eyes open. In case of visual defect, ensure testing is done in intact visual field. The finger-nose-finger and heel-shin tests are performed on both sides, and ataxia is scored only if present out of proportion to weakness. Ataxia is absent in the patient who cannot understand or is paralyzed."

(d) With respect to sensory function, "a score of 2 […] should only be given, when a severe or total loss of sensation can be clearly demonstrated. […] Stuporous or aphasic patients will, therefore, probably score 0 or 1. If the patient does not respond and is quadriplegic, score 2. Patients in coma […] are automatically given a two on this item."

(e) In order to evaluate for dysarthria in a patient with aphasia, rate the "clarity of articulation of spontaneous speech." The patient has a severe dysarthria and scores 2, if the speech is "so slurred as to be unintelligible in the absence of or out of proportion to any dysphasia, or [if the patient] is mute/anarthric."

3.10   Examination of the Patient with an Epileptic Seizure

The patient presenting with an acute generalized epileptic seizure should be assessed immediately according to the ABC approach. Secure the airway and give oxygen. If possible, place the patient in the lateral recovery position to prevent him from harming himself. Do not attempt to put anything in the patient's mouth. Most seizures are self-limiting. However, if convulsions continue for more than 5 min (or the precise onset of the seizure is unknown, e.g., if the patient is admitted to the emergency department while having seizures), the protocol for status epilepticus as outlined in Chap. 6 must be followed. Ask for immediate anesthesiological assistance, if necessary. Do not leave the patient unattended after the seizure has stopped; decreased consciousness and postictal confusion may put the patient at risk.

3.10.1   Taking the History of a Patient with a Seizure

The neurologist assessing the patient presenting with a seizure or with a history of a recent seizure should attempt to answer three essential questions:

- Did the patient have a true epileptic seizure, or was it a nonepileptic event?
- If it was an epileptic seizure, was it an acute symptomatic (provoked) or an unprovoked (spontaneous) seizure?
- If it was an epileptic seizure, was it a primarily generalized or a focal seizure (with or without secondary generalization)?

An accurate and detailed description of the course of the seizure (seizure semiology) is key to the diagnosis and classification of the epilepsy syndrome. The presence or absence of the following features needs to be clarified:

- Motor symptoms (localized or generalized; symmetric or asymmetric; tonic, clonic, atonic, myoclonic)
- Sensory symptoms (olfactory, gustatory, auditory, visual, proprioceptive)
- Psychic symptoms (e.g., fear, depression, euphoria, déjà vu, jamais vu, twilight state)
- Autonomic symptoms (e.g., palpitations, diaphoresis, facial flushing)
- Automatisms (e.g., oroalimentary automatism, stereotypical hand movements)

Importantly, sensory and psychic symptoms are called *aura* and can only be described by the patient himself. Often the patient is not aware that these symptoms represent an epileptic seizure or are part of an epileptic seizure and therefore does not report them spontaneously, hence the need to actively enquire about them.

If the patient has amnesia for the seizure itself, it is useful to ask about the last memory before losing consciousness and the earliest memory upon regaining it. However, as important as the account from the patient is, the information that a witness can provide is also essential. Therefore, a detailed description of the event from paramedics, relatives, and other witnesses is crucial. If a witness is not present at the emergency department, the neurologist should ask for cell phone numbers and make phone calls as early after the event as possible. Due to the well-known shortcomings of the human memory, important information may be missed if questioning of witnesses is postponed. A detailed history and description of the seizure event has to be established before the patient is discharged because reports by the patient during a later follow-up visit in the outpatient clinic are usually less exact. The following questions should be posed:

- When did the seizure happen? What exactly did the patient do in the minutes preceding the seizure?
- What happened at the beginning of the seizure? Was there an onset with focal symptoms, suggesting a focal lesion?
- Did the patient experience any discomfort, nausea, light-headedness, vertigo, chest pain, palpitations, or aura? Nonepileptic events must always be considered in the differential diagnosis. With simple fainting, for instance, the typical symptoms progress from dizziness, sweating, dimming of vision, possibly tinnitus, and leg weakness to loss of vision and consciousness (blackouts) and physical collapse.
- What happened later during the seizure? Was there a spreading of convulsions? How long did the seizure last? Was consciousness impaired or lost? Did the patient hurt himself? Did the patient experience urinary or fecal incontinence, postictal confusion, and muscle pain? Did the patient bite his tongue, and if so, are the bite marks on the side of the tongue (suggesting a true epileptic seizure) or at its tip (suggesting a syncope or psychogenic nonepileptic seizure)?

If the patient does not have a prior diagnosis of epilepsy, it is important to establish whether the present seizure indeed was the first seizure or if the patient has had earlier events suggestive of epileptic seizures. Importantly, the patient may have had several focal seizures without impairment of consciousness during the days or weeks preceding the first seizure with secondary generalization. Often the patient is not aware that these events have been due to epileptic activity and indeed are the key to establishing the diagnosis of epilepsy. Therefore, the neurologist must make every attempt to enquire about them:

- If the patient has had earlier epileptic events, when did they happen, how many times and in which situations?
- Are earlier events consistent with the semiology of the present seizure, or does the patient have two or even more seizure types? Again, witnesses such as spouses, friends, parents, and colleagues should be questioned.

The neurologist should enquire for possible predispositions to epilepsy, including a positive family history, perinatal or postnatal brain injuries, prolonged fever seizures during childhood, and abuse of alcohol or illicit drugs. Metabolic disturbances and intoxications are "accepted" as possible provoking factors, but importantly, sleep deprivation, hunger, and emotional stress are not. A detailed general medical history is important. Also, if the patient *has* an established diagnosis of epilepsy, it is crucial to know about the presence of antiepileptic therapy, possible drug interactions, and recent treatment modifications, as well as patient compliance. Of note, one should never make a diagnosis of "probable epilepsy" because the circumstances of the seizure "were unclear"—this simply suggests that the history taken by the neurologist was inadequate.

3.10.2 The Examination and Management of a Patient with a Seizure

Following a seizure, the patient is assessed for signs of trauma, dental injuries, (lateral) tongue biting, drug or alcohol withdrawal (tachycardia, tremor, sweating), and infection (fever, nuchal rigidity), as well as impairment of consciousness and orientation. The neurological examination may reveal a focal deficit (e.g., Todd's paresis), suggesting an underlying structural cause. Cardiological evaluation is necessary to rule out orthostatic hypotension, cardiac arrhythmias, congestive heart failure, and valvular pathology.

Routine laboratory investigations include electrocardiography, blood tests (e.g., glucose, electrolytes, hematology, infectious parameters, and liver, kidney, and thyroid function tests), and neuroimaging (preferably MRI with epilepsy protocol). CSF analysis should be performed if the possibility of a subarachnoidal hemorrhage or neuroinfection cannot be ruled out. All patients with suspicion of an epileptic seizure require evaluation by EEG at some point; early assessment following the seizure may increase the diagnostic yield (Chap. 5). Measurement of serum levels of antiepileptic drugs (AED) can be useful under certain circumstances (Chap. 5).

Patients with an alarming seizure frequency, new focal deficits, or prolonged impairment of consciousness should be admitted to the ward. Also patients with acute symptomatic epileptic seizures usually require in-hospital evaluation because of the underlying pathology. In addition, patients with possible cardiac arrhythmias require telemetry and timely cardiological follow-up. Driving is prohibited for all patients following an acute seizure, and this should be discussed with the patient prior to discharge and documented in the charts. The regulations of driving prohibition vary from country to country, and the clinician should be familiar with the national laws and rules.

The *differential diagnosis* and *treatment* of epilepsy and nonepileptic events are discussed in Chaps. 4 and 6, respectively.

3.11 Examination of the Patient with Functional/Nonorganic Deficits

The examination of the patient with functional deficits requires rather extensive experience. Opportunities for gaining practice, however, are plenty. It has been suggested that one-third of all outpatients and 10% of all inpatients presenting to a general neurological department have symptoms that are mainly or exclusively functional. Patients with a functional disorder often have some sort of psychological condition or problem in their past or present history. Be careful when diagnosing functionality in patients lacking such a history, especially in the elderly.[12] However, a psychological condition can be difficult to detect; alexithymia may contribute to functional symptoms in patients who apparently lack any psychological problem.[13]

Even though all kinds of people regardless of socioeconomic background present with functional deficits, two types of behaviors are encountered particularly often:

- *La belle indifference* describes the patient who seems happy and unconcerned despite an apparently severe handicap. This patient smiles and involves the physician in a friendly chat even though he is unable to walk and has been bound to a wheelchair since yesterday. Such a patient tends to give a highly vague history, drifting away during conversation, forcing the examiner to constantly remind him to focus on the questions being posed. Complaints vary from one conversation to the next. A bewildering feature is that the most severe complaints are often referred to in passing or during the very end of the conversion. ("Oh, of course, you must know that I can't walk anymore, haven't they told you?")
- The other extreme is the *highly concerned* patient (who usually has fierce support from a relative), who is perseverating, completely fixed in his view of the situation, and stubbornly blocks any attempts by the examiner to focus on positive issues. ("Hey doc, you see that I can't walk, how can you tell me you're

---

[12]Developing a functional disorder out of the blue in later life would be unusual. In the elderly without a history of a psychological condition of any kind, vague complaints about physical symptoms often mask a depressive disorder or a beginning dementia.

[13]Alexithymia (Greek, "not being able to read emotions") is impaired processing of emotions at the cognitive level; e.g., patients report physical signs of panic or anxiety, but they are not *aware* of any stressful feelings.

certain this will improve?") The patient usually shows an overtly hostile attitude toward the healthcare system despite constantly consulting new physicians.

As with any other patient, the examination starts with the history. Take a *social history* but make sure to be entirely empathetic and tactful because making up for lost confidence is nearly impossible. Always search for *positive findings*, e.g., clues to a former or present psychological conflict, and *inconsistency* in the way the patient communicates his problems. Do not take all prior medical diagnoses for granted. Ask about *sleep disturbance, fatigue, chronic pain*, and *concentration difficulties*. However, not all patients suffer from these symptoms; exceptional patients with (overlooked) functional disorders are energetic enough to compete in the Paralympics (David, 2016).

Although the patients usually are eager to give the examiner detailed descriptions of their deficits, it is often even more informative to find out what they actually still *can* do. How is it possible for a patient with complete paraplegia to go to the bathroom without any great difficulties despite lack of a wheelchair and personal assistance?

If the working diagnosis is one of a functional disorder, the neurological examination serves three purposes:

1. To demonstrate the integrity of the nervous system and its function
2. To demonstrate, if possible, that symptoms are not compatible with the rules of anatomy and physiology
3. To demonstrate, if possible, that symptoms are accessible for suggestibility and vanish or improve with distraction

Findings on the examination that are *incompatible with nervous system anatomy and physiology* are, e.g., claims from the patient that numbness is projected precisely in the body midline despite the fact that the examiner pulls the skin a few centimeters over to the other body side. Further, it is incompatible with nervous system physiology when the examiner grasps the patient's trembling hand in order to fixate the forearm, and the tremor immediately becomes worse and "jumps over" to the upper arm. (This is the so-called chasing the tremor phenomenon.) Distraction such as counting backward, in contrast, will usually make parkinsonian tremor worse, but tremor of nonorganic origin better. Also, functional tremor tends to change frequency when the patient is asked to make a rhythmical movement with the other limb. Both limbs will then synchronize. Balance problems *often improve with distraction* or when the patient believes that he is *no longer under observation*. For instance, a patient who is not able to perform Romberg's test may stand perfectly still despite closed eyes if the neurologist asks him at the same time to decipher the numbers that he "writes" with his finger on the patient's forehead.

Functional disorders can *mimic even complex dysfunctions* such as oculomotor palsies, an example being convergent spasm that simulates uni- or bilateral CN VI palsy. Functional disorders have a tendency to *wax and wane*. This is also true for nonorganic gait disorders. Always try to observe the patient before or after the consultation when he believes he is not being watched; it is amazing how often a gait disorder suddenly can disappear. Severe functional gait disorders may at times confine the patient to bed. *Astasia-abasia* denotes a condition in which the patient is unable to walk and stand despite normal bedside examination of power, sensation, and balance. Occasionally symptoms may *vanish with magic words* from the examiner. ("If I press on this point on your right shoulder you will be able to lift your arm again.") The patient with functional paresis characteristically has normal muscle tone and normal reflexes. Often the examiner will find an inverted pyramidal pattern of weakness in the legs; i.e., the extensors will be weaker than the flexors. The patient will often say that plantar flexion of the foot (mediated by the tibial extensor muscles) is not possible during formal power testing at the bedside, but he will have no problem walking on his toes.

During formal testing of muscle power, many patients demonstrate the *give-way phenomenon*, which occurs when the examiner suddenly exerts force on the patient's limb and the patient reacts intuitively with powerful resistance that, however, immediately fades away. In addition, a limb that is left hanging in the air may hover for a second or so above the bed before collapsing. Another highly useful sign is *Hoover's sign*, which can unveil functional palsy of the lower extremities. The following is a variant of Hoover's sign that is somewhat more reliable than the original examination technique. Consider a patient with a functional paresis of the left leg who lies supine on the examination table. Stand before the patient and put both hands between the table and the patient's feet. Ask the patient to press the weak (left) leg down on the examination table and against your right hand. The examiner will feel no muscle contraction and no effort of voluntary hip extension. Then ask the patient to lift his left leg against resistance provided by the examiner's right hand, which is now placed on top of the leg. This should usually evoke simultaneous involuntary hip extension of the contralateral right hip, but the examiner's left hand between the examination table and the right foot will still not feel any pressure. (In contrast, forceful extension of the contralateral hip is felt in patients with true palsy of the left leg who attempt to lift the paralyzed limb.) However, when the patient is asked to lift the right leg against resistance, the examiner will suddenly feel that the patient unintentionally presses the left leg down against the examination table. This is due to the fact that hip flexion always induces contralateral hip extension. Hoover's sign is sometimes easier to elicit with the patient in the sitting position.

In a patient complaining of *sensory disturbances*, it may be helpful to assess vibration on the right and left side of the forehead. Since the tuning fork induces vibration of the whole of the frontal bone, there should be no lateralization of sensation; yet this is precisely what the suggestible patient reports.

In *psychogenic coma*, the patient usually has his eyes closed and often actively resists the examiner's attempt to open them. The examiner should never apply truly painful stimuli in a patient with psychogenic coma (this will only destroy the neurologists further standing); it is sometimes amazing, however, how easily one can wake up "comatose" patients by rubbing their sternum repeatedly. Also, when the examiner holds the hand of a patient in a psychogenic coma above or behind the patient's head, the hand will most often not fall down according to the laws of gravity, but it will "miraculously" find its way back to the side of the body. In addition, a vibrating tuning fork, held at the ear of the patient sounds like a furious wasp, an unexpected stimulus that often will provoke some kind of reaction.

For *PNES* see Chap. 4.

Memory deficits are sometimes also functional. *Worries of developing dementia* are very common. *Prolonged retrograde memory loss with normal anterograde memory* (fugue state), in contrast, is highly unusual and typically due to a functional disorder.

Importantly, many, if not most, patients will remember the neurologist not for what he said but for how it was said. Accept that the patient indeed has a handicap but encourage the patient to continue with their life in an unrestricted manner. Focus on the integrity of the nervous system and the fact that no organic disorder prevents restoration of function. ("This is a software problem, not a hardware problem.") A complete and thorough neurological bedside examination can be of striking therapeutic value in a patient with psychogenic symptoms. Also, the offer to see the patient again in 6 months' time is often helpful. The path between overambitious diagnostic procedures on one side and therapeutic diagnostic procedures on the other is narrow. Any laboratory examination may consolidate the concerns of the patient that something is wrong, but then again, many patients will insist on having an MRI or other tests done, and they might not be able to relax without them taking place. If the neurologist is certain that the diagnosis is a functional disorder, it is usually advisable to either proceed immediately with the relevant laboratory procedures or to set a stop for them altogether. If one agrees to order a diagnostic procedure, it can be wise to make a deal with the patient that no other tests will be conducted. Bear in mind that with neuroimaging, unexpected (and often unpleasant) findings may occur in 10–15% of cases. For instance, an incidental pineal cyst or an unforeseen meningioma can require follow-up controls, and this can have devastating effects on quality of life and social functioning.

The single best *prognostic factor* regarding outcome of functional deficits is whether the handicap still remains after the consultation or discharge from the hospital. Thus, a patient with a functional gait disorder leaving the hospital in a wheelchair has a rather poor prognosis. If the patient has managed to regain a normal gait pattern (usually with help from an empathetic physiotherapist), the long-term outcome is good.

Once again, be humble in light of the fact that all neurologists do mistake organic disorders for functional disorders at some time. The diagnosis of a functional disorder by an experienced neurologist has perhaps a 5–10% likelihood of being false. This of course is not necessarily the same as overlooking a dangerous disease (Case 3.13). There are many examples of disorders that formerly were believed to be functional, classical examples being blepharospasm and other focal dystonias, paroxysmal

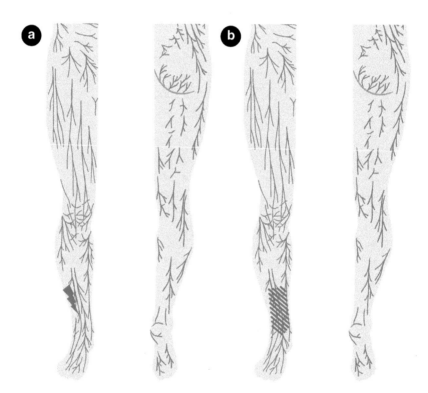

Case 3.13 Wartenberg's migrant sensory neuritis. A 35-year-old female was referred for a second opinion because of transitory sensory symptoms. She had been evaluated at another institution for possible multiple sclerosis, but MRI of the brain, a lumbar puncture, and nerve conduction studies had been normal. Therefore, she had received a diagnosis of functional complaints, which she found very embarrassing. Six months earlier she had experienced intense pain in the right lower limb while walking. For 6 h, the pain occurred with each dorsiflexion of the foot and vanished with plantar flexion (**a**). Following this, an area with decreased sensation remained for several months (**b**). During examination, hypesthesia was found within the distribution of the right superficial peroneal nerve as well as of the digital nerve to the medial border of the right first finger. The remainder of the neurological examination was normal. On follow-up, the patient reported several new episodes of intense but brief pain upon stretching of the extremities, followed by numbness in the respective areas that could last for up to several months (**c**). Repeated nerve conduction studies were normal except for decreased sensory nerve action potentials of the right peroneal nerve. Because of the typical complaints and the characteristic evolution of the symptoms, the patient was diagnosed with WMSN

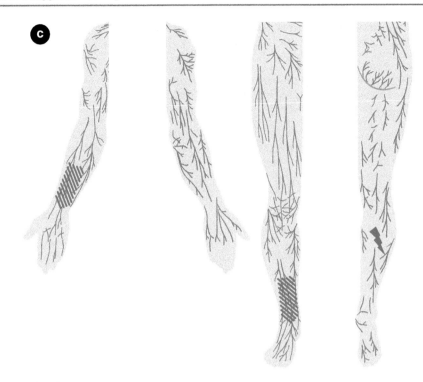

Case 3.13 (continued)

dyskinesias, the restless legs syndrome, and autoimmune disorders such as the stiff limb syndrome. Another typical example is orthostatic tremor in middle-aged women; unsteadiness while standing but not while walking is often believed to be functional in origin (see Chap. 4). Likewise, patients with Ehlers-Danlos syndrome may be diagnosed as having fibromyalgia. Other recent discoveries include the painful Na-channelopathies due to mutations in voltage-gated sodium channels (gain-of-function *SCN9A* mutations), resulting in erythromelalgia and paroxysmal extreme pain disorder. Even a patient with a clear functional deficit may suffer at the same time from an organic disease, and an "organic core" may be hidden beneath nearly every functional symptom. Do not make a diagnosis of a functional disorder just because the patient has a known psychiatric condition. Most patients who exaggerate their symptoms do so because they are anxious that they will not be believed. Malingering and factitious disorders such as Munchhausen syndrome are rare.

References and Suggested Reading

Aerts MB, Abdo WF, Bloem BR. The "bicycle sign" for atypical parkinsonism. Lancet. 2011;377:125–6.

David AS. Paralympics and conversion disorder. J Neurol Neurosurg Psychiatry. 2016;87:217–9.

Demartini B, Petrochilos P, Ricciardi L, et al. The role of alexithymia in the development of functional motor symptoms (conversion disorder). J Neurol Neurosurg Psychiatry. 2014;85:1132–7.

Folstein MF, Folstein SE, McHugh PR. "Mini-mental state": a practical method for grading the cognitive state of patients for the clinician. J Psychiatr Res. 1975;12:189–98.

Giacino JT, Fins JJ, Laureys S, Schiff ND. Disorders of consciousness after acquired brain injury: the state of the science. Nat Rev Neurol. 2014;10:99–114.

Hodges JR, editor. Early-onset dementia. A multidisciplinary approach. Oxford: Oxford University Press; 2001.

Kattah JC, Talkad AV, Wang DZ, et al. HINTS to diagnose stroke in the acute vestibular syndrome: three-step bedside oculomotor examination more sensitive than early MRI diffusion-weighted imaging. Stroke. 2009;40:3504–10.

Kondziella D, Nordenstig A, Mölne A, Axelsson M. Cranial neuropathy in the blue rubber bleb nevus syndrome. J Neurol Neurosurg Psychiatry. 2010;81:1207–8.

Kondziella D, Friberg CK, Frokjaer VG, et al. Preserved consciousness in vegetative and minimal conscious states: systematic review and meta-analysis. J Neurol Neurosurg Psychiatry. 2016;87:485–92.

Krieger DW, Demchuk AM, Kasner SE, et al. Early clinical and radiological predictors of fatal brain swelling in ischemic stroke. Stroke. 1999;30:287–92.

Kurtzhals C, Hansen K, Kondziella D. Spontaneous cerebrospinal fluid leak associated with idiopathic intracranial hypertension. Neurol India. 2011;59:946–7.

Laureys S, Celesia GG, Cohadon F, et al. Unresponsive wakefulness syndrome: a new name for the vegetative state or Apallic syndrome. BMC Med. 2010;8:68.

Mathuranath PS, Nestor PJ, Berrios GE, et al. A brief cognitive test battery to differentiate Alzheimer's disease and frontotemporal dementia. Neurology. 2000;55:1613–20.

O'Brien M. Aids to the examination of the peripheral nervous system. 5th ed. London: Saunders Ltd.; 2010.

O'Regan NA, Dj R, Boland E, et al. Attention! A good screening test for delirium? J Neurol Neurosurg Psychiatry. 2014;85:1122–31.

Owen AM, Coleman MR, Boly M, et al. Detecting awareness in the vegetative state. Science. 2006;313:1402.

Schnakers C, Vanhaudenhuyse A, Giacino J, et al. Diagnostic accuracy of the vegetative and minimally conscious state: clinical consensus versus standardized neurobehavioral assessment. BMC Neurol. 2009;9:35.

Schott JM, Rossor MN. The palmomental reflex: stop scratching around! Pract Neurol. 2016;16:500–1. doi:10.1136/practneurol-2016-001509.

Singman EL, Matta NS, Silbert DI. Use of the Cogan lid twitch to identify myasthenia gravis. J Neuroopthalmol. 2011;31:239–40.

Starmark JE, Lindgren S. Is it possible to define a general "conscious level"? Acta Neurochir Suppl. 1986;36:103–5.

Storey JE, Rowland JT, Basic D, Conforti DA, Dickson HG. The Rowland Universal Dementia Assessment Scale (RUDAS): a multicultural cognitive assessment scale. Int Psychogeriatr. 2004;16:13–31.

Teasdale G, Jennett B. Assessment of coma and impaired consciousness. A practical scale. Lancet. 1974;2:81–4.

Vanhaudenhuyse A, Schnackers C, Bredar S, Laureys S. Assessment of visual pursuit in post-comatose states: use a mirror. J Neurol Neurosurg Psychiatry. 2008;79:223.

Wijdicks EF. The transatlantic divide over brain death determination and the debate. Brain. 2012;135:1321–31.

Wijdicks EF, Bamlet WR, Maramattom BV, et al. Validation of a new coma scale: the FOUR score. Ann Neurol. 2005;58:585–93.

Wijdicks EF, Hijdra A, Young GB, et al. Practice parameter: prediction of outcome in comatose survivors after cardiopulmonary resuscitation (an evidence-based review): report of the Quality Standards Subcommittee of the American Academy of Neurology. Neurology. 2006;67:203–10.

Woo D, Broderick JP, Kothari RU, et al. Does the National Institutes of Health Stroke Scale favor left hemisphere strokes? NINDS t-PA Stroke Study Group. Stroke. 1999;30:2355–9.

Differential Diagnosis: "What Is the Lesion?"

4

Abstract

Following the history and bedside examination, the anatomic localization of the lesion should have been identified, and the neurologist can proceed with a differential diagnosis. This is usually straightforward by taking into account information related to epidemiology, comorbidities, hereditary predispositions, and occupation, as well as the time course of the disorder. For instance, hyperacute onset of deficits is characteristic for cerebrovascular disease, subacute onset for infectious and inflammatory disorders, and prolonged onset over weeks or months for malignancy. A chronic progressive course over years is indicative of neurodegenerative diseases. However, occasionally, a slowly progressing illness comes rather suddenly to the attention of the patient because the declining level of function has been exposed by an unusual activity or event. If important data are unavailable, early fixation on a single differential diagnosis should be avoided due to the risk of overlooking important details. This chapter provides a simple yet comprehensive differential diagnosis of most of the disorders encountered in neurological practice. Further, it makes extensive use of mind maps in order to enable the reader to approach and visualize the differential diagnosis of each neurological field in a structured and intuitive manner.

Keywords

Ataxia • Cognitive impairment • Coma • Dementia • Demyelinating diseases • Differential diagnosis • Encephalopathy • Epilepsy • Headache Head injury • Infectious diseases • Malignancy • Motor neuron disease Movement disorders • Myelopathy • Myopathy • Neuromuscular junction disorders • Peripheral nerve disorders • Sleep disorders • Stroke • Syncope Vertigo

4.1   Introduction to Heuristic Neurological Reasoning

When the anatomic localization of a lesion has been identified, it is often straightforward to deduce its etiology using the available data on the time course, epidemiology, comorbidity, and genetic predispositions, including:

- Hyperacute and acute onset of deficits points toward a cerebrovascular cause.
- Subacute onset over hours or days is characteristic for infectious and inflammatory disorders.
- Prolonged onset over several weeks or months may suggest malignancy.
- A chronic progressive course over many years is indicative of neurodegenerative diseases. A complete family history can be crucial.
- Relapsing-remitting deficits are seen with autoimmune and inflammatory diseases.
- Short-lived phenomena of acute onset with "positive" signs that leave no residual deficits and that may reappear after hours, days, weeks, or even longer periods can be due to epilepsy, migraine, narcolepsy, and other paroxysmal disorders.

The setting in which the illness developed is often as important as the mode of onset and the clinical course. A good rule is to ask the patient precisely what he was doing the exact moment he noticed his symptoms for the first time. However, it is important to be aware of the fact that a slowly progressing illness occasionally comes rather suddenly to the attention of the patient because he has not noticed the declining level of function until it is exposed by an unusual activity or event. Such a "decompensation artifact" (Oluf Andersen, Gothenburg, Sweden, personal communication) might occur, for instance, when a patient with mild cognitive impairment (MCI) due to AD develops a postsurgical delirium or when a patient with a compressive myelopathy due to a thoracic meningioma falls while running for the bus. In both instances, a careful history is crucial in order to avoid believing that symptom onset was sudden and to avoid attributing the cause to an external event. Also, some patients with a chronic, stable deficit present to the neurologist complaining of progressive impairment, but a careful history may reveal that they have simply begun to worry more.

The following rules help to avoid diagnostic confusion:

- The differential diagnoses should be ranked according to their pretest probability, severity, and associated treatment options ("Which diagnosis is most likely?"; "Which diagnoses are particularly serious, and which are treatable?").
- Most diagnostic errors are made not because of limited medical knowledge but because of failure to acquire and correctly analyze basic clinical information. Definitive data from the history and clinical examination should not be diluted by unclear data. In other words, localization and diagnosis should be based on what is reasonably certain.
- When several typical features of a disease are lacking, it is likely that the diagnosis is wrong. Yet, rare manifestations of common diseases are more often encountered than common manifestations of rare diseases. (This is one of the most rephrased statements in clinical medicine but still remains true nonetheless.)
- Overreliance on isolated ancillary investigations, in particular when these are interpreted outside of the clinical context, is another common source of diagnostic error (Case 4.1).
- When all investigations have failed to identify the diagnosis, the tool most likely to help is a better history. In the case that not all necessary data are available, avoid early fixation on a single diagnosis; otherwise, important details may be missed. Time will solve many mysteries.
- Finally, familiarity with Occam's razor, Hickam's dictum, and Crabtree's bludgeon is helpful for neurological differential diagnosis.[1]

---

[1]William Occam (1285–1348) was an English Franciscan friar, philosopher, and theologian; John Hickam (1914–1970) was departmental head of medicine at Indiana University (IN, US) and a pioneer of retinal fluorescein angiography; Crabtree was a fictitious figure created in the 1950s by a group of British scientists and based on Joseph Crabtree (1754–1854), a poet from Gloucestershire, England, UK (Mani et al. 2011).

Case 4.1 Herpes simplex encephalitis misdiagnosed as stroke, stroke misdiagnosed as herpes simplex encephalitis. A 32-year-old female with an unremarkable previous medical history was found unconscious in her apartment and brought to the hospital. A CT showed a right-sided hypodensity which was interpreted as a right MCA stroke by the radiologist. MRI seemingly confirmed this notion as it showed a large area of hyperintense signal change related to the right temporal lobe (**a**, DWI). However, the neurologist on-call correctly noted that the signal change also involved the right anterior lobe (**b**, FLAIR) and that the history of a young patient with no cardiovascular risk factors but with headache and influenza-like symptoms was highly suggestive of herpes simplex encephalitis. Treatment with IV acyclovir was started. A few days later, CSF PCR analysis turned out positive for HSV I. Next, a 82-year-old woman with atrial fibrillation, diabetes mellitus,

and a previous stroke resulting in right-sided hemianopia was admitted with acute onset of left hemiplegia and hemineglect. CT of the brain 2 h after ictus was read as normal except for a previous left occipital infarction. A week later, the patient developed a urinary tract infection and her level of consciousness decreased. An MRI was performed which showed a large area of DWI signal change involving the right temporal lobe (**c**), including some hemosiderin deposits revealed by gradient-echo sequences (**d**). When a lumbar puncture revealed more than 500 cells and 5 g protein, the patient was transferred with a working diagnosis of herpes simplex encephalitis to the department of infectious diseases. The neurology team reviewing the patient a few days later suggested that the inflammatory CSF changes were fully compatible with massive cerebral tissue damage due to brain infarction. Indeed, all blood and CSF cultures turned out to be negative

- Occam's razor ("entities must not be multiplied beyond necessity"; Splade 1999). When evaluating a patient with multiple symptoms, a single diagnosis explaining all features should be sought rather than several unrelated diagnoses. For instance, in a young male with gait ataxia, dysarthria, scoliosis, diabetes, and deafness, a diagnosis of Friedreich's ataxia would elegantly explain the combination of absent tendon reflexes in the lower extremities (suggesting a peripheral lesion) and extensor plantar responses (suggesting a central lesion).
- Hickam's dictum ("a man can have as many diseases as he damn well pleases"; Hilliard et al. 2004). Frequently, patients do not respect Occam's razor and have multiple diagnoses. Hickam's dictum becomes particularly relevant with increasing age of the patient. Thus, upgoing toes combined with loss of Achilles tendon reflexes in an elderly patient might very well be due to degenerative spine disease leading to a cervical compressive myelopathy *and* a diagnosis of diabetic polyneuropathy. Hickam's dictum, however, should be applied only infrequently in younger patients.
- Crabtree's bludgeon ("no set of mutually inconsistent observations can exist for which some human intellect cannot conceive a coherent explanation, however complicated"; Mani et al. 2011). The clinical value of Crabtree's bludgeon is that it cautions against overelaborate explanations. Crabtree's bludgeon is important in those relatively rare situations when patients have several well-established diagnoses that could explain various clinical features, but they suffer from yet another condition, which might easily be overlooked. For instance, in an elderly diabetic patient with a history of degenerative spine disease, who develops subacute progressive extremity weakness, an elevated CSF protein level would not be a surprising finding. But the identification of conduction blocks and significantly reduced nerve conduction velocities on neurophysiological examination would be hard to explain unless the clinician considers a diagnosis of co-occurring CIDP.

Establishing a neurological differential diagnosis can be a most satisfying intellectual delight. There is arguably no other medical specialty with a more extensive differential diagnosis than neurology. This also means that frustration is common in the new beginner. The purpose of the following pages is to provide a simple yet strategic overview of the most important areas in neurology. This chapter will enable the reader to break down the differential diagnosis of each neurological field into manageable entities.

4.2 The Differential Diagnosis of Coma

Wakefulness (or arousal) is mediated by structures in the brainstem, midbrain, and diencephalon, notably the ascending reticular activating system (ARAS) and the rostral dorsolateral pontine tegmentum. Consciousness (or awareness), in contrast, is an exclusive product of higher cerebral activity and therefore depends on the cerebral cortex and its connecting pathways in the subcortical white matter. As a rule, consciousness will be preserved with lesions that only affect one hemisphere. It follows that coma can be due to:

- Structural damage of:
  - The brainstem
  - The cerebral cortex in both hemispheres
- Diffuse brain dysfunction of metabolic-toxic or hypoxic origin

As stated earlier, coma may be defined as a state of non-arousal and unresponsiveness in which the patient is not aware of his surroundings and his own person. Thus, coma must be differentiated from:

- Locked-in syndrome (see Chap. 2)
- Psychogenic coma (see Chap. 3)
- Impairment of consciousness that does not fulfill the criteria of coma, including:
  - Stupor. This is a vague term for patients who are arousable by vigorous and repeated stimulation only.
  - Akinetic mutism. The patient is unresponsive and apparently without any cognitive or spontaneous motor activity despite the fact that the eyes may be open and vocalization present during short periods. Also, the patient with akinetic mutism may occasionally look at the examiner; however, there is no interaction. The sleep-wake cycle is intact. Akinetic mutism may be due to large bifrontal lesions, hydrocephalus, and severe cortical damage.
  - The vegetative state. This is one possible outcome of coma. Coma per se almost never lasts more than a few days or weeks—most patients die, regain their consciousness, or enter a minimal conscious or the vegetative state. In the vegetative state, the patient is arousable to some degree; most of the brainstem and diencephalic functions are intact, including the sleep-wake cycle; thus, eyes are open during periods of wakefulness. However, the patient is not aware of his surroundings or his own person, and therefore, there is lack of any meaningful communication or motor activity. As stated below, chances are high that numerous patients believed to be in the vegetative state indeed are in a minimal conscious state.
  - The minimal conscious state. Striking functional magnetic resonance imaging (fMRI) experiments have shown that many apparently vegetative patients indeed have some degree of preserved consciousness and higher cortical function. In a landmark study, Owen et al. provided auditory cues to a young woman fulfilling the established criteria for a persistent vegetative state following a

traumatic brain injury and studied her brain activity in response to these cues using fMRI. The cues were verbal instructions to imagine performing one of three tasks: playing tennis, going through the rooms of a house, or simply relaxing. Compared to the "relaxed" state, fMRI showed instruction-dependent brain activation akin to that seen in healthy volunteers following the same instructions. The authors concluded that the patient was consciously imagining playing tennis and exploring a house in much the same way control participants did (Owen et al. 2006). This and similar studies are likely to fundamentally change our perception of diagnosis and therapy of patients with chronically decreased consciousness.

When coma or another state of disordered consciousness has been confirmed, the etiology needs to be defined (Fig. 4.1). The following list, although not complete, may help as guidance. Impairment of consciousness and arousal may be due to:

4.2.1   Structural Causes of Coma

- Structural lesions
  - Supratentorial
    - Infectious, e.g., abscess, HSV-1 encephalitis, and bacterial meningitis
    - Postinfectious, e.g., acute demyelinating encephalomyelitis (ADEM)
    - Traumatic, e.g., diffuse axonal injury (DAI) with closed head trauma, penetrating skull trauma, and multiple contusions
    - Vascular, e.g., bilateral thalamic infarctions, multiple cortical infarctions, malignant MCA infarction, intracranial hemorrhage, infectious or noninfectious vasculitis, pituitary apoplexy, anoxic-ischemic encephalopathy, and cerebral venous sinus thrombosis (in particular thrombosis of the straight

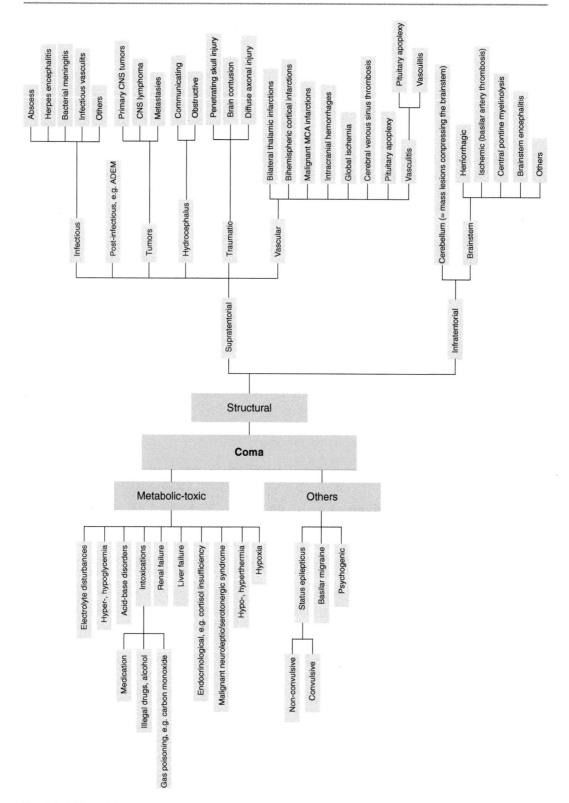

Fig. 4.1 Differential diagnosis of coma

sinus and deep cerebral veins leading to bilateral thalamic venous congestion) (Case 4.2)

○ Tumors, primary or secondary CNS malignancies

○ Hydrocephalus, obstructive or communicating

– Infratentorial
  • Brainstem
    – Hemorrhage
    – Basilar artery thrombosis and other posterior circulation strokes
    – Central pontine myelinolysis
    – Others

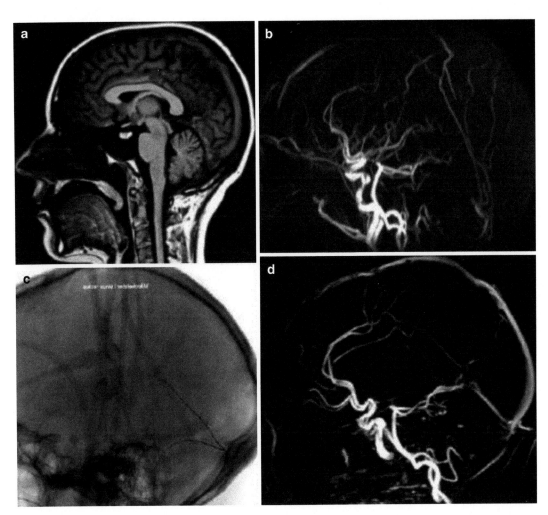

Case 4.2 Cerebral venous sinus thrombosis and hyperthyroidism. A 28-year-old female developed subacute onset of headache and visual disturbances, followed a few days later by focal epileptic seizures, abulia, tetraparesis, and decreased consciousness. Sagittal T1-weighted MRI (**a**) and MR venography (**b**) showed thrombosis of the superior sagittal sinus and straight sinus. The etiology of the CVST was unknown; apparently, the patient did not have any risk factors for a prothrombotic state. Despite immediate administration of IV heparin, her level of consciousness declined, and, therefore, she was treated with local infusion of 60 mg recombinant tissue plasminogen activator for 48 h (figure shows microcatheter in the straight sinus; **c**). After the procedure, MR venography showed that both the superior sagittal sinus and the straight sinus were open again (**d**). Only 3 days later, awake, orientated, and ambulatory, the patient had made a near-complete recovery. However, 10 days after admission, she developed tachycardia, flushing, sweating, and anxiety. Blood results confirmed a thyrotoxicosis and also showed a reactive thrombocytosis. The role of hyperthyroidism as the predisposing factor for CVST is well described in the medical literature, although still not widely acknowledged (Digital subtraction angiography images courtesy of Aase Wagner, Department of Neuroradiology, Rigshospitalet, Copenhagen)

- Cerebellum (cerebellar mass lesions affecting the brainstem)
  - Tumors
  - Hemorrhage
  - Infarctions
  - Abscesses

4.2.2 Nonstructural Causes of Coma

- Metabolic-toxic causes
  - Electrolyte disturbances, e.g., hyponatremia (the reversion of which may lead to central pontine myelinolysis, if performed too quickly) and hypercalcemia
  - Hypoglycemia and hyperglycemia
  - Liver failure
  - Renal failure
  - Acid-base disorders
  - Endocrinological disturbances, e.g., severe hypocortisolism (Addisonian crisis)
  - Poisoning, e.g., illicit and prescription drugs, carbon monoxide, cyanide, and other gases
  - Derangement of body temperature (hypothermia, hyperthermia)
  - Hypoxia
- Others
  - Basilar migraine
  - Status epilepticus, convulsive or nonconvulsive
  - Malignant neuroleptic and serotonergic syndrome
  - Psychogenic coma

When Plum and Posner (Posner et al. 2007) listed the final diagnoses of 500 patients admitted to the emergency department due to "coma of unknown origin,"[2] drug poisoning was by far the most common cause, followed by, in decreasing frequency, anoxia/ischemia, intracerebral hematoma, brainstem infarction, subdural supratentorial hematoma, hepatic encephalopathy, encephalomyelitis and encephalitis, subarachnoid hemorrhage, and endocrinological disturbances, including diabetes, acid-base disorders,

pontine hemorrhage, temperature deregulation, cerebral infarct, uremic encephalopathy, supratentorial brain tumor, supratentorial brain abscess, cerebellar hemorrhage, and supratentorial epidural hematoma.

4.3 The Differential Diagnosis of Traumatic Brain Injury

Head injury leading to penetration of the skull is usually the domain of the neurosurgeon and will therefore not be considered here.

Closed head injury can manifest as or be associated with:

- Minor blows against the head without loss of consciousness, amnesia, or focal neurological signs.
- Skull fracture (with or without CSF fistula).
- Brain concussion. This is a closed head injury that leads to acute loss of consciousness (usually <5 min) and/or amnesia but not to focal neurological deficits.
- Brain contusion. This can be defined as closed head injury with brain tissue damage ("brain bruise") and can lead to impaired consciousness and/or focal deficits, depending on the site and the severity of the injury.
- Diffuse axonal injury (DAI)
- Cerebral traumatic edema/hyperemia
- Intracranial bleeding
  - Epidural hemorrhage
  - Subdural hemorrhage
  - Subarachnoidal hemorrhage
  - Intracerebral hemorrhage
- Vascular damage
  - Dissection, typically involving the extracranial and/or (less commonly) intracranial parts of the carotid and vertebral arteries
  - Traumatic pseudoaneurysm
  - Dural arteriovenous (AV) fistula, e.g., carotid-cavernous sinus fistula

A lucid interval ("talk and die") classically occurs with epidural hematoma but is also frequently associated with other intracranial hemorrhages, e.g., in warfarin-treated patients with subdural or intracere-

---

[2]Thus, obvious cases of poisoning and trauma were not included in this series.

bral hemorrhage. In contrast, DAI typically leads to continuing impairment of consciousness even though the initial CT of the brain may have been interpreted as unremarkable. MRI sequences sensitive to hemosiderin (SWI, T2*) show traumatic microbleeds due to DAI. Unexpected neurological deficits despite an initially normal CT of the brain may also occur with cerebral infarction due to cerebral vascular dissections.

4.3.1   Assessing the Need for Observation and Imaging in Closed Head Injury

The necessity for *observation and imaging* of the patient with closed head injury depends on the severity of the trauma and the presence or absence of risk factors. Loss of consiousness, length of (anterograde) amnesia, and the GCS are the best indices of the severity of the injury.

The following rules apply for adults (≥18 years) presenting within 24 h after a closed head injury (Undén et al. 2013):

- Minimal head trauma (no loss of consciousness, GCS 15): A patient with a simple blow to the head without loss of consciousness, prolonged amnesia, or focal neurological deficits can be discharged without CT scan or observation; oral and written information must be provided. Friends or relatives should be present for subsequent observation.
- Mild head trauma, low risk (GCS 14 or GCS 15 with either short-lasting loss of consciousness or vomiting): These patients should be assessed by measuring serum levels of S100B. They can be discharged with written and oral information, if S100B levels are <0.10 μg/L (assessed within 6 h after the injury) and there is no evidence of significant extracranial injuries. If S100B is ≥0.10 μg/L, a CT scan must be ordered (or, alternatively, the patient is admitted for observation for at least 12 h). The patient can be discharged as outlined above, if CT is normal. Otherwise he or she is admitted for observation for ≥24 h, including neurosurgical consultation if appropriate. The CT scan should

be repeated immediately if the patient's level of consciousness decreases (GCS increase ≥2 points) and/or in case of deteriorating neurological deficits.

- Mild head trauma, moderate risk (GCS 14–15 *plus* age ≥65 years and treatment with platelet inhibitors): These patients require a CT scan (or, alternatively, observation for at least 12 h); they can be discharged home, if the CT of the brain is normal, or must be admitted to the ward as outlined above.
- Mild head trauma, high risk (GCS 14–15; and at least one of the following: treatment with anticoagulation or known coagulation disorder; clinical signs of skull fracture, e.g., crepitations, periorbital hematoma, liquorrhea, bleeding from the nose or ears, or mastoid ecchymosis; focal neurological deficits; seizures; presence of an intracranial shunt, e.g., ventriculoperitoneal): These patients need a CT scan *and* admission for observation as outlined above.
- Moderate head trauma (GCS 9–13): These patients need a CT scan *and* admission for observation as stated.
- Severe head trauma (GCS 3–8): These patients must be transferred to a trauma center with neurosurgical expertise available 24/7.

Obviously, patients require also admission to the ward in case of significant comorbid medical illness or any other factors that the examiner believes are putting the patient at risk.

If a CT of the brain is performed, it should be evaluated for signs of:

- Epidural, subdural, subarachnoidal, intraventricular, and parenchymal hemorrhage
- Brain tissue contusion
- Cerebral edema
- Effacement of perimesencephalic cisterns
- Midline shift and brain incarceration
- Skull fractures
- Pneumocephalus

In case of intracranial hemorrhage, skull fracture, and mass edema or other signs of increased ICP, a neurosurgeon should be contacted without delay.

4.4   The Differential Diagnosis of Headache

The differential diagnosis of headache can be divided into:

- Primary headache syndromes
- Secondary headaches

The two most common primary headache syndromes are migraine and tension-type headache (Fig. 4.2). The annual sex-adjusted prevalence rate of the former has been estimated at 38% and of the latter at 35%. In comparison, the figure for the third most common primary headache syndrome, cluster headache, is only 0.15% (Evers et al. 2007; Steiner et al. 2014). Thus, the odds are very high that the patient with headache seeking medical advice either has migraine or tension-type headache. However, co-occurring medication-overuse headache should not be missed.

4.4.1   Primary Headache Syndromes

Primary headache syndromes include:

- Migraine. This is a throbbing headache with features such as nausea, vomiting, phonophobia, and photophobia. Headache episodes can be preceded by a prodrome (e.g., hunger, agitation, depression, or elevated mood for several hours or up to 3 days prior to a migraine headache) and/or aura (seen in roughly 30% of migraineurs, this is an episode of focal, transitory neurologic dysfunction in the pre-headache phase of a migraine attack, usually developing gradually over 5–20 min and lasting less than 60). There are many migraine variants, e.g., abdominal migraine in children and cyclical or menstrual migraine in young females. Migraine can lead to a number of complications (e.g., chronic migraine, medication-overuse headache, status migrainosus, persistent aura with and without infarction, migraine triggered seizures). The diagnostic criteria of the International

Headache Society for migraine *without* aura include:

- At least five headache attacks lasting 4–72 h (untreated or unsuccessfully treated), which have at least two of the four following characteristics: unilateral location, pulsating quality, moderate or severe intensity interfering with daily activities, and aggravation by walking on stairs or similar routine physical activity.
- During headache episodes at least one of the two following symptoms must occur: phonophobia and photophobia, and nausea and/or vomiting.
- The headache is not attributable to another disorder.

The diagnostic criteria of the International Headache Society for migraine *with* aura include at least two attacks with headache not attributable to another disorder and accompanied by symptoms fulfilling at least three of the following characteristics:

- One or more fully reversible aura symptoms indicating focal cerebral cortical and/or brainstem dysfunction. Symptoms can be positive (e.g., flickering lights, spots, or lines; pins and needles) and/or negative (e.g., loss of vision, numbness). Typical auras are homonymous visual disturbance, unilateral paresthesias and/or numbness, unilateral weakness, aphasia, or unclassifiable speech difficulties.
- At least one aura symptom develops gradually over ≥ 5 min, or two or more symptoms occur in succession.
- The aura lasts less than 60 min (if more than one aura symptom is present, the accepted duration is proportionally increased).
- The aura is followed by headache with a free interval lasting less than 1 h.
- The headache may begin before or simultaneously with the aura.

Observe that the headache symptoms in migraine with aura do not need to meet the criteria necessary in migraine without aura; thus, headache episodes may lack migrainous features.

Headache usually follows the aura symptoms but, as stated above, may begin simultaneously or precede the aura. Less commonly, headache is completely absent.

Several screening tests have been developed for migraine. One of the most practical is "PIN the diagnosis of migraine" (Lipton and Bigal 2007), which is said to have a 93% positive predictive value with two positive questions and 98% positive predictive value with three positive questions out of the following:

- *P*hotophobia: "Does light bother you a lot more than when you don't have headaches?"
- *I*mpairment: "Does the headache limit your ability to study, work, or do whatever you need to do for at least one day?"
- *N*ausea: "Do you feel nauseated or sick to your stomach?"

• Tension-type headache. Together with migraine, this is the most common primary headache syndrome. In contrast to migraine, it is featureless, which means that apart from a squeezing headache, there are no other significant symptoms. Typically, physical activity does not worsen the pain. New-onset daily persistent headache, as suggested by its name, is de novo chronic headache that clinically resembles tension headache. However, it is necessary to exclude secondary headache forms before this diagnosis can be made.
• Headache associated with abuse of painkillers (medication-overuse headache). This is probably the third most common type of headache in the general practice. With time, excessive consumption of triptans, NSAID, and opioids ($\geq$10 days/month) obscures the original headache type. The only acceptable treatment is detoxification combined with correct treatment of the underlying headache syndrome and, if necessary, pain prophylaxis.
• Trigeminal autonomic cephalalgias (TAC). These headaches are characterized by autonomic symptoms such as ipsilateral miosis, ptosis, and nasal discharge that occur together with intense, usually periorbital pain. TAC include:

- Cluster headache (Horton's headache). A typical patient is a middle-aged man (male-to-female ratio 5–10:1) waking in the early morning hours because of exceptionally severe, sharp, orbital, or periorbital pain with localized autonomic features. Attacks typically (but not always) occur in clusters lasting for a few weeks, usually with one to three headache episodes per day. The headache is always unilateral, usually reaches its peak within 15 min, and most episodes are relatively short, often between 30 and 45 min, although they may last for 3 h (or even longer). A useful rule is that the pain is so excruciating that a patient who sits or lies calmly during an attack is not having cluster headache. Indeed, almost all sufferers complain that this is the worst pain they have ever experienced. In roughly 90% of patients, onset of cluster headache is before the age of 50 years. The diagnostic criteria of the International Headache Society include:
  1. Severe or very severe unilateral orbital, supraorbital, and/or temporal pain lasting 15–180 min if untreated.
  2. Headache is accompanied by at least one of the following: ipsilateral conjunctival injection and/or lacrimation, ipsilateral nasal congestion and/or rhinorrhea, ipsilateral eyelid edema, ipsilateral forehead and facial sweating, ipsilateral miosis and/or ptosis, and a sense of restlessness or agitation.
  3. Attacks have a frequency from one every other day to eight per day during most of the cluster period.
- Paroxysmal hemicrania.
- Short-lasting unilateral neuralgiform headache attacks with conjunctival injection and tearing (SUNCT) and short-lasting unilateral neuralgiform headache with cranial autonomic symptoms (SUNA).
• Other primary headache syndromes, e.g., hemicrania continua, primary cough headache, primary exertional headache, primary headache associated with sexual activity, primary stabbing headache, primary thunderclap headache,

and hypnic headache. Hypnic headache is also called alarm clock headache because it starts suddenly during the morning hours and wakes the patient. It is therefore an important differential diagnostic to cluster headache, yet hypnic headache is milder and bilateral and tends to occur later in life (mean age of onset is 62 years). Also, trigeminal autonomic symptoms and remission periods are lacking.

- When thunderclap headache associated with physical exertion and sexual activity occurs for the first time, subarachnoidal hemorrhage, arterial dissection, and arterial hypertension must be excluded.
- Indomethacin-responsive headaches. This category overlaps with the last two. Indomethacin-responsive headaches include hemicrania continua and paroxysmal hemicrania. If in doubt, performing an indomethacin test is always advisable; see Chap. 6.

4.4.2 Symptomatic Headaches

Secondary headache syndromes (Fig. 4.2) may be due to:

- Intracranial causes.
  - Tumors.
  - Hemorrhage.
  - Obstructive hydrocephalus.
  - Vascular disorders, including:
    Cerebral venous sinus thrombosis.
    Vascular malformations.
    CNS vasculitis.
    Intracranial artery dissection.
    Excessively high blood pressure, with or without posterior reversible encephalopathy syndrome (PRES).
    Reversible cerebral vasoconstriction syndrome (RCVS). Due to improved neuroimaging, RCVS has become a common vascular headache diagnosis. Thunderclap headaches with or without physical activity occur repetitively during days or weeks. CT or MR angiograms reveal generalized cerebral vasospasm, and other causes such

as primary CNS angiitis and systemic vasculitides are ruled out (e.g., CSF analysis is normal). Usually this condition is self-limiting and the prognosis good (see Chap. 6 for treatment); although rarely, vasospasms can lead to ischemic and hemorrhagic infarctions, usually borderzone infarcts, as well as cortical subarachnoidal hemorrhage (Case 4.3). Fatal cases are uncommon but well described (Case 4.4).

- Idiopathic intracranial hypertension (pseudotumor cerebri), usually encountered in obese young women.
  - Hypoliquorrhea syndrome.
    Spontaneous CSF fistula. Note that with long-standing hypoliquorrhea, the characteristic orthostatic feature of the headache (better in the supine position) may be replaced by constant headache that is independent of the position of the body (Case 4.5).
    Post-lumbar puncture headache. Risk factors include younger age, female sex, lean body shape, and a history of migraine. Using atraumatic spinal needles decreases the risk of post-lumbar puncture headache. Although the evidence is weak, performing the lumbar puncture in the lateral decubitus position may also be associated with less frequent headaches. Normohydration is important, but hyperhydration and bed rest after the procedure can no longer be recommended. If invasive treatment of the headache is warranted, an epidural blood patch may be helpful.
- Infectious processes (e.g., abscess, cerebritis, meningitis, meningoencephalitis).
  - Headache with neurological deficits and CSF lymphocytosis (HaNDL), also called pseudomigraine with pleocytosis. This condition is discussed in more detail with the differential diagnosis of transitory ischemic attack (TIA)/stroke.
- Extracranial causes.
  - Trauma (e.g., post-commotio headache; typically, the severity of the pain is not proportional to the degree of the trauma)

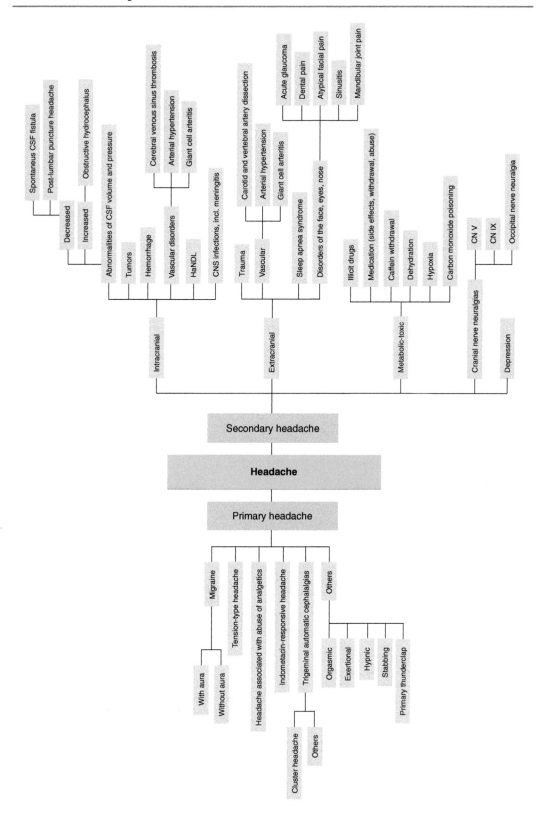

Fig. 4.2 Differential diagnosis of headache

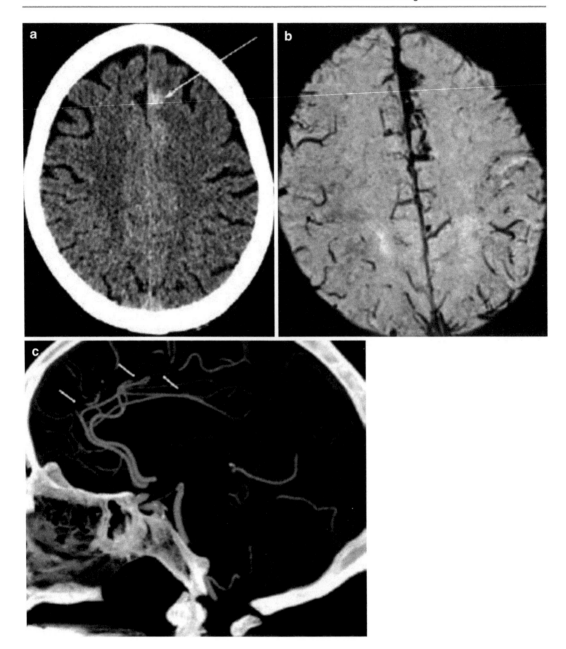

Case 4.3 Reversible cerebral vasoconstriction syndrome (RCVS). A 60-year-old female presented with a 5-day history of multiple episodes of thunderclap headache. A CT of the brain showed a small cortical area with hyperintense signal change (*arrow*) (**a**), and gradient-echo MRI (SWI) revealed hemosiderin deposits consistent with a gyral SAB (**b**). CTA revealed spasms of multiple cerebral vessels, including the ACA (*arrows*; **c**). CSF analysis was normal. The patient was diagnosed with RCVS. Treatment with nimodipine was initiated, the headaches vanished, and 3 months later on the follow-up angiography, spasms were no longer seen

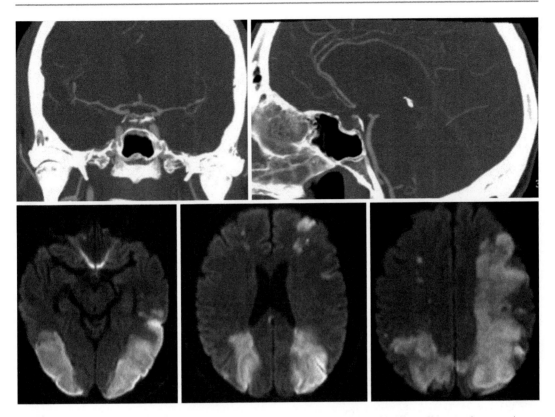

Case 4.4 Reversible cerebral vasoconstriction syndrome (RCVS) with fatal outcome. A 58-year-old male with chronic obstructive pulmonary disease and alcoholic neuropathy was admitted with repeating thunderclap headaches over a period of 48 h. Neurological examination was normal. Non-contrast head CT and lumbar puncture, including CSF analysis for xanthochromia, were unremarkable. CT angiography revealed widespread vasospasms in the anterior and posterior intracranial circulation. A working diagnosis of RCVS was made, and treatment with 60 mg oral nimodipine six times daily was started. Over the next 2 days, episodes of confusion, blurred vision, and speech problems occurred and subsequently, the patient became obtunded (GCS 9: e2, m5, v2; FOUR 12: e1, m3, b4, r4). The patient developed a right-sided hemiparesis with bilaterally extensive toes. A second CT angiography showed progressive vasospasms (above). Treatment with epoprostenol 1 ng/kg/min in a central IV line was started 3 days after admission. However, there was no change in the clinical condition. MRI of the brain revealed widespread infarctions in both hemispheres (below). The patient died on day 7. The significance of this case is twofold. First, it shows that RCVS can be fatal despite the "R" in its name ("R" stands for "reversible"). Second, the posterior location of the infarctions is well in line with recent data indicating that RCVS and PRES are manifestations of similar underlying pathophysiologic mechanisms and that both conditions frequently coexist in a given patient (adapted with permission from Thydén et al. (2016))

- Vascular disorders (e.g., giant cell or temporal arteritis, extracranial artery dissection)
- Disorders involving the face, eyes, and oral cavity (e.g., acute glaucoma, dental pain, sinusitis, atypical facial pain, mandibular joint dysfunction). Atypical facial pain is a relatively common condition with a recognizable clinical presentation; it most often occurs in middle-aged women following dental procedures. The pain is more or less constant, moderately intense, and described as deep, aching, or boring. Typically, multiple visits to the dentist and ENT specialist have been unrewarding, neuroimaging is normal, the pain has been resistant to various analgesics, and the patient feels very distressed. Treatment consists of antidepressants and counseling, including possibly behavioral therapy, but is often unsatisfactory.

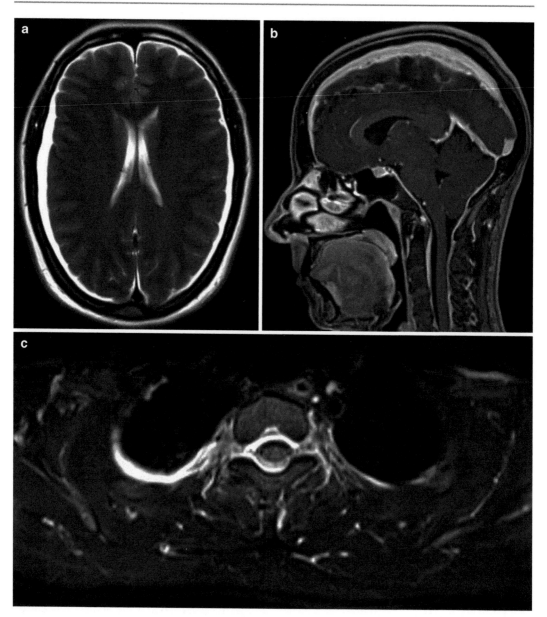

Case 4.5 Spontaneous intracranial hypotension and spinal CSF leak. This 43-year-old male presented with a 6-month history of dull headache of moderate severity. The pain was consistent with an orthostatic headache, as it improved in the supine position, although the patient had noticed that lying flat did no longer alleviate symptoms to the same degree. His medical history was unremarkable, but he had suffered moderate back pain following a traffic accident 2 years prior to admission. MRI of the brain showed findings suggestive of intracranial hypotension ("brain sagging"), including bihemispheric subdural effusions (**a**, T2 weighted), pachymeningeal and pituitary gland contrast enhancement, a downward drooping splenium of the corpus callosum, distortion of the upper brainstem structures, and cerebellar tonsillar herniation (**b**, T1 weighted, gadolinium enhanced). An MRI of the spinal column revealed a fluid collection around the right pulmonary apex consistent with a cervicothoracic spinal CSF leak (**c**). Two blood patches were ineffective. Following discussions with the spinal surgery team, it was decided to opt for a conservative approach. Amitriptyline was slowly titrated to 75 mg once daily at bedtime with excellent clinical response

- Hypercapnia. This typically leads to generalized moderate to severe throbbing headaches in the morning. Hypercapnia is often associated with sleep apnea; thus, the sleep partner should be inquired about snoring, gasping, or choking sounds and whether breathing appears interrupted; daytime sleepiness is frequent. Also, it is important to take complaints of headache in a patient with a primary myopathy such as Pompe's disease or myotonic dystrophy very seriously. Such complaints may point to hypercapnia because of respiratory muscle failure. Does the patient need continuous positive airway pressure (CPAP) at night?
- Metabolic-toxic causes, e.g., use of prescription drugs (dipyridamole, many others), use or withdrawal of illicit drugs, dehydration, caffeine withdrawal, carbon monoxide poisoning, and other causes of hypoxia.
- CN neuralgias (e.g., CN V, CN IX, occipital neuralgia).
- Depressive and other psychiatric disorders.

Red flags suggesting that a headache is not due to a benign cause include focal neurological deficits, worst-ever headaches, new-onset headaches, new onset of unusual headache features, migrainous headache that is always unilateral and never occurs on the other side, systemic features (meningism, weight loss, fever, diarrhea, skin rash), general malaise, and prior history of malignancy.

It is crucial not to miss the following conditions associated with acute or subacute headache:

- Brain tumors, metastasis, and other mass lesions.
- Parenchymal hemorrhagic stroke.
- Subarachnoidal hemorrhage, including warning leaks and growing aneurysms.
- Ischemic stroke, when leading to headache, is usually due to arterial dissection and/or posterior circulation infarction.

- Cerebral sinus venous thrombosis.
- Posterior fossa processes, e.g., cerebellar hemorrhage and Arnold-Chiari malformation (downward displacement of the cerebellar vermis and medulla through the foramen magnum).
- CSF outflow obstruction, which occasionally may be intermittent, e.g., due to a colloid cyst at the foramen of Monro.
- Pituitary apoplexy.
- Bacterial meningitis.
- Lymphomatous or carcinomatous meningitis.
- HSV type I encephalitis.
- Other meningoencephalitic syndromes.
- Giant cell arteritis (temporal arteritis).
- Acute glaucoma.
- Hypercapnia (see above).

Importantly, except for the first two, all of the conditions listed above may be associated with a CT that has been read as unremarkable ("CT-negative headaches").

4.5   The Differential Diagnosis of Cognitive Impairment and Dementia

Dementia is usually defined as acquired cognitive decline that involves memory and at least one other cognitive domain that is severe enough to affect social or occupational functioning. A diagnosis of dementia cannot be established in patients with disturbed consciousness. With the increased awareness of dementia in the population and the advent of techniques for early diagnosis, patients with very mild subjective symptoms are often referred to the neurologist, and to wait for dementia criteria to be fulfilled is no longer appropriate. However, some patients presenting with mild cognitive complaints represent the "well and worried," often young or middle-aged individuals complaining of unspecific episodes of memory slips that are described in a highly detailed manner. Characteristically, these episodes have not had any impact on performance in professional or private life except for the fact that the patient feels rather embarrassed. These patients are usually very thankful for clear reassurance that they do not fulfill the criteria of dementia or other any other cognitive impairment and that there are no findings suggesting an underlying cerebral disease. However, in some patients, a program with thorough cognitive tests, ancillary examinations, and follow-up is the only way to make sure that subtle symptoms do not represent the initial phase of a degenerative brain disorder.

When examining patients with cognitive impairment, it is important to identify and treat psychiatric conditions, by differentiating between the three "Ds":

- Depression[3]
- Delirium[4]
- Dementia

The differentiation may be challenging, and sometimes a treatment trial with antidepressant therapy and follow-up are needed to separate depression with cognitive symptoms from

---

[3]Depression is defined as a cluster of symptoms that may include depressed mood; anhedonia; changes in eating, appetite, or weight; hypersomnia or insomnia; psychomotor agitation or retardation; impaired self-esteem and self-confidence; ideas of guilt and unworthiness; bleak and pessimistic view of the future; tiredness; impaired concentration and memory; and in some cases thoughts of death. For a diagnosis of depression, at least two of the core symptoms (depressed mood, anhedonia, and reduced energy) must be present, plus two of the other symptoms mentioned above (ICD10 2010, WHO 2010).

[4]Delirium is defined as an acute or subacute condition with reversible and fluctuating decreased consciousness due to organic brain disease or metabolic-toxic impairment. Common causes are polypharmacy, electrolyte derangements, hypo- and hyperthyroidism, kidney and liver failure, and hypo- and hyperthermia, as well as urinary tract and other infections. Patients are disoriented in time and space, incoherent, and perseverative, with agitation or apathy, and they may have visual hallucinations and asterixis.

early-phase AD or FTD with prominent affective symptoms. Delirium, more common in patients with dementia, is potentially fatal and should be identified and treated immediately. Clarify and treat the underlying cause (e.g., urinary tract infection), and treat the symptoms of delirium appropriately.

Only when the "mimics" of dementia—depression and delirium—have been excluded, is it safe to diagnose the patient with dementia, but it is important to remember that dementia is a syndrome, not a diagnosis, which is why the underlying etiology must be defined (Fig. 4.3). Furthermore, patients with cognitive impairment not meeting the criteria for dementia often present to the neurologist and should be examined as thoroughly as patients with dementia. MCI is defined as impairment in memory or in a single non-memory cognitive domain, which does not (yet) impair social functioning (Petersen et al. 1999). In fact, many of the systemic conditions that may cause cognitive impairment are most often associated with mild cognitive dysfunction rather than dementia. With the advent of biomarkers, it may be possible to establish a diagnosis of a neurodegenerative disorder, e.g., Alzheimer's disease, in the pre-dementia (MCI) stage. Of note, in their new edition of the *Diagnostic and Statistical Manual of Mental Disorders* (DSM-5), the American Psychiatric Association recently introduced the terms "major neurocognitive disorder" and "minor neurocognitive disorder" as alternatives to "dementia" and "MCI" (American Psychiatric Association 2013).

4.5.1 Potentially Reversible Conditions

In the differential diagnosis of cognitive impairment, pay particular attention to identifying potentially reversible conditions before considering a diagnosis of a (irreversible) neurodegenerative disorder, including:

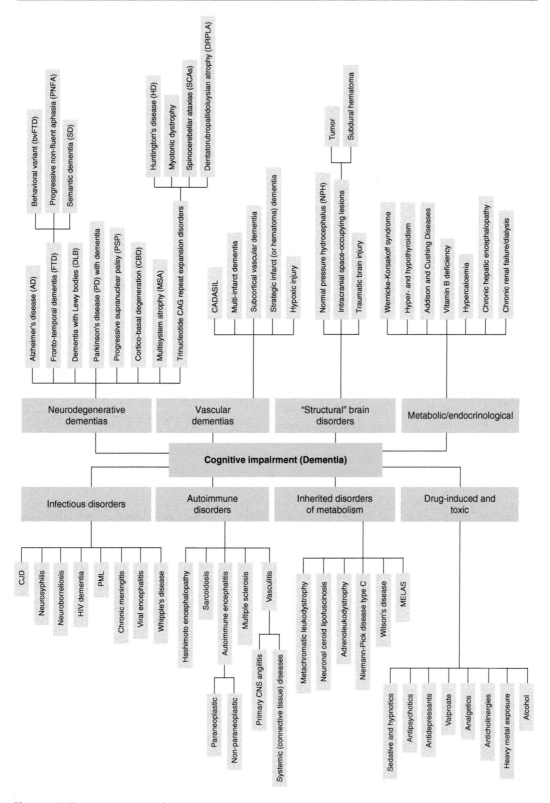

Fig. 4.3 Differential diagnosis of cognitive impairment and dementia

- Drug or alcohol abuse.
- Side effects of drugs (most CNS active drugs may impair cognition, but other drugs, such as aspirin (high doses), may also give rise to cognitive symptoms).
- Partial complex seizures leading to episodic impairment of cognition in a patient with unidentified epilepsy.
- Chronic infections (e.g., *Borrelia*, neurosyphilis).
- Inflammatory brain diseases (autoimmune encephalitis, sarcoidosis, vasculitis, Hashimoto's disease).
- NPH, characterized by a triad of gait ataxia, mental slowing, and urinary incontinence.
- Subdural hemorrhage in a patient with a (unrecognized) head trauma, a frontal meningioma, or other space-occupying lesions may occasionally present with cognitive impairment or personality change.
- Metabolic impairment, including hyper- and hypothyroidism, vitamin deficiencies (B12, B1, and B6), hyponatremia, hyperparathyroidism, hypercalcemia, Cushing disease, Addison disease, and chronic hepatic and renal failure.
- Chronic sleep apnea syndrome.

4.5.2 The Amnestic Syndrome

Because neurologists often see patients with amnesia, who do not meet criteria for dementia, it is helpful to know the potential underlying causes. When isolated amnesia is thought to be a precedent to AD, it is named amnestic MCI, MCI due to AD, or prodromal AD. Amnesia may also be seen early in the course of other neurodegenerative disorders. However, there are several other causes of amnesia (Fig. 4.3):

4.5.2.1 Transient
- Epileptic amnesia
- Wernicke's encephalopathy
- Transient global amnesia
- Concussion of the brain
- Electroconvulsive therapy
- Alcohol and drugs

4.5.2.2 Chronic
- Traumatic brain injury
- Anoxic brain damage
- Limbic encephalitis
- Herpes encephalitis
- AD (and other neurodegenerative disorders)
- Korsakoff's syndrome
- Ruptured AComA aneurysm
- Infarcts, tumor, and hemorrhage

4.5.3 Chronic Dementia Disorders

The term dementia disorder usually refers to the chronic and progressive degenerative brain disorders, where dementia is one of the main symptoms. Few other fields in neurology are presently undergoing such rapid changes in classification as cognitive neurology. New pathophysiological insights change the way dementias are being understood and categorized. For instance, based on different abnormal protein aggregations found in the brain, neurodegenerative disorders associated with parkinsonism and dementia can be broadly classified into tauopathies (FTD, AD, PSP, CBD) and synucleinopathies (Parkinson's disease, DLB, multiple system atrophy, neurodegeneration with brain iron accumulation (NBIA) type I). With the application of neuroimaging (MRI with assessment of total brain and hippocampal volumes, FDG PET, DAT-SPECT, and amyloid PET) and CSF biomarkers for AD, it is possible to differentiate the most common neurodegenerative disorders and to establish an accurate diagnosis early in the course of the disease, even before dementia evolves. The most commonly used current clinical criteria for the neurodegenerative dementia disorders are listed in Table 4.1.

Chronic dementias may be further divided into:

- Primary cortical dementias
- Primary subcortical dementias
- Dementias that are both cortical and subcortical from the onset

Thus,

- *Primary cortical dementias* are those that, at least in the beginning, tend to affect either

Table 4.1 Clinical criteria for dementia disorders

Condition	Criteria	References
Dementia (as a syndrome)	ICD 10	World Health Organization (2010)
Major neurocognitive disorder	DSM-5	American Psychiatric Association (2013)
Mild cognitive impairment (MCI)	Petersen criteria	Petersen et al. (1999)
Minor neurocognitive disorder	DSM-5	American Psychiatric Association (2013)
MCI due to Alzheimer's disease (AD)	NIA-AA workgroup	Albert et al. (2011)
Alzheimer's disease (prodromal)	International Working Group	Dubois et al. (2007, 2010)
Dementia due to AD	NIA-AA workgroup	McKhann et al. (2011)
Posterior cortical atrophy	International Working Group	Crutch et al. (2013)
Vascular dementia	NINDS-AIREN	Román et al. (1993)
Vascular cognitive impairment	VASCOG	Sachdev et al. (2014)
Dementia with Lewy bodies (DLB)	DLB consortium	McKeith et al. (2005)
Behavioral variant FTD (bvFTD)	International bvFTD consortium	Rascovsky et al. (2011)
Semantic dementia (SD)	International primary progressive aphasia working group	Gorno-Tempini et al. (2011)
Progressive nonfluent aphasia (PNFA)	International primary progressive aphasia working group	Gorno-Tempini et al. (2011)

higher cognitive domains such as memory, language function, visuospatial orientation, praxis, gnosis (e.g., AD), and/or personality (e.g., FTD). As a rule of thumb, early in the course of the disease, there are little or no non-cognitive neurological deficits. Primary cortical dementias include AD and FTD.

- *Primary subcortical dementias*, in contrast, tend to leave higher cortical functioning relatively spared early in its course, but there is characteristic psychomotor retardation and often depressive symptoms. Moreover, patients with primary subcortical dementias tend to have more focal neurological deficits revealed during bedside examination. These dementias include, for instance, subcortical vascular dementia and NPH.
- However, most dementias have elements of both cortical and subcortical symptoms with a mixture of cognitive and noncognitive neurological and psychiatric symptoms.

The most common dementia disorders are:

- *Alzheimer's disease*. Its cognitive deficits are prominent, whereas personality is largely preserved until the late stages (Albert et al. 2011; McKhann et al. 2011). Episodic memory

impairment is very characteristic in the early phase, but atypical presentations with specific deficits in other non-memory cognitive domains are also seen (Case 3.1). Familial autosomal dominant AD is rare, as compared to sporadic AD, and is associated with mutations in the amyloid precursor (*APP*), presenilin (*PSEN*)-1 or *PSEN-2* genes. *Posterior cortical atrophy* is a variant of AD, with isolated disruption of visual processing but reasonable day-to-day memory. Patients with posterior cortical atrophy may have partial Balint's syndrome, simultanagnosia, visual inattention, topographical disorientation, impaired face and object recognition, or isolated deficits in writing, reading, and praxis (Crutch et al. 2013) (See Case 5.5).

- *Frontotemporal dementias*. The categorization of FTD syndromes and underlying pathologies is rather complex. Specific syndromes are associated with the familial autosomal dominant FTDs: FTD with mutation in the *MAPT*, progranulin, chromosome 9 open reading frame 72 (*C9ORF72*), and *CHMP2B* (FTD-3) genes. Some of these patients develop FTD in combination with MND or PD. The general neurologist should be able to identify the most common syndromes because counseling and rehabilitation differ:

- *Behavioral variant frontotemporal dementia* (bvFTD, sometimes still known as Pick dementia). It is characterized by striking personality and behavioral changes, executive dysfunction, impaired sympathy and empathy, perseverate, stereotypic or compulsive behavior, apathy or disinhibition, and lack of insight but relatively intact memory early in the course of the disease (Cases 2.15 and 4.6) (Rascovsky et al. 2011).
- *Primary progressive aphasia* is often used as a term for degenerative disorders with aphasia at onset, which comprise *progressive nonfluent aphasia* (PNFA), *semantic dementia* (SD), and *logopenic aphasia* (Gorno-Tempini et al. 2011).
- *Progressive nonfluent aphasia (PNFA)*. Personality and cognitive domains other than expressive language function are usually spared until late in its course. Characterized by effortful halting speech, phonological errors, and agrammatism, PNFA is often associated with impaired comprehension of complex sentences (but spared comprehension of words, object knowledge and repetition, and relatively intact insight) (Case 4.7).
- *Semantic dementia (SD)*. This is a condition of primarily severe fluent aphasia with relatively intact episodic memory function. Characterized by impaired confrontation naming and single-word comprehension, often associated with impaired object knowledge and surface dyslexia but with spared repetition and speech production. Patients with SD may have bizarre delusions and hyper-religious thoughts. Recent studies indicate that their semantic deficits may improve with training (Case 2.17).

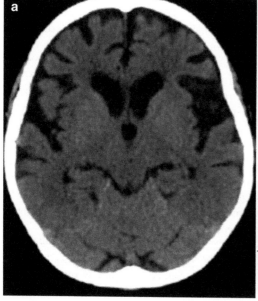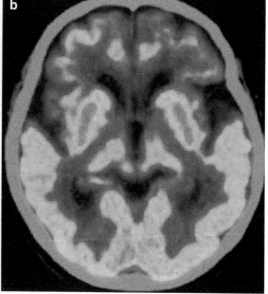

Case 4.6 Behavioral variant frontotemporal dementia (bvFTD). A 68-year-old female was referred to the memory clinic for evaluation of behavioral changes and functional decline during the past 2 years. She had gradually withdrawn from social activities, had developed a preference for candy, was apathetic, and lacked empathy. There were no focal deficits, but she had difficulties cooperating during the neurological examination. Neuropsychological testing revealed lack of insight, pronounced apathy, and impaired naming, abstraction, and executive functions, but no amnesia. CSF and EEG were normal. CT of the brain showed bilateral frontotemporal atrophy (**a**), and FDG PET revealed hypometabolism in the same area (**b**). She was diagnosed with bvFTD (PET images courtesy of Ian Law, Department of Clinical Physiology and Nuclear Medicine, Rigshospitalet, Copenhagen)

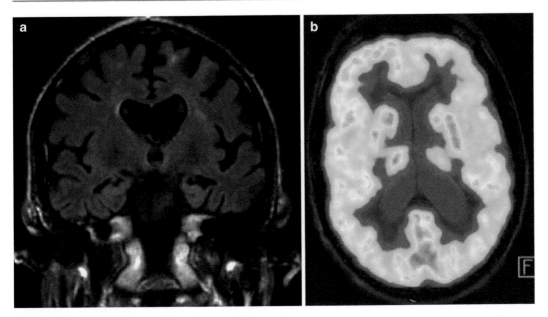

Case 4.7 Progressive nonfluent aphasia (PNFA). A 64-year-old male complained of increasing word-finding and pronunciation difficulties over the previous 2–3 years. He was still able to work as a carpenter. The MMSE score was 26/30. The neurological examination was unremarkable except for disturbed word fluency and naming, as well as mildly impaired psychomotor speed and executive functions. CSF analysis and EEG were normal. MRI demonstrated global cortical atrophy, which was most severe in the left frontal and anterior temporal lobe (**a**). FDG PET showed frontotemporal-parietal hypometabolism, which was most pronounced on the left side (**b**). He was diagnosed with PNFA (PET images courtesy of Ian Law, Department of Clinical Physiology and Nuclear Medicine, Rigshospitalet, Copenhagen)

- – Characterized by hesitant speech and anomia, *logopenic aphasia* is a language disorder which is sometimes seen in early-phase AD.
- *Vascular dementias*. Cognitive disorders of vascular etiology are a heterogeneous group of disorders with diverse pathologies (e.g., dementia following strategic infarctions, small vessel disease, and cerebral autosomal dominant arteriopathy with subcortical infarcts and leukoencephalopathy (CADASIL)) and clinical manifestations (e.g., acute onset, a stepwise progression, or a gradual progression). For a diagnosis of vascular dementia to be made, there must be neuroradiological evidence of significant vascular disease. The vascular lesions must be related in terms of localization to the extent and severity of cognitive impairment (Román et al. 1993). For patients with strategic infarcts, the vascular lesions must be related to the onset of dementia. Patients with cognitive impairment due to cerebrovascular disease have a characteristic clinical profile and may not always meet criteria for dementia (or major neurocognitive disorder), which was taken into account by the International Society for Vascular Behavioral and Cognitive Disorders in their recently published clinical criteria for vascular cognitive impairment (Sachdev et al. 2014).

- Note that many elderly patients with AD also have small subcortical vascular lesions (and these patients may be classified as having mixed AD dementia).
- *Dementia with Lewy bodies (DLB)* is characterized by fluctuations of wakefulness and cognitive impairment, prominent visuospatial deficits (and less prominent memory impairment) in the early phase of the disease, vivid visual hallucinations, REM sleep disorders, parkinsonism, and sensitivity for antipsychotic drugs (which should be avoided or prescribed with minimal doses and short duration) (McKeith et al. 2005).
- *Parkinson's disease with dementia*. Up to 70% of patients with PD develop cognitive

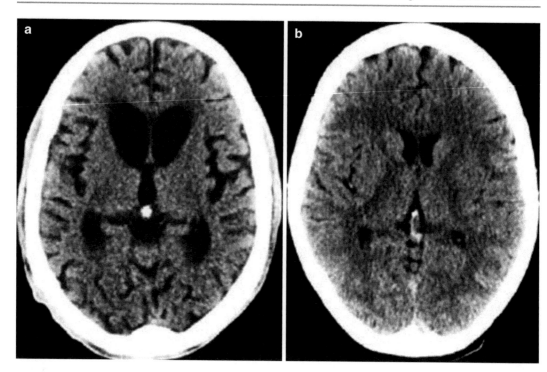

Case 4.8 Huntington's disease. A 45-year-old female had been dismissed from her job because of inappropriate sexual behavior. Her family history was noticeable insofar as her father had developed late life chorea. Examination showed subtle choreiform movements of her hands and feet. Genetic testing revealed that the patient carried the gene mutation for HD with 47 CAG repeats on the expanded allele. CT of the brain showed marked bilateral caudate atrophy (**a**). An image of a normal brain is shown for comparison (**b**)

impairment with a similar profile to DLB during the course of their disease. The distinction between DLB and PD with dementia is somewhat arbitrary. When cognitive impairment occurs at least 1 year prior to parkinsonism, the diagnosis is DLB; otherwise, it is classified as PD with dementia (Emre et al. 2007).

- *The so-called Parkinson plus disorders* such as MSA, CBD, PSP, and DLB. CBD is characterized by a combination of frontal dysfunction (e.g., personality change, impaired reasoning), speech and language impairment, and asymmetric motor features with alien limb, myoclonus, limb apraxia, rigidity, and/or akinesia. PSP is associated with cognitive impairment in combination with frequent falls and (vertical) gaze palsy, often with axial rigidity, gait disorder, and retropulsion. For more information, see Sect. 4.14.

- *Huntington's disease* (*HD*). This is an autosomal dominant trinucleotide repeat disorder with characteristic neuropsychiatric symptoms, dementia, and chorea leading inevitably to death. HD may present with cognitive impairment, personality change, or psychiatric symptoms years before chorea (Case 4.8).

Other causes of cognitive impairment or dementia (see also potentially reversible dementias above):

- Chronic psychiatric diseases:
  - Schizophrenia
  - Bipolar disorder
- MS
- Heavy metal poisoning
- Mitochondrial encephalomyopathy with lactic acidosis and stroke (MELAS)
- Myotonic dystrophy
- Lysosomal and peroxisomal storage diseases
- Wilson's disease
- Chronic CNS infections:
  - HIV dementia, associated with a low CD4+ T-cell count and long duration of immunosuppression

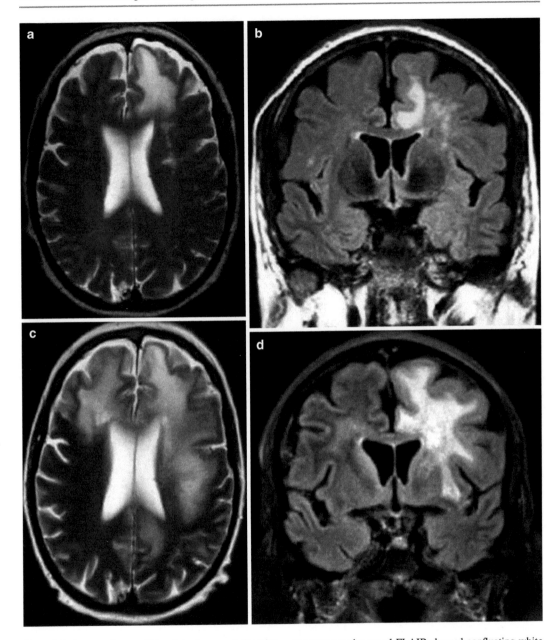

Case 4.9 Progressive multifocal leukoencephalopathy (PML). A 61-year-old female presented with a 6-week history of progressive aphasia, right-sided hemiplegia, gait ataxia, and focal epileptic seizures. She was receiving immunosuppressive therapy for a kidney transplantation undertaken 10 years earlier. MRI with axial T2-weighted sequences and coronal FLAIR showed confluating white matter signal changes in the left frontal lobe (**a**, **b**). Cerebrospinal fluid PCR was positive for JC virus, and a diagnosis of PML was made. An MRI 2 months later showed progressive white matter involvement (**c**, **d**), and the patient died 4 months later

- CJD, the most common prion disease characterized by rapidly progressive dementia, ataxia, and myoclonus
- Progressive multifocal leukoencephalopathy (PML), due to John Cunningham (JC) virus (Case 4.9)

- Whipple's disease
- Subacute sclerosing panencephalitis (SSPE)
- Alcohol-related dementia
  - Korsakoff's syndrome and Wernicke's encephalopathy. Acute thiamine deficiency

that is not immediately reversed may lead to permanent anterograde and retrograde amnesia with confabulation (Korsakoff's syndrome). Although other cognitive domains remain relatively spared, this is a devastating condition.

- Decreased cognitive performance related to long-term alcohol abuse and brain atrophy on neuroimaging may be partially reversible (but represents a controversial entity).

4.5.4   Rapidly Progressive Dementias

As stated above, cognitive impairment of acute or subacute onset must be differentiated from chronic dementias. Rapidly progressive dementias may develop within a few months, weeks, or even days. Compared to chronic dementias, the spectrum of rapidly progressive dementias is quite different. Many of these disorders are fatal, but some are treatable, which is why it is of the utmost importance to evaluate patients presenting with fast cognitive decline without delay. Although far from being complete, the following section is useful as a diagnostic guideline for the assessment of rapidly progressive dementias when the preliminary diagnostic procedures have been unrewarding. When initial diagnostic procedures, including neuroimaging, CSF exam, routine blood tests, and medication review, have been without obvious explanation, the most common rapidly progressive dementia is CJD (Case 4.10).

Of 178 patients referred to a tertiary center in the USA with a working diagnosis of suspected prion disease or rapidly progressive dementias, 62% had CJD (75% sporadic CJD, 22% familial CJD, 3% vCJD or iatrogenic CJD) (Geschwind et al. 2008).

- Thirty-eight percent had a non-prion disease:
  - Neurodegenerative disorders (in order of frequency: CBD, FTD, AD, DLB, PSP)
  - Autoimmune disorders (steroid-sensitive encephalopathy with antithyroid autoantibodies, also known as Hashimoto's encephalopathy; antibody-mediated autoimmune encephalitis, including paraneoplastic and non-paraneoplastic; MS; neurosarcoidosis)

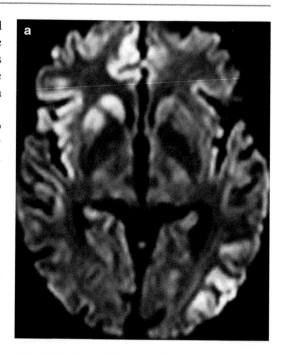

Case 4.10 Creutzfeldt-Jakob disease. A 59-year-old female complained of visual disturbances with altered color perception, stating, for example, that the sky was no longer blue but greenish. During the following 2 months, she developed progressive cognitive deficits, aphasia, and confusion. In addition, neurological examination revealed lead pipe rigidity in the limbs, dystonic posturing of the right arm, and gait ataxia. CSF analysis showed normal cell count and protein levels but highly increased total tau protein and CSF 14-3-3 protein levels. Serial EEG revealed increasing abnormalities and, finally, typical periodic triphasic sharp wave complexes (not shown). MRI of the brain included normal T1- and T2-weighted images, but there were bilateral hyperintense signal changes in the cortex and in the basal ganglia on DWI (a). Because of slightly increased thyroid antibodies levels, the patient was treated with high-dose steroids for 10 days but, as anticipated, subsequently became mutistic and developed generalized myoclonus. She died 1 month after admission. Autopsy confirmed the diagnosis of CJD. Isolated visual impairment at onset, including blurred vision, visual field restriction, metamorphopsia, cortical blindness, and/or hallucinations, is seen in roughly 20% of CJD patients and reflects neuronal loss and gliosis in the occipital lobes (Heidenhain variant) (adapted with permission from Kondziella et al. (2012)). Figures (b) and (c) show the serial EEG of another patient, also ultimately diagnosed with CJD. Six weeks after onset of depressive mood symptoms, confusion, and word-finding difficulties, EEG showed regional slowing of background activity and sharp waves in the left temporal region (b). In the following 2 weeks, he became mutistic and bedridden, and EEG revealed generalized periodic epileptiform discharge activity (c). He died 2 days later (EEG images courtesy of Hans Høgenhaven, Department of Clinical Neurophysiology, Rigshospitalet, Copenhagen)

Case 4.10   (continued)

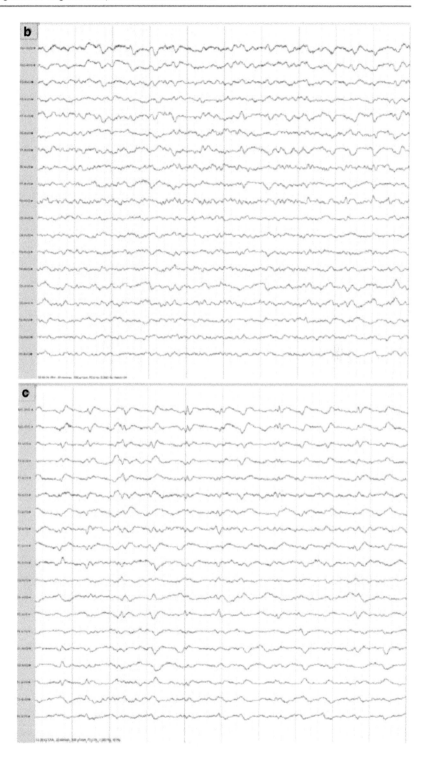

– Infectious causes (viral meningoencephalitis of unknown origin)
– Psychiatric diagnosis
– Malignancy (including primary cerebral lymphoma and antibody-negative paraneoplastic syndromes)
– Toxic-metabolic   reasons   (ethanol, methotrexate)
– Vascular findings not further specified
– Unclassified disorders

Obviously, this list is biased insofar as the referring institutions had excluded most of the malignant, infectious, vascular, and drug-induced causes for rapidly progressive dementias prior to referral. Diagnoses that are not reported by Geschwind et al. but by others who have performed similar studies at tertiary referral centers include:

- HIV dementia.
- PML (see Case 4.9).
- Neuronal ceroid lipofuscinosis.
- Neuroborreliosis.
- MELAS (see Case 4.26).
- In the young, Wilson's disease and Niemann-Pick's disease should always be excluded.
- Elderly men with GI symptoms, weight loss, ataxia, and dementia may have Whipple's disease.
- Valproate encephalopathy, which usually develops in the elderly after prolonged valproate use, is reversible upon discontinuation of valproate.
- Hereditary storage diseases may occasionally first manifest during adulthood.

It is mandatory not to miss the treatable mimics of CJD. In particular, Hashimoto's encephalitis and certain forms of antibody-mediated limbic encephalitis can imitate CJD and respond within days to corticosteroids or plasma separation. A steroid trial seems reasonable in any very rapidly progressive dementia patient with the slightest diagnostic uncertainty.

Brain biopsy may be useful in rare and atypical cases of (rapidly) progressive dementia (see Chap. 5).

4.6   The Differential Diagnosis of Encephalopathy

Encephalopathy is a state of global brain dysfunction with acute or subacute onset, and it has a variety of underlying etiologies (Fig. 4.4). Most of these were discussed previously or will be discussed in the following chapters in the sections on coma, dementia, epilepsy, infections, and malignancies. As a result, no further comments will be made here, apart from a short review of autoimmune encephalitis and posterior reversible encephalopathy syndrome (PRES).

Autoimmune encephalitis (AIE) is a group of inflammatory antibody-mediated CNS diseases with neurological and psychiatric symptoms. Patients often have deficits compatible with affection of the limbic system (e.g., amnesia, confusion, and epileptic seizures), but the inflammatory process frequently involves extra-limbic brain structures as well. Symptom onset is usually subacute, ranging from days to weeks. A more insidious onset with depression or hallucinations may lead to a misdiagnosis of psychiatric illness. Previously, AIE was considered a very rare paraneoplastic condition associated with intracellular antibodies and a very poor prognosis (e.g., anti-Hu syndrome). However, during the last two decades, it has become evident that AIE is much more frequently associated with antibodies directed against synaptic/cell membrane proteins and that, more often than not, an underlying malignancy is absent. The two most frequent conditions are AIE with antibodies against glutamate receptors of the N-methyl-D-aspartate (NMDA) type and AIE with antibodies against a protein associated with the voltage-dependent potassium channel (leucine-rich glioma-inactivated 1; LGI1). The former is typically seen in children and young adults, whereas the latter occurs more frequently in the elderly. Of note, prognosis in AIE with synaptic surface protein antibodies can be good, if aggressive immunomodulatory treatment is initiated early. Treatment (see Chap. 6) consists of high-dose steroids plus IVIG or plasmapheresis, occasionally followed by treatment escalation using rituximab or cyclophosphamide, and tumor removal where appropriate. However, chronic cognitive deficits are frequent.

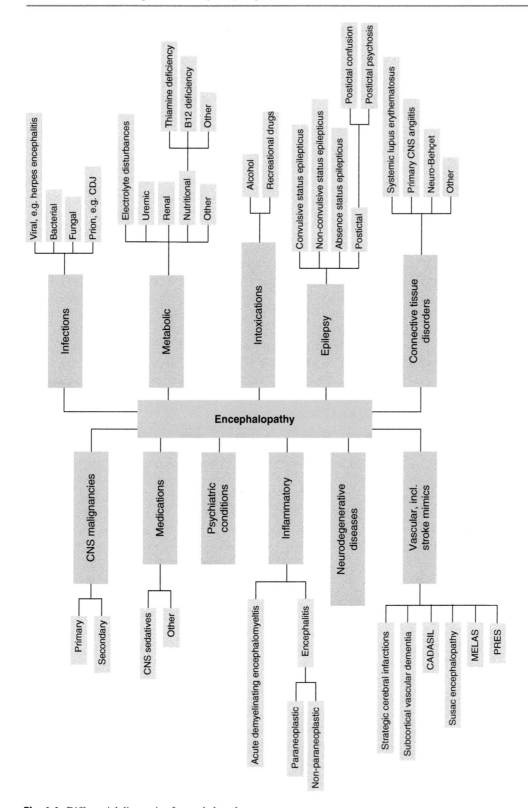

Fig. 4.4 Differential diagnosis of encephalopathy

- AIE associated with intracellular paraneoplastic antibodies. These conditions are rare. The diagnosis of paraneoplastic AIE requires the demonstration of cancer within 5 years of the diagnostic neurological symptoms or the detection of well-characterized onconeuronal, intracellular antibodies, e.g.:
  - Ri (breast, small cell lung cancer, (SCLC))
  - Yo (breast, ovarian)
  - Hu (SCLC)
  - Ma2 (testis)
  - Amphiphysin (breast, lung)
  - CV2 (SCLC, thymoma)
  - Antibodies against glutamic acid decarboxylase (GAD), which is also an intracellular protein, are only occasionally associated with paraneoplastic limbic encephalitis, and their pathogenic properties remain unclear. Of note, anti-GAD antibodies are seen with stiff person syndrome.
- AIE associated with antibodies against neuronal surface or synaptic antigens. These conditions are relatively common. They occur more often than not without malignancy, although searching for an underlying neoplastic process is always mandatory.
  - Voltage-gated potassium channel (VGKC) complex:
    Leucine-rich glioma-inactivated 1 (LGI1). This is one of the two most frequent AIE. It is typically seen in middle-aged people and the elderly (>40 years). Men are twice as often affected as women. Less than 5% of cases are associated with malignancies. Characteristically, anti-LGI1 encephalitis is associated with hyponatremia and faciobrachial dystonic seizures, an epileptic syndrome preceding the onset of limbic encephalitis. Anti-LGI1 encephalitis is a classical limbic encephalitis, leading to mesial temporal lobe inflammation and related neurological symptoms, including amnesia, neuropsychiatric features, and epilepsy. Increased signal activity on MR T2-weighted and fluid-attenuated inversion recovery (FLAIR) sequences may be seen in the temporal lobes corresponding to inflammatory infiltrates (although these imaging changes can be subtle or even missing in the early and late stages of the disease), and

FDG PET of the brain typically shows focal hypermetabolism in one or both temporal lobes. EEG reveals focal slowing and/or epileptic activity involving the temporal lobes. CSF is usually slightly inflamed with pleocytosis, increased protein levels and/or oligoclonal bands, and IgG index, but occasionally can be normal (Case 4.11).

Contactin-associated protein-like 2 (CASPR2). This antibody is associated with Morvan's syndrome, consisting of neuromyotonia, autonomic dysfunction, hallucinations, and severe insomnia.

- N-Methyl-D-aspartate (NMDA) receptor. This is the other of the two most frequent AIE. It typically affects children and young adults who present with sudden neuropsychiatric features followed by seizures, encephalopathy, and oral automatisms. A prodromal phase with fever and headache often occurs a few days to 2 weeks before manifestation of neurological symptoms. The majority of patients are female, and 20–50% of cases are associated with ovarian teratoma. Anti-NMDA encephalitis may be fatal because of autonomic failure including central hypoventilation, catatonia, and cardiac arrhythmia. In contrast to other AIE, NMDA receptor encephalitis may be associated with a relatively high CSF cell count (up to 200 cells/mm^3) and a characteristic EEG pattern termed extreme delta brush (Case 4.12). Cases of NMDA receptor encephalitis following herpes simplex encephalitis are increasingly recognized (Case 4.13).
- α-Amino-3-hydroxy-5-methyl-4-isoxazolepropionic acid (AMPA) receptor.
- mGluR5, associated with Ophelia syndrome (a form of limbic encephalitis occurring together with Hodgkin's lymphoma).
- GABAa receptor and GABAb receptor.
- Glycine receptor and many others.
- Seronegative. In seronegative AIE no antibodies can be detected, but new antibodies are described at an astonishing pace, and many of these patients will probably harbor antibodies that are yet to be isolated. As stated above, in all patients with AIE, including those who are

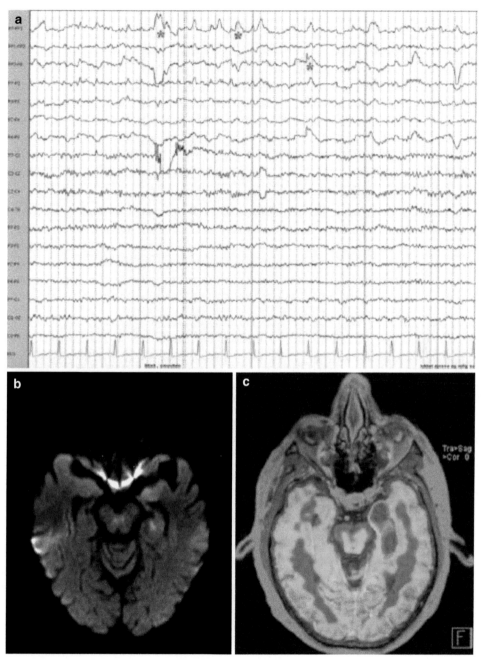

Case 4.11 Limbic encephalitis with anti-LGI1 antibodies. A 69-year-old previously healthy male presented with a 2-week history of behavioral disturbances, including anxiety, hypochondriac complaints, and motor hyperactivity. The neurological examination was unremarkable except for slight motor agitation. Over the next few days, the patient had several episodes of sudden onset of unresponsiveness and orofacial automatisms, including frequent jerks of the right side of the face and ipsilateral arm (faciobrachial dystonic seizures). The episodes lasted for 30–60 s. Routine blood tests showed hyponatremia. An EEG revealed epileptic spike-and-wave activity bilaterally with predominance in the left prefrontal lead (**a**; *asterisk*). MR of the brain revealed slight hyperin-tense signal change on FLAIR sequences in the left mesial temporal lobe (**b**). FDG PET showed an area of increased metabolism in the same area (**c**). Analysis of CSF was notable for slightly increased protein (0.66 g/L) but was otherwise normal. A whole-body PET CT did not reveal signs of systemic malignancy. When CSF analysis revealed anti-LGI1 antibodies, the patient was diagnosed as having limbic encephalitis associated with anti-LGI1 antibodies. Treatment with high-dose steroids, IVIG, and lamotrigine resulted in significant clinical improvement, although moderate neuro-psychiatric disturbance and memory deficits remained (EEG image courtesy of Hans Høgenhaven, Department of Clinical Neurophysiology, Rigshospitalet, Copenhagen)

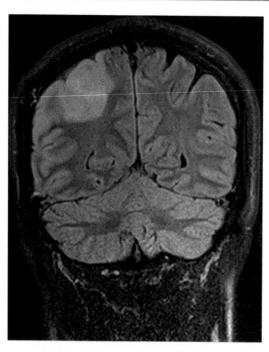

Case 4.12 *N*-Methyl-D-Aspartate receptor (NMDAr) encephalitis. A 26-year-old previously healthy woman had a 2-week history with progressive signs of disorientation, disorganized speech, altered behavior, and disturbances of sleep and memory. She was admitted to a psychiatric department where she stayed for a total of 3 weeks. Upon admission, she presented with varying and fluctuating behavioral symptoms (screaming, aggression, inappropriate sexual behavior), formal thought disturbance (vague or incoherent speech), and delusions (e.g., paranoia and somatic delusions). She also had prominent perceptual disturbances (arms felt like clay, the consistency of food felt altered) and auditory hallucinations (rhythms), as well as fluctuating catatonic symptoms (e.g., staring, verbal stereotypies, bizarre movements and actions, waxy flexibility, mutism, and stupor). She was treated with atypical (olanzapine) and typical (haloperidol) neuroleptics as well as benzodiazepines (oxazepam), with no or very limited response. She then received six electroconvulsive treatments (ECT). Due to the lack of treatment response, development of convulsive seizures, increasing catatonia, and autonomic dysfunction (central hypoventilation), she was transferred to the department of neurology with a working diagnosis of autoimmune encephalitis. EEG showed an encephalopathic pattern with excess of delta activity, including "brief ictal rhythmic discharges" (BIRD; but no "extreme delta brushes"). MR FLAIR revealed a cortical parietal lesion on the right. Empirical treatment with high-dose steroids and plasmapheresis was initiated with excellent response, both with respect to the psychiatric and the neurological symptoms. Her lesion had vanished on follow-up MRI 2 weeks later. CSF analysis showed a mild lymphocytic pleocytosis (45 cells) and a strong IgG anti-NMDAr antibody titer, confirming the diagnosis of NMDAr encephalitis. Screening for malignancy, including ovarian teratoma, was negative. The patient was put on maintenance prednisolone which was slowly tapered, while azathioprine was commenced as a steroid-sparing agent. Three years later, when it was decided that withdrawal of immunosuppressive treatment was safe, she was fully independent in her activities of daily living. Yet she suffered from cognitive sequelae, including decreased levels of concentration and short-term memory deficits, which had forced her to abandon her job as a nurse

seronegative, it is crucial to look for a systemic malignancy.

PRES is characterized by subacute onset of seizures, headache, confusion, and visual disturbances, often even cortical blindness. Arterial hypertension plays a role in two-thirds of all patients, but other causative factors include pregnancy (preeclampsia/eclampsia), allogenic or solid organ transplantation, autoimmune disorders, cytotoxic medication, and sepsis. The posterior circulation has relatively poorer sympathetic innervation than the anterior circulation, probably because it is phylogenetically much older. Thus, harmful stimuli such as severe hypertension may lead to breakdown in cerebral autoregulation, predominantly in the parietal and occipital lobes (and infratentorially), which explains the clinical

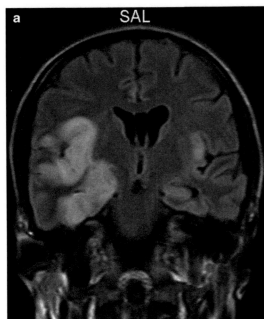

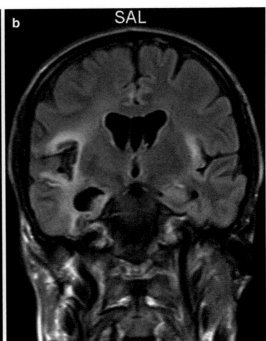

Case 4.13 Post-herpetic NMDAr encephalitis. A 44-year-old male, the owner of a large chain of stores with several hundred employees, developed headache and tiredness but did not seek medical advice. After 5 days, he appeared confused during a business meeting and his colleagues called an ambulance. On admission, he had a focal seizure, starting with a blank facial expression and lip smacking, evolving into twitching of the left corner of his mouth and finally leading to generalized tonic-clonic convulsions. His body temperature was elevated. CT showed a right temporal hypodensity. CSF analysis revealed a lymphocytic pleocytosis (500 cells, 0.91 g protein). Treatment with intravenous aciclovir was commenced immediately. Herpes simplex type 1 DNA was identified by polymerase chain reaction (PCR), thereby confirming the diagnosis of herpes simplex encephalitis. MRI showed severe inflammatory edema primarily involving the right temporal lobe; minor lesions were seen affecting the left insula, the left mesial temporal lobe, as well as the cingulate cortex (**a**; FLAIR). His condition improved during the next 4 weeks and he was discharged home, albeit with moderately severe amnestic dysfunction. Back at work, he felt unable to fulfill the requirements of his former position as CEO and started as a sales assistant in one of his own stores. Two weeks later, he experienced an episode of paranoid hallucinations and agitation, leading to admission to a psychiatric department. Although his agitation quickly subsided, visual and auditory pseudohallucinations (i.e., he was able to recognize that these vivid sensory experiences were not real) persisted which were both pleasant and unpleasant. For instance, on one occasion, he saw his little son lying in bed next to him involving him in a friendly chat, while on another occasion, he saw black thick hair growing from the walls and the ceiling. The patient was fully awake and responsive; his MMSE was 26/30. There was no suspicion of subclinical seizure activity, and no paroxystic activity was noted during EEG. MRI showed moderately severe atrophy and hippocampal sclerosis, predominantly involving the right hemisphere (**b**). Lumbar puncture revealed six cells and normal protein; HSV DNA was negative. However, CSF IgG anti-NMDAr antibody titer was strongly positive. A diagnosis of post-herpes NMDAr encephalitis was made. Following treatment with high-dose steroids and IVIG, pseudohallucinations ceased within a few days. The patient was put on oral prednisolone maintenance therapy. He was back to baseline with moderate cognitive deficits within 2 weeks, fully able to cope with his activities of daily living but unable to take responsibility for the management of his business (mRS 2)

symptoms. The diagnosis is based on clinical presentation and T2-weighted or FLAIR MR. The treatment includes blood pressure treatment, withdrawal of offending agents, and treatment of sepsis and other causes and usually requires admission to a neuro-ICU. PRES is largely reversible, although infarcts and intracerebral hemorrhages (ICH) do occur. Of note, PRES can be associated with RCVS, and vice versa. Prognosis is mainly related to the underlying disease (Case 4.14).

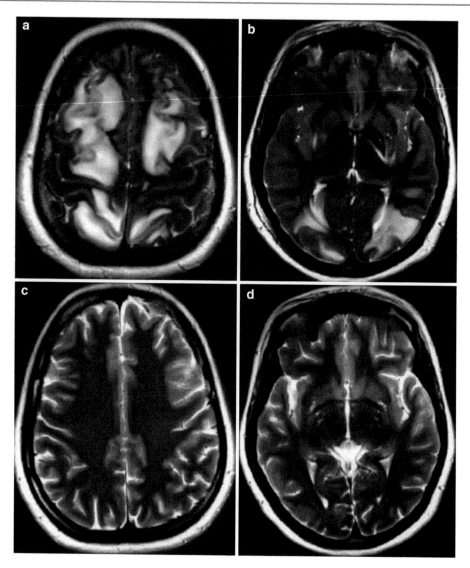

Case 4.14 Posterior reversible encephalopathy syndrome (PRES). A 35-year-old female with SLE and chronic renal failure complained of severe headache and cloudy vision. Three hours later she became unconscious with eyes and head deviating to the left and upward, followed by generalized tonic-clonic convulsions, urinary incontinence, and lateral tongue biting. Her blood pressure was 243/134 mmHg. T2-weighted MRI showed hyperintense signal involving the occipital and parietal lobes bilaterally, consistent with severe vasogenic edema and a diagnosis of PRES (**a, b**). Following aggressive blood pressure control and symptomatic treatment, she made a full recovery within a few days. MRI 2 months later showed complete resolution of the white matter abnormalities (**c, d**)

4.7   The Differential Diagnosis of Epilepsy

It is mandatory to clearly distinguish between the terms *epilepsy*, *epileptic seizures*, *epileptic syndromes*, and *status epilepticus*. The epilepsy community, under the framework of the International League Against Epilepsy (ILAE), is continually reviewing and revising definitions, according to the latest developments in the field. This effort is particularly admirable as every community member is invited to make their voice heard, and all comments are posted openly on the ILAE's website.[5] Admittedly, for the non-epileptologist neurologist,

---

[5] Visit *http://www.ilae.org/visitors/centre/Class-Seizure.cfm* for an impression of the lively discussions concerning a revision of seizure classifications (accessed November 2016).

these rapidly changing definitions can sometimes appear somewhat confusing. However, it is important to understand that this is work in progress with the final vision of providing clinically practical classifications that reflect current pathophysiological knowledge and that are endorsed by the entire epilepsy community.

4.7.1   Practical Clinical Definition of Epilepsy

According to an official report published by the International League Against Epilepsy (ILAE) in 2014, epilepsy is "a disease of the brain defined by any of the following conditions: (1) At least two unprovoked (or reflex) seizures occurring >24 h apart; (2) one unprovoked (or reflex) seizure and a probability of further seizures similar to the general recurrence risk (at least 60%) after two unprovoked seizures, occurring over the next 10 years; (3) diagnosis of an epilepsy syndrome."

The report specifies further that "epilepsy is considered to be resolved for individuals who had an age-dependent epilepsy syndrome but are now past the applicable age or those who have remained seizure-free for the last 10 years, with no seizure medicines for the last 5 years" (Fisher et al. 2014).

The perhaps most significant clinical implication of this revised definition (as opposed to the traditional definition, which required a mandatory number of at least two unprovoked seizures) is the fact that epilepsy now can be diagnosed (and treated!) in a patient presenting with a first-time focal seizure due to an acquired brain lesion.

4.7.2   Epileptic Seizures

An epileptic seizure is the clinical manifestation of abnormal and excessive hypersynchronous electrical discharge of a population of cortical neurons. The semiology of the epileptic seizure reflects the cortical representation and possible seizure spread to other brain regions, including the contralateral hemisphere. Depending on the involved cortical areas, an epileptic seizure leads to motor, sensory, autonomic, and/or psychic symptoms. Sensory and psychological symptoms can only be experienced and described by the patient and are called *aura*. It is important to understand that the aura represents epileptic cortical activity; its presence suggests a defined cortical lesion; thus, when occurring unprovoked and repeated, the patient is having partial (or focal) epilepsy. Although structural lesions account for <50% of all cases of epilepsy, this proportion is much higher in patients with partial epilepsies and in those with a later onset, in particular those over the age of 60. As a result, the etiology is structural in most new-onset epilepsies.

Epileptic seizures must be distinguished from syncope, psychogenic nonepileptic attacks, and other causes of paroxysmal events (Fig. 4.5). Epilepsy is suggested by unprovoked stereotyped and repeated events occurring with (or without) aura, automatisms, convulsions, lateral tongue biting, posturing, incontinence, postictal confusion, and muscle soreness. As stated above, it is mandatory to assess whether a generalized tonic-clonic seizure has a focal start or not; this is done by asking the patient and witnesses about a possible focal seizure onset and if there have been prior episodes consistent with partial seizures. The latter is particularly important because the patient may not volunteer this information, believing that these episodes are not related to the present event. Most epileptic seizures last no longer than 2–3 min. If a patient describes intermittent spells of symptoms lasting for more than 30 min, it is unlikely that these are epileptic seizures.

In 1981, the ILAE put forward a classification scheme for seizures, and in 1989, it introduced a classification scheme for epilepsies and epileptic syndromes. Both classifications remain in common use. Yet, modern neuroimaging, genomic technologies, and molecular biology are providing new insight into the pathophysiology of seizures and epilepsies. As a result, the ILAE Commission on Classification and Terminology issued a revised classification called *ILAE Proposal for Revised Terminology for Organization of Seizures and Epilepsies 2010*, which is shown in Table 4.2. However, because this update is once again under revision, many general neurologists still rely on the classifications from 1981 for seizures and from

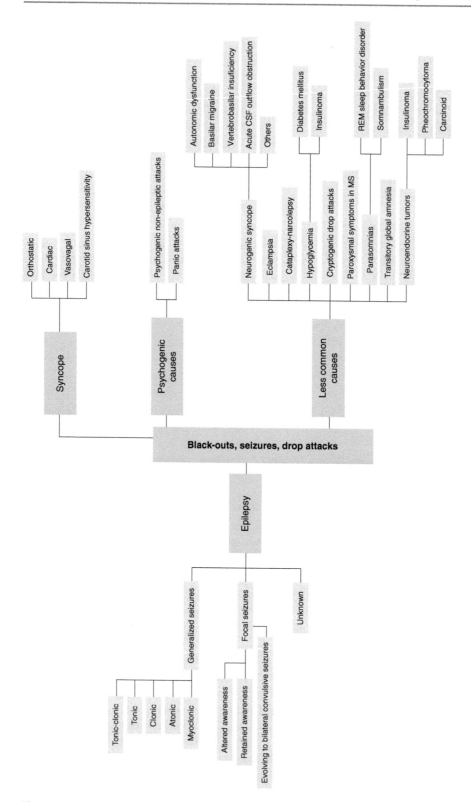

Fig. 4.5 Differential diagnosis of blackouts, seizures, and drop attacks

Table 4.2 International League Against Epilepsy (ILAE) Proposal for Revised Terminology for Organization of Seizures and Epilepsies 2010

Classification of seizures
Generalized seizures
Tonic-clonic
Absence
Typical
Absences with special features (myoclonic absence, eyelid myoclonia)
Atypical
Clonic
Tonic
Atonic
Myoclonic (myoclonic, myoclonic-atonic, myoclonic-tonic)
Focal seizures
Focal seizures are characterized according to one or more features:
Aura, motor, autonomic, and altered or retained awareness/responsiveness
Focal seizures may evolve to bilateral convulsive seizures (previously termed "secondarily generalized")
Unknown (insufficient evidence to classify as generalized, focal, or both)
Epileptic spasms
Others
Classification of seizure etiology
Genetic
Structural-metabolic
Unknown
Electroclinical syndromes and other epilepsies grouped by specificity of diagnosis
Electroclinical syndromes; they may be arranged by, for example, age of onset: benign neonatal seizures (neonatal period), Dravet syndrome (infancy), CAE (childhood), JME (adolescence-adulthood)
Distinctive constellations/surgical syndromes, e.g., mesial temporal lobe epilepsy with hippocampal sclerosis
Nonsyndromic epilepsies; they do not meet criteria for specific syndromes or constellations and are attributed to and organized by structural-metabolic causes, e.g., due to tumor, infections, and vascular malformations
Epilepsies of unknown cause

1989 for epilepsies and epileptic syndromes. According to these, seizures are categorized as generalized, focal, or unclassified based on clinical grounds and EEG evaluation.

- Partial (focal, local) seizures
  - Simple partial seizures (seizures without impairment of consciousness).
  - Complex partial seizures (seizures with impairment of consciousness).
  - Focal seizures may generalize secondarily. This is usually the case when epileptic activity in one hemisphere spreads to the other hemisphere.
- Generalized seizures
  - Absence seizures
  - Atypical absence seizures
  - Tonic seizures
  - Tonic-clonic seizures
  - Clonic seizures
  - Atonic seizures
  - Secondary tonic-clonic generalized seizures
- Unclassifiable seizures, usually due to lack of clinical data

Most generalized convulsions starting in adulthood are secondarily generalized. Convulsions in sleep are mostly secondarily generalized, whereas convulsions following awakening are usually primary generalized.

Figure 4.5 provides a diagram of the differential diagnosis of epileptic seizures.

4.7.3 Epileptic Syndromes

After classifying seizures as described above, the neurologist attempts to define the epilepsy syndrome. This is done by analyzing the following:

- Site of seizure onset (focal, generalized, or unclassifiable)
- Presumed etiology
  - Symptomatic, a structural or metabolic cause is known.
  - Cryptogenic, likely to be symptomatic; a structural cause is assumed but not identified.
  - Idiopathic, implies a presumed genetic cause with age-specific seizure onset, normal brain imaging, and usually responds well to AED therapy.

Table 4.2 shows the classification of epileptic syndromes as suggested in the *ILAE Proposal for Revised Terminology for Organization of Seizures and Epilepsies 2010*.

There are dozens of epilepsy syndromes, too many to list them all here. Localization-related epilepsy syndromes in adults may be caused by, e.g., trauma, hippocampal sclerosis, brain tumors, cortical dysplasias, and vascular CNS malformations. Some of these syndromes include:

- Temporal lobe seizures. Can be very frequent and may occur several times per day. Hippocampal sclerosis is the most common cause of adult epilepsy. Chapter 2 discusses the semiology of mesial and cortical/lateral temporal lobe epilepsy.
- Frontal lobe seizures. Since the frontal lobes are large, the semiology of frontal lobe seizures is varied. The so-called Jacksonian "march of convulsion" is the spreading of seizure activity along the primary motor cortex with characteristic sequence of motor phenomena in the arm and face. Occasionally, postictal transient focal weakness may occur (Todd's phenomenon). Supplementary motor area seizures are characteristically adverse seizures characterized by head and eyes turning away from the seizure focus and jerking or elevation of the arm contralateral to the focus (fencing, the sign of four). Frontal lobe epileptic seizures associated with

sleep tend to be short-lasting (<1 min), are secondarily generalized, and postictal confusion is generally lacking. There is bizarre motor activity such as cycling, punching, running, and shouting (hypermotor seizures). Frontal lobe seizures are therefore often mislabeled as psychogenic. Speech arrest or dysphasia suggests focus in the dominant hemisphere; the opposite is true if speech is rather unaffected during ictus.

- Occipital seizures. Often provoke contralateral visual (pseudo-) hallucinations and ipsilateral eye deviation to the side of the focus (see Chap. 2).

Idiopathic generalized epilepsies include, among others:

- Juvenile myoclonic epilepsy (JME). This epilepsy syndrome is associated with myoclonus in the early morning hours, generalized tonic-clonic seizures on awakening, and (to a lesser degree) absences and photosensitivity. Seizures occur particularly often following sleep deprivation and alcohol withdrawal. JME usually manifests in teenage years and, despite its name, is usually a lifelong disorder. Only one-third or less of all JME patients are seizure-free after 25 years and no longer need AED treatment (Cramfield and Cramfield 2009).
- Juvenile absence epilepsy (JAE). There is clinical overlap with JME. Absences are characterized by sudden onset and offset of impaired consciousness, sometimes accompanied by eyelid myoclonus or automatisms, and brief duration (5–10 s). Absences may be mild or severe and may occur several hundred times per day. They can be distinguished from complex partial seizures by their short duration, lack of postictal confusion, and their characteristic EEG pattern (sudden onset and termination of generalized 3 Hz spike-and-wave activity). Also, a typical absence seizure can often be reproduced by 1 or 2 min of hyperventilation, whereas a complex partial seizure cannot. Occasionally, absence status epilepticus leads to a "twilight" state in which patients are amnestic and not interacting normally but may remain able to perform basic activities.

- Childhood absence epilepsy (CAE), also known as pyknolepsy, is differentiated from JAE mainly by the age of onset.
- Generalized tonic-clonic seizures on awakening, without absence or myoclonus, also belong to the so-called idiopathic generalized epilepsies.

Idiopathic focal epilepsies are predominantly encountered in children:

- Benign epilepsies of childhood, such as benign childhood epilepsy with centrotemporal spikes, are usually self-limiting and do not always require treatment.
- Monogenic focal epilepsies. Although representing only a tiny proportion of all epileptic syndromes, more and more monogenic focal epilepsies are recognized, examples being autosomal dominant nocturnal frontal lobe epilepsy (NFLE) and epilepsy associated with glucose transporter type 1 (GLUT1) deficiency syndrome.

Symptomatic and cryptogenic generalized epilepsies are typically severe epilepsies with childhood onset and associated with intellectual disability, e.g.:

- West syndrome
- Lennox-Gastaut syndrome
- Myoclonic astatic epilepsy

For differential diagnosis of myoclonic epilepsies, please consult Sect. 4.15.2.

4.7.4 Status Epilepticus

Status epilepticus occurs because of failure of cellular mechanisms to terminate seizures. Ongoing seizure activity promotes drug resistance, neuronal energy failure, and accumulation of reactive oxygen metabolites, subsequently leading to neuronal death. Convulsive status epilepticus is associated with a high morbidity and mortality; the three most important prognostic factors are age, etiology, and seizure duration. Long-term consequences may include chronic epilepsy (because of enhanced epileptogenesis) and cognitive decline.

Traditionally, status epilepticus has been defined as a period of 30 min of continuous epileptic activity or repeated epileptic seizures without regaining of consciousness in between. Again, the ILAE has recently published revised criteria. According to these, status epilepticus is

"a condition resulting either from the failure of the mechanisms responsible for seizure termination or from the initiation of mechanisms, which lead to abnormally, prolonged seizures (after time point t1). It is a condition, which can have long-term consequences (after time point t2), including neuronal death, neuronal injury, and alteration of neuronal networks, depending on the type and duration of seizures. This definition is conceptual, with two operational dimensions: the first is the length of the seizure and the time point (t1) beyond which the seizure should be regarded as 'continuous seizure activity.' The second time point (t2) is the time of ongoing seizure activity after which there is a risk of long-term consequences. In the case of convulsive (tonic–clonic) SE, both time points (t1 at 5 min and t2 at 30 min) are based on animal experiments and clinical research" (Trinka et al. 2015).

For all practical purposes, since most epileptic seizures terminate within a few minutes, prolonged seizure activity exceeding 5 min should be regarded as status epilepticus and treated as such. Further, it is important to note that in many instances, status epilepticus is an acute symptomatic event occurring in patients without a previous diagnosis of epilepsy.

- A generalized tonic-clonic status epilepticus is always life-threatening. Its recognition is usually easy, but difficulties can arise in patients with prolonged status epilepticus. These patients may no longer have generalized convulsions but may exhibit only subtle signs of seizure activity such as twitching of the eyelids or corners of the mouth, as well as impaired consciousness. Also *psychogenic (nonepileptic) convulsions* may provide diagnostic difficulties, but typically, there are no signs of cardiorespiratory distress such as cyanosis or lactic acidosis, and EEG and serum levels of myoglobin and creatine kinase are normal. (Importantly, the rise of serum prolactin peaks at 20 min postictally and remains elevated for 60 min following a single generalized tonic-clonic seizure, but serum prolactin levels are normal in generalized tonic-clonic status epilepticus and, therefore, cannot be used to distinguish status epilepticus from prolonged psychogenic nonepileptic convulsions.)

- Nonconvulsive status epilepticus may follow a generalized tonic-clonic seizure or may arise by itself; it can be nonconvulsive generalized or focal. In nonconvulsive generalized status epilepticus, the patient typically exhibits bizarre behavior and has impaired consciousness. Focal nonconvulsive status epilepticus (sometimes termed epilepsia partialis continua) is a condition in which a patient has continuous focal motor seizures such as twitching in the face and the ipsilateral arm; it can be especially resistant to antiepileptic treatment and is always due to an underlying structural pathology, e.g., a brain tumor.
- Absence status epilepticus is a complication of absence epilepsy and affects children, only very occasionally adults.

All forms of status epilepticus are medical emergencies and require immediate antiepileptic therapy (Chap. 6) as well as evaluation and treatment of the underlying cause.

4.8   The Differential Diagnosis of Nonepileptic Seizures, Blackouts, and Drop Attacks

As stated in the previous chapter, the primary aim of the neurologist evaluating a seizure is to distinguish epileptic seizures from nonepileptic events (Fig. 4.5), including:

- Syncope
- Psychogenic nonepileptic attacks
- Other causes (Case 4.15)

Generations of physicians have remembered the differential diagnosis of epileptic seizures, syncope, and psychogenic attacks by using the mnemonic "fits, faints, and funny turns." As a rule, the likelihood of psychogenic attacks is higher in young patients, while syncope and TIA are common in the elderly. A good history, preferentially from both the patient and witnesses, as soon after the event as possible, is the best initial tool to settle the differential diagnosis. When evaluating a patient with a first-time seizure in the emergency room, it is advisable to ask for mobile phone numbers to call witnesses. Unprovoked events, aura, automatisms, convulsions, lateral tongue biting, posturing, incontinence, and postictal confusion all point toward epilepsy. If the diagnosis is uncertain, *ex juvantibus* prescription of AED is never a good idea as it exposes the patient to potentially dangerous and unnecessary medication. The chance is also very high that the problem will remain unsettled. Video-EEG monitoring, if available, is especially helpful in this situation.

Syncope is usually characterized by a specific history, as outlined below. In contrast to a generalized epileptic seizure, syncope is typically not associated with postictal confusion. Consequently, patients with syncope tend to wake up before the ambulance arrives, whereas following an epileptic seizure patients often regain full consciousness only in the ambulance or upon arrival at the hospital. Bear in mind that, due to temporary cortical hypoxia, syncope can lead to short-lasting myoclonic paroxysms in the extremities (convulsive syncope) and bladder emptying. A convulsive syncope is release of brainstem activity from cortical influence rather than an electrocortical seizure, but this is easily misinterpreted by the layman as signs of an epileptic seizure. Also, a minor tongue bite at the tip of the tongue may occasionally occur with syncope but not lateral tongue biting. (The explanation for this is that with syncope, sudden loss of muscle tone leads to protrusion of the tongue, and when the patient falls, the front teeth hit the tip of the tongue. In contrast, patients with a generalized tonic-clonic seizure "chew" on their tongue leading to the typical injuries of the lateral aspects of the tongue.)

Syncope can be divided into:

- Vasovagal syncope. This diagnosis is normally suggested by the situation (e.g., bathroom, public transport, and hot summer days), prodrome (sensation of blackout, pallor, tachycardia, sweating, and tremor), and short unconsciousness with or without random muscle twitching

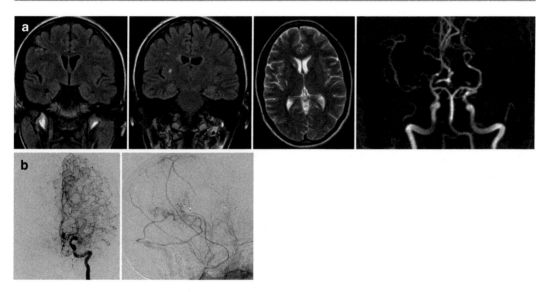

Case 4.15 Moyamoya disease. Within a year, a 25-year-old female experienced up to 100 spells of sensorimotor symptoms involving the left side of her body. These spells lasted only a few seconds. Sensory symptoms ("pins and needles") were roughly three times as frequent as motor spells ("funny twitches"). In addition, she had roughly one episode per month during which she suddenly felt close to fainting, although she never did. Neurological examination was normal. MRI showed a few scattered lesions within the territory of the right MCA, consistent with small infarcts (**a**, coronal FLAIR to the left and in the middle, axial T2 to the right). MR angiography revealed bilateral proximal MCA stenosis (observe that this was even more pronounced on the asymptomatic left MCA). Digital subtraction angiography (DSA) revealed a fine network of small collateral vessels (**b**). The patient was diagnosed with Moyamoya disease (which is a cryptogenic condition and requires exclusion of secondary factors such as sickle cell anemia; see also Case 4.23, Moyamoya phenomenon associated with Fanconi's anemia). She was referred for bilateral IC-EC bypass (**d**, DSA shows the bypass graft on the right). Following surgery, the frequency of her symptoms decreased dramatically (roughly 1–2 sensory spells per year)

and occasionally urinary incontinence (both of which can be mistaken as signs of epileptic seizure), followed by fast reorientation and a feeling of general exhaustion. Vasovagal syncope variants are cough and micturition syncope; the latter typically occurs in men who urinate at night while standing.

- Cardiac syncope comes suddenly and usually lacks a prodromal phase, although sometimes the patient may report cardiac palpitations, chest pain, and shortness of breath. Brief unconsciousness is followed by rapid recovery as in other forms of syncope. Often arrhythmias and other abnormal ECG signs are present. Cardiac monitoring, including telemetry/Holter ECG and echocardiography, is mandatory. Syncope and near-syncope due to the long QT syndrome tends to be misdiagnosed as epilepsy, often with fatal consequences for the patient—and his relatives who may suffer from the same condition.

- Orthostatic syncope. This is the typical syncope associated with dizziness and blackout after sudden change from the supine to the upright position. It occurs especially often in the young and the elderly and in those on antiparkinsonian medications and beta-blockers.
- Carotid sinus syncope. When due to hypersensitivity of the carotid sinus, it occurs in the elderly. Shaving, wearing a tight collar, or turning the head can trigger a sudden syncope.

Psychogenic nonepileptic seizures (PNES) and other attacks of unresponsiveness due to psychological reasons can be very difficult to distinguish from true epileptic seizures, but much of what has been said about the patient with functional palsy and psychogenic coma (see Sect. 3.11) is also true for the patient with PNES. Patients with functional seizures often have a characteristic way of presenting their history; they may refer extensively to their "seizures," but when the examiner inquires about the nature of these phenomena, they try to avoid giving detailed descriptions.

- PNES, or dissociative convulsions, may account for about 20% of referrals to epilepsy clinics. Seizure duration longer than 5 min, gradual seizure onset with fluctuating course, closure of eyes and the mouth, resistance to passive eye opening, violent movements with trashing of the head from side to side, opisthotonus and pelvic thrusting, hyperventilation, exclusive occurrence of witnessed seizures, and recall of the period of unresponsiveness are all common features in dissociative seizures but are rare to exceptional in epileptic seizures.[6]
- Panic attacks are suggested by the circumstances (e.g., shops, crowds, and claustrophobic situations), slow buildup with increasing anxiety, breathlessness, tingling, blurred vision, long duration, and tearfulness.

Other, usually far less common causes of acute unresponsiveness and paroxysmal motor phenomena include:

- Hypoglycemia. This is usually encountered in patients with diabetes mellitus. An unusual cause of hypoglycemic attacks is insulinoma, which often remains unrecognized for a long time.
- Neurocardiogenic syncope due to primary autonomic insufficiency, acute inflammatory demyelinating polyneuropathy, adrenal insufficiency, basilar migraine, cerebrovascular insufficiency (dominant vertebral artery and/or basilar artery stenosis, vertebral artery compression, subclavian steal), CSF flow obstruction (including ventriculoperitoneal shunt malfunction), multiple system atrophy (MSA) (in particular, MSA with predominantly autonomic features), postganglionic insufficiency, and syringomyelia.
- Eclampsia.
- Parasomnias such as REM sleep behavior disorder and sleep walking.
- Other neuroendocrine tumors (besides insulinoma) with paroxystic systemic symptoms include pheochromocytoma and carcinoid (Case 4.16).

The following phenomena, sometimes confused with epileptic seizures, occur by definition without loss of consciousness:

- Drop attacks. These may be due to vertebrobasilar ischemia (either due to stenosis of the basilar/vertebral arteries or associated with a subclavian steal syndrome), posterior fossa lesions (including Arnold-Chiari malformations), hydrocephalus, intraventricular tumors, inner ear disorders (e.g., Ménière's disease, migrainous vertigo), and intermittent cervical cord compression. Cryptogenic drop attacks are relatively frequent and mainly affect middle-aged women.[7]
- Cataplexy is triggered most often by laughter, although any emotional stimulus can induce it. Occasionally, cataplexy may also occur in situations devoid of any specific emotional content but associated with certain postures such as bending forward. Loss of muscular tone may be complete or discrete and unremarkable to anyone other than the patient. A patient with narcolepsy may suffer from cataplexy several times a day or only once or twice during a lifetime, and therefore, a careful history is crucial to detect the presence of mild cataplexy. The duration of hypotonia in cataplexy ranges from several seconds to a few minutes (rarely longer), followed by complete recovery. It is useful to check tendon reflexes when observing a

---

[6] Beware of the fact that coexistent epilepsy is found in up to 20% of those with dissociative seizures. Also, many bizarre motor features such as pelvic thrusting and bicycling, while commonly seen in PNES, may occur in frontal lobe seizures. Further, it must be borne in mind that panic and other emotions may be part of a temporal lobe seizure. In addition, resistance to passive eye opening is frequently seen in patients with NMDAR encephalitis. Lastly, the "teddy bear sign" (referring to adults who bring stuffed toy animals to an epilepsy monitoring unit), often suggested to be associated with PNES, is not a very reliable sign.

[7] In elderly patients with sudden falls and presumed drop attacks, however, the absence of a history of loss of consciousness is unreliable. More often than not, syncope is the correct diagnosis.

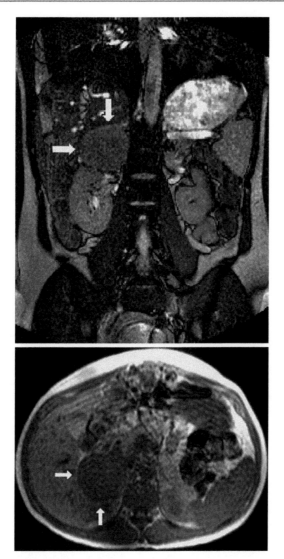

Case 4.16 Pheochromocytoma. A 30-year-old previously healthy woman in the 26th week of her first pregnancy was referred from her gynecologist because of new-onset episodic frontal throbbing headaches of moderate to severe intensity, accompanied by nausea, vomiting, and hyperventilation. Episodes occurred up to five times daily and lasted from a few minutes to 1 h. On two occasions, the patient had noted a scintillating scotoma in her left visual field. She had no history of migraine. Since proteinuria and edema were absent, preeclampsia had been ruled out by her gynecologist prior to referral. Neurological examination, including fundoscopy, was unremarkable. The patient had no fever and blood pressure was 130/85 mmHg in both arms. MRI of the head including MR angiography and a lumbar puncture were normal. However, on day 3 after admission, the patient was observed during a severe headache with marked tachycardia, sweating, pallor, tremor, and anxiety. Blood pressure was 220/110 mmHg, pulse rate 115 beats/min. A working diagnosis of pheochromocytoma was made. Repeated 24 h urinary catecholamine testing revealed increased levels of norepinephrine, epinephrine, metanephrines, and vanillylmandelic acid. MRI of the abdomen showed a 6 × 6 cm solid right adrenal mass (**a, b**). Genetic testing for mutations in the *RET*, *VHL*, *SDHB*, and *SDHD* genes was negative. Using a multidisciplinary approach involving endocrinologists, anesthesiologists, surgeons, and neonatologists, it was decided to treat the patient with phenoxybenzamine (α-adrenoceptor antagonist) and await fetal maturity. Headaches vanished completely. In the 31st week of pregnancy, the patient underwent an uncomplicated cesarean section combined with removal of the adrenal mass. Release of catecholamines from a pheochromocytoma is related to changes in blood flow or necrosis within the tumor and to any activity that mechanically compresses it. Thus, pregnancy may uncover a pheochromocytoma due to fetal movement, uterine growth, or delivery. Undiagnosed pheochromocytoma is associated with maternal and fetal mortality of up to 58% and 56%, respectively. With an established antenatal diagnosis, maternal mortality decreases to 2% and fetal mortality to 15% (adapted with permission from Kondziella et al. (2007a, b))

possible cataplexy attack; reflexes are absent during an attack but present in between. Status cataplecticus ("limp man syndrome") is excessive daytime sleepiness associated with frequent episodes of sudden buckling of the knees without falls. It is a rare, but important, differential diagnosis because it may be confused with a functional gait disorder. For all practical purposes, cataplexy is pathognomic for narcolepsy, although there have been case reports of cataplexy in Niemann-Pick type C disease. (See also Sect. 4.10.)

- Some paroxysmal symptoms in the young are highly characteristic for MS; these include brief (seconds-minutes) and very frequent (50–100/day) paroxysms of dysarthria and/or ataxia or unilateral dystonia responding to carbamazepine. The paroxysms are due to ephaptic transmission at sites of demyelination, often at the brainstem level.

- TGA, although frightening for the patient, is usually harmless, and there is no increased risk of developing stroke. When a reliable account from a witness is available, TGA is easy to diagnose (see Case 2.18).

- Transient ischemic symptoms, including, for instance, the rare syndrome of limb-shaking TIA (usually seen with high-grade contralateral ICA stenosis) and the capsular warning syndrome (transient lacunar ischemia that typically precedes a capsular infarction).

- Transient sensorimotor symptoms associated with cerebral amyloid angiopathy ("amyloid spells") (Case 4.17).

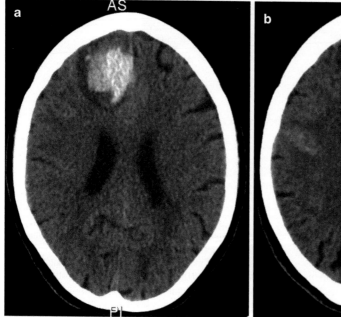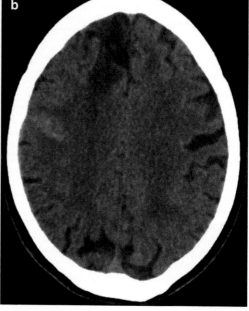

Case 4.17 Amyloid spells: Jacksonian sensory march due to cerebral amyloid angiopathy (CAA). A 71-year-old male with a history of hypertension and chronic obstructive lung disease had sudden onset of bizarre behavior and headache. CT of the brain revealed a right frontal lobar hematoma (**a**). The patient made an uneventful recovery. Four years later, he presented with complaints of sensory spells starting in the fingers of his left hand, progressing to the arm and finally spreading to the left side of his face within 10 min. He had had nine such episodes within the previous 8 days. Neurological examination was unremarkable except for slight spasticity in both legs. In addition, despite a normal Mini-Mental State Examination score (29/30), he showed the "head-turning sign," that is, he frequently addressed his wife when being asked questions, suggestive of a mild cognitive deficit. CT of the brain showed a right post-central sulcal hemorrhage, compatible with his Jacksonian sensory marches (**b**). Apart from the previous lobar hemorrhage, T2-weighted magnetic resonance imaging revealed multiple atraumatic convexal hemosiderin deposits, confluent white matter hyperintensities (**c**) and microbleeds (not shown). According to the modified Boston criteria, the patient was diagnosed with probable cerebral amyloid angiopathy ("definitive" CAA requires a full postmortem examination). The pathophysiology of recurrent paresthesias or "amyloid spells" remains not fully understood, but cortical spreading depolarizations (as opposed to focal epileptic seizure activity) are a likely mechanism

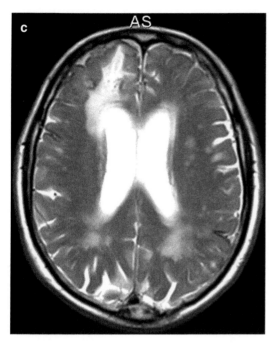

Case 4.17 (continued)

4.9   The Differential Diagnosis of Vertigo and Dizziness

Although many patients use the terms vertigo and dizziness synonymously, the neurologist should carefully distinguish between vertigo on one hand and dizziness or light-headedness on the other. Vertigo is best defined as an illusion of motion, the false sensation of movement (Chap. 2), and it is either of central (brainstem, cerebellopontine angle, cerebellum) or peripheral origin (inner ear, vestibular system) (Fig. 4.6). Dizziness or light-headedness, in contrast, is far more unspecific, and the patient may use these terms to describe problems of gait and balance, an experience of presyncope, a feeling of being unwell, visual impairment, or even a state of depressed mood.

4.9.1   Vertigo of Central Origin

As described earlier (Chaps. 2 and 3):

- A patient with vertigo due to a brainstem lesion will almost always have other signs and symptoms of impaired CN and sensorimotor pathway function.

- Likewise, a patient with vertigo due to a cerebellopontine lesion (e.g., a vestibular schwannoma) will typically have signs and symptoms referable to the cerebellum and/or the adjacent CNs (e.g., decreased corneal sensation, peripheral facial palsy, sensory hearing loss).
- However, a patient with a cerebellar lesion may occasionally exhibit monosymptomatic vertigo, and then, the key to the correct diagnosis is careful examination of the eye movements as outlined in Chap. 3 ("three-step oculomotor bedside examination").
- Monosymptomatic vertigo has also been described with certain supratentorial lesions, including the anterior insula and the parietal lobes, and of course, it may reflect a focal seizure in patients with temporal lobe epilepsy.
- Vertigo may also occur with migraine, MS, and other neurological disorders, as well as due to medication side effects and intoxications.
- Rupture of an intracranial demoid cyst is another differential diagnosis of acute vertigo of central origin (Case 4.18).

4.9.2   Vertigo of Peripheral Origin

The hallmark of peripheral vertigo is the distinct sensation of relative motion with the visual world (Fig. 4.6). Peripheral vertigo typically comes in spells and usually lasts seconds as benign positional vertigo, minutes as in Ménière's disease, or hours as in vestibular neuritis. Frequent accompanying symptoms are hearing loss, tinnitus, and aural fullness. A diagnosis of benign positional vertigo, for instance, is very likely in patients with short vertigo brought on by a change of position such as rolling over in bed. The onset is sudden, while the offset is usually less well defined.

The most common associated disorders include:

- BPPV
- Vestibular neuritis
- Ménière's disease
- Infections (labyrinthitis)
- Motion sickness
- Labyrinthine fistula
- Trauma
- Intoxications (e.g., alcohol, quinine, aminoglycosides, NSAID)

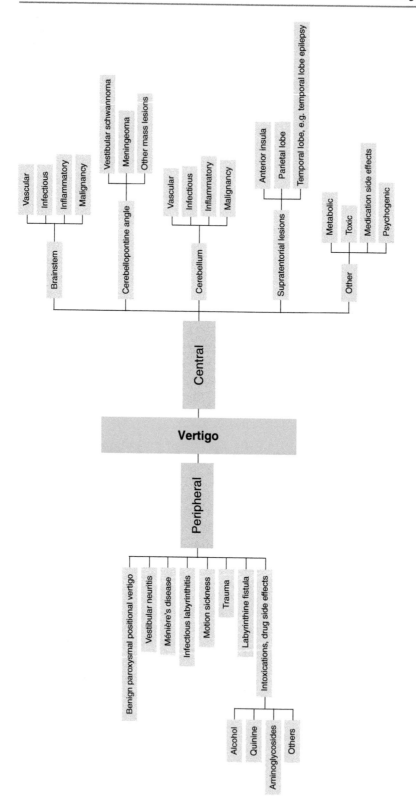

Fig. 4.6 Differential diagnosis of vertigo

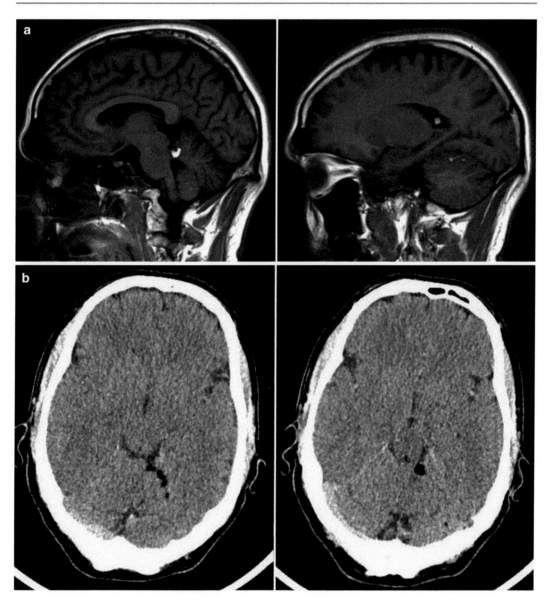

Case 4.18 Ruptured intracranial dermoid cyst. A 51-year-old male with a history of anxiety was admitted because of sudden onset of vertigo and headache. The ENT team had reviewed the patient and had not found evidence of a peripheral vertigo. Neurological examination revealed saccadic pursuit, difficulties with finger-nose and heel-shin tests, and moderate gait ataxia. The attending neurologist ordered an MRI, suspecting an acute cerebrovascular event from the posterior circulation. However, MR angiography and DWI were normal. Instead, T1-weighted imaging revealed a midline cystic lesion at the level of the midbrain and scattered bright signal in several cerebellar sulci (**a**). Whereas the cystic lesion was enhancing with gadolinium contrast, the cerebellar lesions were spontaneously hyperintense. On CT, the latter lesions appeared very dark (−100 Hounsfield units), which was consistent with fat (**b**). The patient made an uneventful recovery. Intracranial dermoid cysts are benign congenital lesions of ectodermal origin and comprise less than 1% of all intracranial tumors. They typically occur in the midline, often in the sellar/parasellar region, but may also be found in the posterior fossa. With the accumulation of epithelial desquamation and glandular secretion, they may gradually enlarge and suddenly rupture. Their material is spread around adjacent brain regions and appears as fat on MRI (spontaneous bright signal on T1) and CT (very dark signal). Most patients present with acute neurological complaints. Imaging reveals the ruptured cyst, but a previous scan showing the *intact* cyst is usually not available. The diagnosis is therefore based on the history, the typical neuroradiological appearance, and the exclusion of other conditions. Prognosis is excellent, although some patients may develop aseptic chemical meningitis due to inflammation related to lipid contents circulating in the CSF

4.9.3 Dizziness and Light-Headedness

The differential diagnoses of dizziness and light-headedness are vast and include (Fig. 4.6):

- Postural hypotension, e.g., dehydration and autonomic dysfunction
- Cardiological disorders, e.g., congestive heart failure and arrhythmias
- Psychiatric disorders, e.g., depression and anxiety
- Trauma, e.g., concussion and whiplash
- Medication, e.g., antidepressants, AED, aminoglycosides and other antibiotics, antihypertensive drugs, anxiolytics, sedating drugs, chemotherapeutic agents, diuretics, and salicylic acids

4.10 The Differential Diagnosis of Sleep Disorders

Sleep disorders are best categorized into those that are common and those that are not.

- The most common sleep disturbances are due to poor sleep hygiene, simple worries, depression, anxiety, alcohol, medication side effects, shift work, jet lag, sleep apnea syndrome, chronic pain, restless legs syndrome, periodic leg movements in sleep, and chronic diseases of neurological (MS, parkinsonism), and non-neurological origin (e.g., anemia, congestive heart failure, hepatitis, diabetes, hypo- and hyperthyroidism).
- Somewhat less common are:
  - REM sleep behavior disorder. Patients have vivid dreams, and during the stage of REM sleep, they may violently act out their dreams. Following a prolonged interval that may last years or even decades, most patients with idiopathic REM sleep behavior disorder will eventually develop a neurodegenerative disorder, most commonly one of the synucleinopathies (Parkinson's disease, DLB, and MSA). The prevalence of REM sleep behavior disorder is approximately 0.5% but

is much higher among patients with neurodegenerative disease or narcolepsy and among patients taking antidepressants.

  - Epileptic seizures arising from sleep, e.g., nocturnal frontal lobe epilepsy (NFLE).
  - Parasomnias (e.g., somnambulism, sleep automatism, and sleep terrors). Accurately diagnosing sleep-related events, and particularly distinguishing parasomnias from other sleep disorders such as NFLE, can be challenging. Important clues from the history pointing to a parasomnia include the time of onset during the night (NREM parasomnias typically occur 1–2 h after falling asleep, whereas seizures tend to occur soon thereafter or just before wakening in the morning), the number of events per night (only once or twice for parasomnias), and duration (several minutes, whereas typically less than 1 min for seizures). Patients (exceptionally) reporting a clear recall of events are more likely to have NFLE, and while both groups of disorders frequently arise during childhood, onset from mid-teens to age 50 years suggests NFLE. Even later onset raises the possibility of REM sleep behavior disorder. Lastly, whereas complex motor phenomena can occur with both NFLE and parasomnias, prominent bipedal ("cycling") automatisms strongly suggest NFLE. Using the Frontal Lobe Epilepsy and Parasomnias scale (Derry et al. 2006) and admitting the patient to the epilepsy monitoring unit (if available) may help to clarify the situation.
  - Narcolepsy has a prevalence of approximately 0.025–0.05%. The symptoms of narcolepsy are due to instability of the transition of sleep and wake, as well as of REM sleep and non-REM sleep. The classic tetrad consists of excessive daytime sleepiness with imperative sleep attacks, cataplexy, sleep paralysis, and hallucinations upon falling asleep or upon awaking. Cataplexy is triggered by sudden emotions and can be socially stigmatizing (e.g., jaw sagging and facial slackening with laughter). However, the degree of cataplexy

ranges from frequent, complete loss of muscle tone leading to sudden collapse to very mild symptoms, hardly noticed by the patient and only occurring a few times in a lifetime. (See Sect. 4.8 for a detailed description of cataplexy.) Further, some patients with otherwise typical features of narcolepsy lack cataplexy entirely (the so-called monosymptomatic narcolepsy or narcolepsy without cataplexy). Indeed, the complete tetrad of symptoms is present in only a minority of patients (ca. 15%).

It is less well appreciated that narcoleptics may experience episodes of automatic behavior and amnesia, lasting for seconds to hours, usually when the patient is alone and performing monotonous tasks such as driving. The patient gradually loses track of what is going on but continues to perform routine tasks automatically, until he is interrupted by a concerned observer. Characteristically, the patient has complete amnesia for the attack.

In addition, narcolepsy can occasionally be associated with psychosis exceeding the usual hypnagogic hallucinations. This association can be threefold: a "psychotic form" of narcolepsy, narcolepsy and an unrelated psychiatric disorder, or narcolepsy and drug-induced psychosis (due to treatment with stimulants such as amphetamines). The differential diagnosis is rather straightforward. If treatment of narcolepsy abolishes psychotic features, the diagnosis is a "psychotic form" of narcolepsy; if daytime sleepiness and other features of narcolepsy improve following treatment but psychotic features remain, it is likely that the patient has both narcolepsy and an unrelated psychiatric disorder; if psychosis occurs after initiation of amphetamine treatment, it is likely a drug-induced psychotic disorder (Case 4.19).

- Rarities include Kleine-Levin syndrome (usually male adolescents with periodic hypersomnia, hyperphagia, hypersexuality, aggression, and confusion; see Chap. 2), idiopathic hypersomnia (a diagnosis of exclusion), fatal familial insomnia (a hereditary

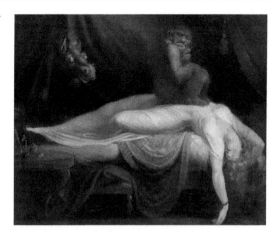

Case 4.19 Narcolepsy. A 35-year-old female was referred by her psychiatrist with a working diagnosis of epilepsy with focal seizures with altered awareness. From the age of 15, she had experienced recurrent episodes of depression, anxiety, psychosis, and persecutory delusions. She also complained of visual, auditory, and tactile hallucinations, such as the perception of men and animals sitting on her chest, preventing her from breathing freely, and pulling on her arms and legs. She was on aripiprazole (a second-generation atypical antipsychotic) and a benzodiazepine at bedtime. MR of the brain and EEG were normal. A more detailed history revealed that the hallucinations involving men and animals sitting on her chest occurred when the patient was falling asleep or during the morning upon awakening. In these situations, she was unable to move or talk. Strong emotions could lead to sudden loss of muscle tone. The patient also complained of daytime sleepiness and of suddenly falling asleep in monotonous situations. Because of hypnagogic hallucinations, sleep paralysis, sleep attacks, and cataplexy, she was diagnosed as having narcolepsy. A multiple sleep latency test showed an overall sleep latency of less than 3 min and an average latency of REM sleep of 1 min in four out of four naps, corroborating the clinical diagnosis. (Supplementary measurement of the CSF hypocretin level was not available at that time.) Despite treatment for narcolepsy, paranoid delusions and mood disturbances persisted, and consequently, the patient was diagnosed with both narcolepsy and a schizoaffective disorder. The patient's hypnagogic hallucinations and sleep paralysis strikingly resemble *The Nightmare* by Johann Heinrich Füssli (Swiss painter, 1741–1825), on exhibition at the Detroit Institute of Arts (reproduced with permission from The Bridgeman Art Library Ltd.)

prion disease characterized by progressive loss of deep sleep, abnormal REM sleep, dysautonomia, neuropsychological features, and motor signs), and African trypanosomiasis (the classic sleeping sickness).

4.11 The Differential Diagnosis of TIA and Stroke

Stroke is due to (Fig. 4.7):

- Ischemia in 80–85% of cases
- Intraparenchymal hemorrhage in 10–15%
- Subarachnoidal bleeding in 2–5%

The frequency of etiological causes of ischemic stroke varies somewhat according to different sources and population-based series, but roughly, ischemic stroke is due to:

- Cardiac embolism in 30% of cases.
- Large vessel disease in 25%.
- Small vessel disease in 20%.
- Unusual causes in 5%.
- The rest are of undetermined origin (20%).[8]

Intraparenchymal hemorrhage can occur with:

- Hypertensive bleeds
- Vascular malformations
- Coagulation disturbances
- Malignancy (usually hemorrhagic tumor necrosis)
- Other conditions

Subarachnoidal bleeding may be:

- Aneurysmal
- Non-aneurysmal

4.11.1 Ischemic Stroke: Clinical Presentation and Classification

Focal neurological symptoms consistent with the diagnosis of stroke include acute development of:

- Motor signs (e.g., complete or incomplete hemiparesis).

- Sensory impairment (e.g., numbness in a complete or incomplete hemi-distribution), visual disturbances (monocular blindness, visual field defects, cortical blindness).
- Loss of specific higher cognitive functions (fluent, nonfluent aphasia, visuospatial neglect).
- Brainstem signs such as dysphagia, diplopia, dysarthria, vertigo, and ataxia usually suggest stroke when they occur acutely and together with long tract signs.

In contrast, light-headedness, syncope, confusion, drop attacks, hearing impairment, tinnitus, and acute fatigue almost never indicate stroke, if occurring in isolation. As stated above (Chap. 3), analysis of eye movements is crucial for the clinical differential diagnosis of otogenic vertigo vs. a cerebellar stroke.

When evaluating a patient with stroke at the bedside, it is advisable to try to classify the origin of the present deficits as belonging to the lacunar syndromes (LACS), the posterior circulation syndromes (POCS), the partial anterior circulation syndromes (PACS), and the total anterior circulation syndromes (TACS). Classification of stroke syndromes according to the Oxfordshire Community Stroke Project is easy to memorize and has reasonable positive and negative prediction when compared with brain imaging.

- LACS are characterized by the presence of motor and/or sensory signs that involve at least two out of three areas (face, arm, leg; the limbs should be completely involved). Importantly, higher cortical deficits and visual field defects are lacking. LACS include:
    - Pure motor hemiparesis (pure motor stroke)
    - Pure hemi-sensory deficit (pure sensory stroke)
    - Sensorimotor hemiparesis (sensorimotor stroke)
    - Ataxic hemiparesis (including the so-called dysarthria-clumsy hand syndrome and limb-shaking TIA)

LACS may be associated with the capsular warning syndrome ("stuttering lacune"), i.e., clusters of TCI due to a single vascular lesion of the internal capsule, usually preceding manifest stroke.

---

[8] Most cases of cryptogenic ischemic stroke are probably due to undetected paroxysmal atrial fibrillation, hence the need for prolonged cardiac monitoring using telemetry/Holter ECG monitor.

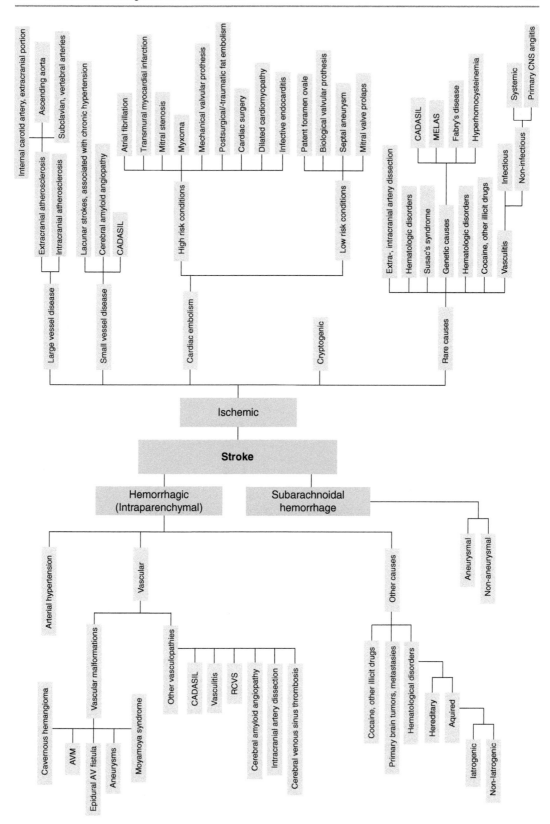

Fig. 4.7 Differential diagnosis of stroke

- POCS are suspected when the patient presents with impairment of one or more CNs, diplopia, dysphagia, dysarthria, cerebellar dysfunction, homonymous hemianopia, and cortical blindness. Motor and/or sensory deficits may be unilateral or bilateral.
- PACS include one or more of the following: unilateral motor or sensory deficits, aphasia, or visuospatial neglect (which may or may not be combined with homonymous hemianopia). Motor or sensory deficits are sometimes less extensive than in LACS, e.g., restricted to the hand.
- TACS involve hemiplegia and homonymous hemianopia contralateral to the lesion and either aphasia or visuospatial neglect. There may or may not be a sensory deficit contralateral to the lesion

The patient with stroke or TIA is investigated in order to define the etiology of the event. As already stated, *cerebral ischemia and TIA* may be due to:

- Large vessel atherosclerosis:
  - Extracranial, proximal aorta, vertebral and subclavian arteries, and ICA
  - Intracranial, traditionally regarded as being somewhat more common in patients of African and Asian descent: ICA, MCA, ACA, PCA, vertebral arteries, basilar artery, and Circle of Willis
- Embolism from the heart:
  - High risk: atrial fibrillation, mitral stenosis, acute myocardial infarction, intracardiac thrombus, myxoma, mechanical valve prosthesis, cardiac surgery, severe dilated cardiomyopathy, and infective endocarditis
  - Low risk: patent foramen ovale, interatrial septal aneurysm, mitral valve prolapse, and tissue valve prosthesis
- Intracranial small vessel occlusion:
  - Small vessel disease of the deep perforators due to hypertension
  - Others, e.g., cerebral autosomal dominant arteriopathy with subcortical infarcts and

leukoencephalopathy (CADASIL) (Case 4.20) and Susac's syndrome (Case 4.21)[9]
- Other examples include:
  - Extra- and intracranial artery dissection. Together with cardioembolism, this is the most common stroke etiology seen in young patients (20%). Intracranial artery dissection is much rarer than extracranial dissection but is associated with risk of secondary subarachnoidal bleeding.
  - Vasculitis, either as primary CNS angiitis or due to secondary causes such as infections, drugs, and systemic inflammatory disorders.
  - Migraine.
  - Venous infarctions due to sinus venous thrombosis or dural venous fistulas.
  - Metabolic disorders such as MELAS, Fabry disease, and homocysteinuria.
  - Hematologic disorders, including polycythemia rubra vera, leukemia, and sickle cell disease.
  - Various intracranial vascular malformations.
  - Heat stroke, if severe, can lead to large bilateral cerebellar infarcts due to particular susceptibility of cerebellar Purkinje cells to heat, and subsequent brain herniation can be fatal.

See Sect. 4.11.4 for a detailed account of rare causes of ischemic stroke.

4.11.2 Space-Occupying Ischemic Stroke

Space-occupying focal brain edema because of ischemic stroke occurs in the anterior circulation (often referred to as malignant MCA infarction) and in the posterior circulation. The prognosis is poor without treatment; the mortality in malignant MCA infarction approaches 80%. Twelve to 72 h after stroke onset, patients with large MCA infarction may develop head-

---

[9] Susac's syndrome involves microangiopathy of the brain, retina, and cochlea; it usually affects young women (female/male ratio 3:1) and leads to encephalopathy, retinopathy, and hearing loss.

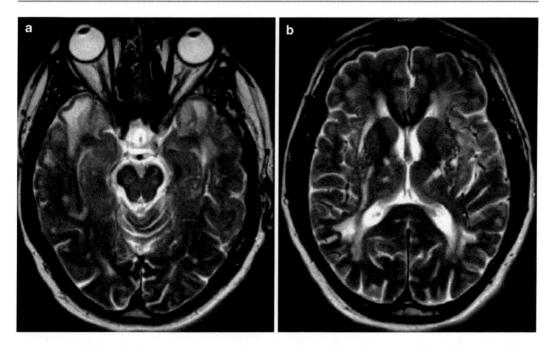

Case 4.20 Cerebral autosomal dominant arteriopathy with subcortical infarcts and leukoencephalopathy (CADASIL). A 44-year-old female presented with an acute episode of confusion, decreased consciousness, seizures, and elevated body temperature but spontaneously recovered within 7 days. Her former medical history included migraine-like headaches since her twenties and repetitive stroke-like events in her late 30s. Her mother had developed cognitive impairment in her 50s.

T2-weighted MRI showed confluating white matter signal changes (**a**, **b**). The presence of white matter hyperintensity in both anterior temporal poles (**a**) and external capsules (**b**) is highly specific for CADASIL. The diagnosis was confirmed by genetic testing showing a mutation of the *NOTCH 3* gene located on chromosome 19. The initial episode of acute encephalopathy was consistent with "CADASIL coma," an under-recognized feature of the disease

ache, decreased consciousness, worsening pyramidal signs, and third nerve palsy because of cerebral herniation. Death occurs typically between 2 and 7 days after stroke onset. Clinical risk factors include younger age (because of lesser degree of cerebral atrophy and intracranial space reserve) and severe clinical deficits (NIHSS ≥20 with dominant and ≥15 with non-dominant hemisphere stroke). Radiologic risk factors are large infarction (early hypodensity of >50% MCA territory, additional involvement of ACA and PCA territory) and developing mass effect with anteroseptal shift of more than 5 mm and pineal shift of more than 3 mm. Patients with high likelihood of developing malignant MCA infarction should be admitted

to a neurointensive care unit for observation; fatal brain herniation can develop within a few hours.

Space-occupying ischemic stroke in the cerebellum is often fatal because of brainstem compression and acute obstructive hydrocephalus. Admission to a neurointensive care unit is mandatory. Ominous signs include progressive CN and pyramidal tract deficits, vomiting, hypertension, bradycardia, and especially a decreasing level of consciousness. Radiologic predictors for developing space-occupying edema are hypodensity of two-thirds or more of the cerebellar hemisphere, compression and/or displacement of the fourth ventricle, brainstem, and basal cisterns, supratentorial hydrocephalus, and hemorrhagic infarct transformation.

Case 4.21 Susac's syndrome. Characterized by the triad of perceptive hearing loss, branch retinal artery occlusions, and encephalopathy; Susac's syndrome occurs mainly in young women. In 80% of patients, the complete triad is initially lacking. This was also the case for a 28-year-old female with a 3-month history of visual disturbances, confusion, incontinence, and gait difficulties but normal hearing. Coronal and axial T2-weighted MRI showed characteristic multifocal lesions, predominantly of the white matter, and including the corpus callosum (**a**). Lesions of the corpus callosum are typically centrally located and appear circular ("snowballs"), while the lesions in MS involve the undersurface at the septal interface and have a fingerlike appearance (hence, the term Dawson fingers). Ophthalmological evaluation, including fluorescence angiography, revealed visual field defects, retinal infarctions, and branch retinal artery occlusion (here shown for the left eye, **b**; courtesy of Marianne Wegener, Department of Ophthalmology, Rigshospitalet, Copenhagen, Denmark). Following immunosuppressive treatment, the patient fully recovered except for lasting visual field defects (adapted with permission from Wegener et al. (2009))

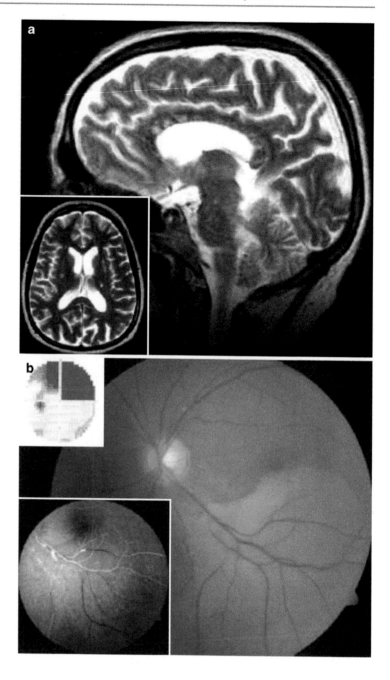

4.11.3 Transitory Ischemic Attacks: Definitions and Risk Assessment

In contrast to stroke, TIA is traditionally defined as focal deficits of cerebrovascular origin that are reversible within 24 h, although in practice nearly all TIAs last less than 1 h. With the advent of DWI, it has become clear that many cerebrovascular events defined clinically as TIAs indeed are manifest cerebral infarctions. Therefore, a recent task force group suggested dropping the time criterion and adapting the following "tissue-based definition of transient ischemic attack (TIA): a transient episode of neurological dysfunction caused by focal brain, spinal cord, or retinal ischemia, without acute infarction" (Easton et al. 2009). The pathophysiology behind TIA and ischemic cerebral infarction is identical. Therefore, every TIA should be diagnosed and treated according to the same principles that apply for ischemic stroke.

The risk of stroke following TIA is much higher than previously thought, and it is highest immediately after the event. The following numbers show that stroke and TIA need immediate diagnostic and therapeutic attention. In a pooled analysis, the early risk of stroke was 3.1% at 2 days, 5.2% at 7 days, 8.0% at 30 days, and 9.2% at 90 days (Giles and Rothwell 2007). Yet, when only studies with active outcome ascertainment were considered, risk of stroke increased to 9.9%, 13.4%, and 17.3% at day 2, 30, and 90, respectively. Stroke risk has been lower in studies from specialist stroke services offering emergency treatment and higher in population-based studies without urgent intervention (Wu et al. 2007). Emergent diagnostic evaluation and initiation of secondary prevention in TIA patients treated at specialist centers is associated with an impressive stroke risk reduction of 80% (Rothwell et al. 2007; Lavallée et al. 2007).

The ABCD2 score, first published by Johnston et al. (2007), is an excellent way to assess the risk of a subsequent stroke in the days immediately following initial presentation with TIA. The score has a minimum score of 0 and a maximum score of 7. It is based on five components:

- Age (≥ 60 year =1 point)
- Blood pressure (systolic ≥ 140 mmHg and/or diastolic ≥ 90 mmHg =1 point)
- Clinical features (unilateral weakness =2 points; speech disturbance without weakness =1 point)
- Duration of symptoms in minutes (≥ 60 = 2 points; 10–59 = 1 point)
- Diabetes (present =1 point)

High-risk patients have an ABCD2 score of 6–7 (8.1% risk of stroke occurrence within 2 days), moderate-risk patients of 4–5 (4.1%), and low-risk patients of 0–3 (1.0%).

4.11.4   Rare Causes of Ischemic Stroke and Transitory Ischemic Attacks

Although rare causes only account for a minor proportion of all ischemic strokes, they comprise a plethora of diagnoses, including cardioembolic, inflammatory, and genetic disorders. The differential diagnosis is challenging but of particular importance because these disorders often affect young individuals (e.g., monogenetic disorders such as *COL4A1* mutations); they typically require sophisticated diagnostic methods (e.g., fluorescence angiography in Susac's syndrome), and many of them are treatable (e.g., enzyme replacement for Fabry disease). Similar to the more common causes of ischemic stroke, rare ischemic stroke syndromes can be classified into cardioembolic, large and small vessel disorders, and others.

- Rare causes of cardioembolic stroke
  - Depending on the virulence of the causative agent, infective endocarditis may or may not be associated with systemic symptoms such as fever, malaise, and weight loss. Petechial rash, including subungual splinter hemorrhages are highly indicative but may easily be overlooked. The radiological hallmark is multi-territorial cerebral infarctions due to septic emboli. The definite diagnosis requires echocardiography showing valvular vegetations and positive blood cultures. Of note, mycotic aneurysms may arise during the ensuing weeks and months due to inflammatory vessel wall changes secondary to septic material. In contrast to classical aneurysms that typically arise around the Circle of Willis, mycotic aneurysms are located in distal artery branches (Case 4.22). Due to their high bleeding risk, endovascular treatment by coiling might be considered.
  - Myxoma is a myxoid tumor of primitive connective tissue. It is usually benign and the most common primary cardiac tumor in adults. Like infective endocarditis, it is

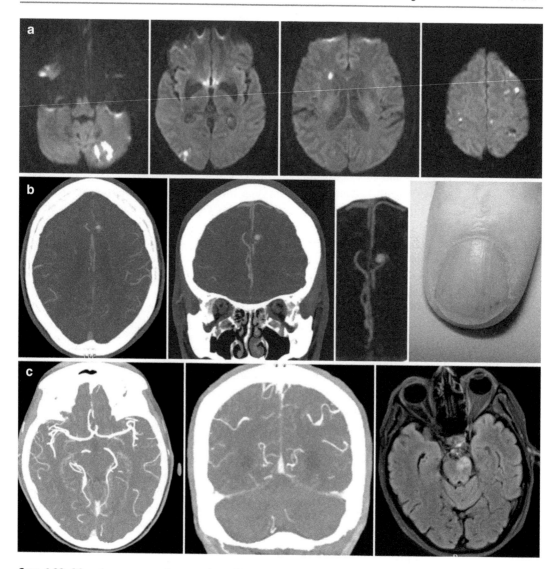

Case 4.22 Mycotic aneurysms due to endocarditis and myxoma. A 64-year-old female presented subacutely over 7 days with fever, confusion, and gait disturbance. Examination revealed petechia, including subungual splinter hemorrhages, cerebellar ataxia of the left extremities (note the infarction in the left cerebellar hemisphere), and a cardiac murmur. MR DWI showed a typical embolic stroke pattern with multiple lesions both in the anterior and posterior circulations on both sides (**a**). On CT angiography, a mycotic aneurysm was noted in the left ACA territory (**b**). A 71-year-old female presented with a comparable history of subacute neurological deficits, low grade fever, and a cardiac murmur, although her blood cultures were negative. MRI revealed a left-sided pontine ischemic stroke (**c**, right). The patient was diagnosed with

myxoma following echocardiography and was referred for immediate thoracic surgery to prevent further embolism. On follow-up, CT angiography revealed mycotic aneurysms of distal branches within the left distal PCA and both MCA territories (**c**, left), and digital subtraction angiography documented additional aneurysms (**d**). Mycotic aneurysms can arise during the ensuing weeks and months due to inflammatory vessel wall changes secondary to septic or tumorous material. In contrast to classical saccular or "berry" aneurysms that typically occur at vessel bifurcations due to local vessel wall degeneration, mycotic aneurysms are located in distal artery branches as seen here in both cases. Due to their high bleeding risk, endovascular treatment of aneurysms by coiling may be considered

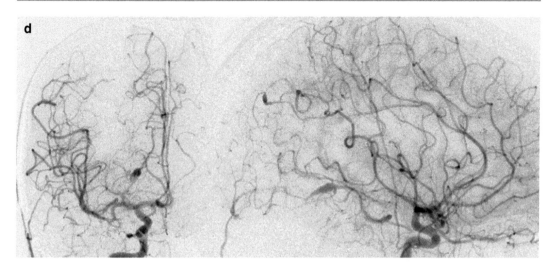

Case 4.22 (continued)

associated with systemic symptoms such as low-grade fever, multi-territorial cerebral infarctions, as well as mycotic aneurysms (see Case 4.22). Echocardiography may also reveal even less common benign primary tumors such as papillary fibroelastomas, fibromas, rhabdomyomas, teratomas, and lipomas. Malignant primary tumors include sarcoma, lymphoma, and mesothelioma.

– Whereas infective endocarditis and myxoma have a high risk for embolization, low-risk sources of cardiac embolization include atrial septum defects such as a patent foramen ovale (PFO) and pulmonary AV fistulas. Stroke may occur due to paradoxical cerebral emboli passing through a right-to-left shunt. In general, it is notoriously difficult to prove that a PFO (prevalent in roughly 20% of the population) is indeed causative. In addition to searching for a deep venous thrombosis, agitated saline may be injected intravenously in order to demonstrate passage of air bubbles through a cardiac right-to-left shunt by echocardiography. It should be noted, however, that pulmonary right-to-left shunting cannot necessarily be verified using this technique but requires transcranial Doppler which may reveal micro-embolic signals in the middle cerebral artery.

• Rare causes of large vessel stroke
  – Moyamoya disease is an idiopathic disorder leading to progressive stenosis of (usually both) the proximal internal carotid arteries and middle cerebral arteries (Suzuki grade 1). Consequently, a fine collateral network of compensatory capillaries arises at the site of occlusion ("rete mirabile") (Suzuki grades 2–5). Following injection of contrast medium during digital subtraction angiography, this network appears and vanishes like a puff of smoke, hence the Japanese term *moyamoya*. When the internal carotid arteries become fully occluded, moyamoya collateral vessels disappear again (Suzuki grade 6) (See Case 4.15). More common in Asia, moyamoya disease is encountered in people of many ethnic backgrounds, including American and European. Moyamoya disease predominantly affects children around 5 years of age and adults in their mid-forties. Symptoms and signs of moyamoya can be attributed to changes in cerebral blood flow resulting from stenosis of the internal carotid arteries, predisposing patients on one hand to ischemic strokes, TIA, headaches, and paroxysmal events with sensorimotor symptoms (which may be mistaken as epileptic seizures and can sometimes be

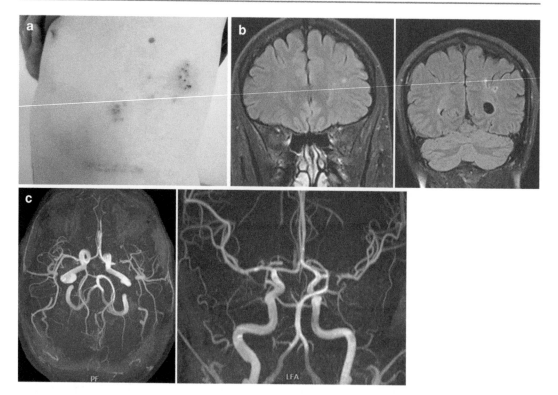

Case 4.23 Moyamoya phenomenon due to Fanconi anemia. A 41-year-old male had a diagnosis of Fanconi's anemia, a rare inherited bone marrow failure syndrome; possible complications include hemorrhages, infections (note herpes zoster rash in left dermatome T7, **a**), leukemia, myelodysplastic syndromes, liver tumors, and other cancers (note the scar following excision of a malignant melanoma, **a**). He experienced sudden onset of right arm and facial weakness, which resolved within half an hour. MR FLAIR showed scattered lacunar infarctions in the left MCA territory (**b**). MR angiography revealed left distal ICA/proximal MCA stenosis (**c**). DSA confirmed the presence of a rete mirabile (not shown). Although the blood disorder typically seen with Moyamoya is sickle cell anemia, the association with Fanconi's anemia has been described in a few case reports as well. Hence, the patient was diagnosed as having a Moyamoya phenomenon (as opposed to cryptogenic Moyamoya disease; see Case 4.15). Following discussion of his situation, he opted for a conservative approach and was started on aspirin. He experienced one relapse when he forgot to take his medication for a few days but has been stable since (3 years follow-up)

induced by hyperventilation), and intracranial hemorrhage on the other.

- Idiopathic moyamoya disease must be differentiated from a secondary moyamoya syndrome associated with various conditions, including Down syndrome, sickle cell anemia, neurofibromatosis type 1, intracranial atherosclerosis, and cranial radiation (Case 4.23). Direct and indirect revascularization techniques, including, but not limited to, extracranial-intracranial bypass techniques may halt secondary progression.

- Certain conditions such as Marfan syndrome, Ehlers-Danlos type 4, and fibromuscular dysplasia (FMD) predispose to neck vessel dissections. Diagnosis is typically not difficult and is based on recognizing key features of the diseases, e.g., the typical long and slender body habitus of a Marfan patient or the angiographic string-and-pearls appearance of the carotid arteries with FMD. Diagnostic opportunities are limited, but screening for and treatment of other organ involvement is mandatory (e.g., renal artery angiography and nephroprotection for FMD).

- Inflammatory conditions include postherpetic infarcts ipsilateral to a recent ophthalmic zoster and giant cell arteritis, both of which typically affect the elderly, whereas

Takayasu arteritis predominantly occurs in young women. In the latter, the inflammation damages the aorta and its main branches leading to stenosis and, besides stroke, to ischemic symptoms such as arm or chest pain.

- Rare causes of small vessel stroke. Due to advances in genetic technologies (so-called next-generation sequencing; see Sect. 5.7.2), hereditary forms of small vessel disease due to monogenic disorders are increasingly recognize d. Genetic counseling is essential for all patients with a monogenic stroke disorder and their relatives. Treatment is supportive, except for Fabry disease for which enzyme replacement is available.

  - The best known and most frequent of these disorders is cerebral autosomal dominant arteriopathy with subcortical infarcts and leukoencephalopathy (CADASIL) due to mutations of the *NOTCH 3* gene, which encodes the NOTCH 3 protein that plays a key role in the function of vascular smooth muscle cells. Patients typically develop migraine headaches with prolonged aura during their twenties, followed by stroke-like episodes during their forties and fifties, dementia of a subcortical type 10 years later, and ultimately, premature death. So-called CADASIL coma, a subacute onset encephalopathy with decreased consciousness and confusion that may last several days, is an under-recognized presentation (See Case 4.20). Penetrance is high and there is usually a positive family history, although de novo mutations may occur. The clinical history is highly characteristic and so is the MRI, showing subcortical infarcts and a diffuse leukoencephalopathy with anterior temporal lobe and external capsules being predilection sites. Diagnosis is by genetic analysis or skin biopsy. The latter reveals granular osmiophilic deposits in vascular smooth muscle cells vessel as demonstrated by electron microscopy, although skin biopsy may have a suboptimal sensitivity. Occasionally, a NOTCH 3-negative CADASIL phenotype may be encountered.

  - Cerebral autosomal recessive arteriopathy with subcortical infarcts and leukoencephalopathy (CARASIL) is an autosomal recessive variant due to mutations of the *HTRA1* gene. Neuroimaging features are very similar to those of CADASIL. However, CARASIL is associated with a more aggressive deterioration with dementia occurring by 30–40 years of age, lumbago and alopecia may be seen as additional features, and a family history is often less obvious due to the recessive inheritance pattern.

  - A history of repetitive ischemic and hemorrhagic strokes in a young patient with an MRI revealing leukodystrophic changes and hemispheric cysts and cavities is highly suggestive of mutation of the *COL4A1* gene, which encodes the alpha-1 subunit of collagen type IV (Case 4.24).

  - Males with *Fabry disease*, an X-linked lysosomal storage disorder due to deficiency of alpha-galactosidase A, often complain of episodes of burning pain in their hands and feet due to a small fiber neuropathy. Cutaneous angiokeratomas, corneal opacity, and progressive renal and cardiac failure may arise in addition to ischemic strokes. The latter may occur due to small vessel disease, embolism because of cardiac involvement, as well as large vessel disease which is associated with a predilection for posterior circulation infarcts and elongated and ectatic vertebral and basilar arteries. In males the diagnosis can be made by demonstrating alpha-galactosidase A deficiency in plasma and leukocytes, whereas in heterozygote females (who usually have a less severe phenotype due to residual enzyme activity) genetic testing for a mutation of the *GLA* gene is mandatory.

  - Retinal vasculopathy with cerebral leukodystrophy (RVCL), an autosomal dominant disorder due to mutation of the *TREX1* gene, is characterized by vascular retinopathy, Raynaud's phenomenon, and kidney and liver dysfunction.

  - Among the non-hereditary microangiopathies, *Susac's syndrome* deserves special attention (see Case 4.21). The complete triad of visual field defects, sensory hearing

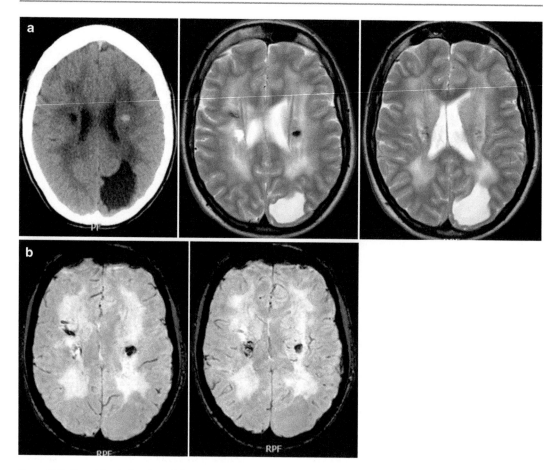

Case 4.24 Repetitive ischemic and hemorrhagic strokes due to COL4A1 mutation. Since the age of 20, this female had suffered repetitive focal neurological deficits. She was able to walk without a walking aid and attended university despite a mild spastic hemiparesis and slight difficulties with concentration and memory. Her family history and genetic testing for CADASIL and Fabry disease were negative. At the age of 24, she complained of sudden onset of slurred speech and pins and needles in her face. Neurological examination revealed novel signs, including a right-sided facial weakness, dysarthria, and tongue deviation to the right. CT and MRI of the brain showed a hyperdense spot in the left corona radiate, a lacunar lesion at exactly the same location in the contralateral hemisphere, as well as a large occipital hypodensity (**a**). While the first lesion was compatible with an acute hemorrhage and consistent with the new focal deficits, the last two lesions suggested previous infarctions. In addition, periventricular white matter disease ("leukoaraiosis") was noted. Within a few days, dysarthria worsened and she developed dysphagia. MR T2-weighted (**a**) and gradient-echo (**b**) imaging revealed a hemorrhage in the right hemisphere (the dark spot just above the right lacunar stroke). Bilateral lesions affecting the corticobulbar tracts were consistent with the patient's pseudobulbar palsy. Repetitive hemorrhagic and ischemic strokes in a young person with white matter disease are highly suggestive of *COL4A1* or *COL4A2* gene mutations, and indeed, genetic analysis confirmed a relevant mutation of the *COL4A1* gene

impairment, and encephalopathy may take several months to develop. Females are much more commonly affected. The diagnosis primarily relies on ophthalmologic evaluation demonstrating branch retinal artery occlusions by retinal fluorescence angiography. *Sneddon syndrome* is another non-hereditary microangiopathy, associated with livedo reticularis and (often, but not always) antiphospholipid antibodies.

- Other rare causes of ischemic stroke
  - Screening for an underlying malignancy (e.g., intravascular B-cell lymphoma or upper gastrointestinal tract tumor) should be considered in all middle-aged patients with a negative initial workup (Case 4.25).

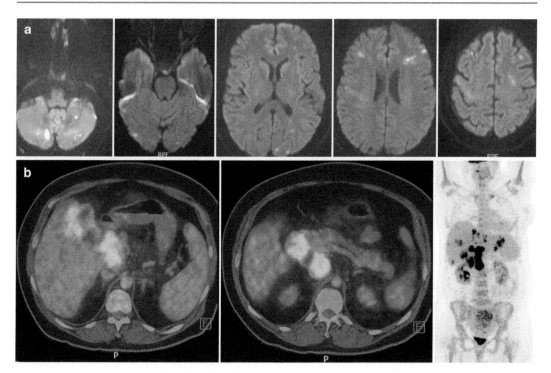

Case 4.25 Paraneoplastic stroke. A 49-year-old female was admitted because of subacute onset (hours) of unstable gate and short-lasting left-sided arm weakness. Her previous medical history was nonsignificant; of note, she did not have any modifiable cardiovascular risk factors. MR DWI showed scattered infarctions in the anterior and posterior circulation of both hemispheres, suggesting an embolic stroke pattern, mostly likely of cardiac origin (**a**). However, cardiac workup was unremarkable, including telemetry and echocardiography. Blood tests showed slightly increased C-reactive protein and liver parameters. A whole body PET/CT scan was ordered. This showed an upper gastrointestinal malignancy, which had metastasized primarily to the liver (**b**). Biopsy revealed a gall bladder cancer. Paraneoplastic hypercoagulability is a well-recognized cause of stroke, in particular in association with lymphoma or malignancies of the upper gastrointestinal tract such as gall bladder or pancreas. Paraneoplastic stroke should be high on the list of differential diagnoses in middle-aged persons with an embolic stroke pattern and negative routine workup

- A history of migraine with prolonged aura together with mitochondrial stigmata such as a short stature, sensory deafness, early cataracts, diabetes, and proximal weakness due to a myopathy should prompt evaluation for mitochondrial myopathy, encephalomyopathy, lactic acidosis, and stroke-like episodes (MELAS) (Case 4.26).
- Inflammatory causes include systemic and primary CNS vasculitides.
- Air embolism may be associated with a history of Valsalva maneuver, sexual activity during pregnancy or postpartum, cesarean section, and iatrogenic catheter-based interventions. Fat embolism may occur following major trauma or orthopedic surgery and causes decreasing consciousness, petechia,

  disseminated intravascular coagulation, shock, and multiorgan failure (see Case 3.8). Amniotic fluid embolism may lead to an identical clinical picture and is seen in the third trimester of pregnancy.
- Blood disorders include acquired coagulopathies (e.g., antiphospholipid antibody syndrome), hereditary coagulopathies (e.g., protein S and C deficiencies, factor V Leiden), and hemoglobinopathies (e.g., sickle cell anemia).
- Intravascular B-cell lymphoma has a predilection for the brain, leads to accumulation of cerebral infarcts, and is usually rapidly fatal (within weeks).
- Traumatic brain injury may occasionally lead to stroke associated with intracranial vessel dissection (Case 4.27).

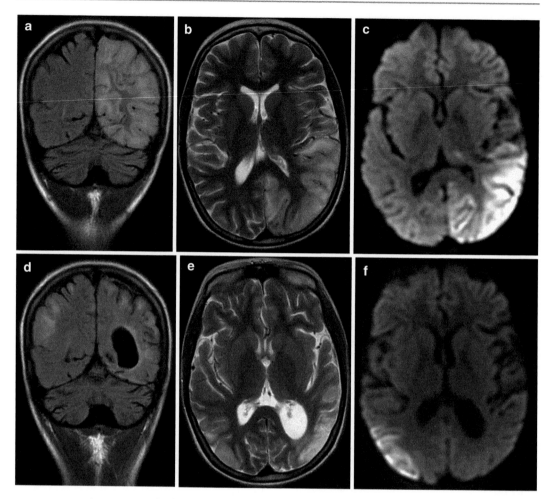

Case 4.26 Mitochondrial Encephalomyopathy, Lactic Acidosis, and Stroke-like episodes (MELAS). An 18-year-old woman with a slender stature, myopathic facial features, proximal more than distal weakness in the extremities, mildly decreased IQ, and a history of migraine headaches had been diagnosed with MELAS (mtDNA 3243A> G point mutation). Her mother had died from complications arising from the same condition at the age of 50 years. The patient presented with relatively sudden onset (hours) of gait disturbance and confusion. Examination also revealed a right-sided hemianopia. MRI of the brain showed cortical posterior edema on the left (coronal FLAIR, **a**; axial T2 weighted, **b**). There were hyperintense signal changes on MR DWI in the same area, indicative of cytotoxic edema (**c**). Blood tests were unremarkable except for increased serum lactate. Gait disturbances and confusion resolved within a few days. However, 12 months later, she suffered from a complex partial seizure with secondary generalization. MRI now showed left parietal lobe atrophy (note the enlarged posterior horn of the left lateral ventricle; coronal FLAIR **d**; axial T2 weighted, **e**) and a new zone of DWI signal changes in the right occipital lobe (**f**). MELAS often leads to migraine with prolonged aura and stroke-like episodes. Strokes more often occur posteriorly but do not respect arterial territories (as shown here) because they are due to mitochondrial energy failure and not occlusive vessel disease

4.11.5 Ischemic Stroke Mimics

In the acute setting, the three most common stroke mimics are migraine with aura, focal epilepsy, and functional (nonorganic) deficits. The *differential diagnosis of TIA and ischemic stroke mimics* includes:

- Focal epilepsy, e.g., postictal paralysis.[10]
- Migraine usually affects a much younger patient group, and there is often a family history. Aura symptoms are frequently "posi-

---

[10]However, limb shaking because of a lacunar TIA or hemodynamic carotid artery stenosis may be misdiagnosed as an epileptic seizure.

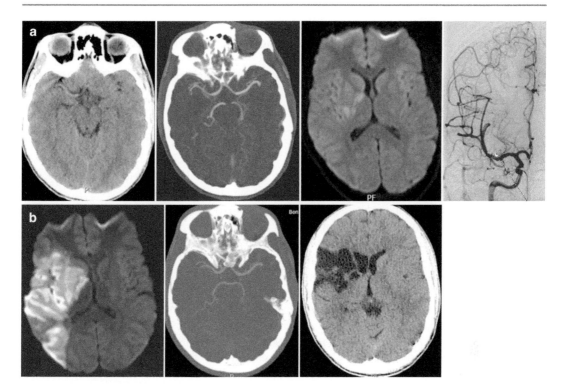

Case 4.27 Intracranial dissection following traumatic brain injury. An 18-year-old male presented with stroke in progression 5 days after a head trauma. He had been diagnosed with Tourette's syndrome a few years earlier. Unfortunately, his obsessive compulsive behavior had captured the attention of a group of teenagers who beat him in the street. He was discharged from the emergency room on the day of the trauma with a diagnosis of mild concussion after a normal neurological exam and an unremarkable CT of the brain (not shown). However, a few days later, he experienced transient left-sided weakness. On readmission (**a**), his NIHSS was 5. CT of the brain now showed a right-sided dense MCA sign, and CT angiography revealed tapering of the M1 segment suggesting dissection of the right MCA. He was given IV thrombolysis. One hour later, MR DWI revealed mild ischemia of the right nucleus lentiformis, suggesting damage to the right lenticulostriate arteries arising from the distal M1 segment. Digital subtrac-

tion angiography (DSA) showed a tiny vessel wall defect located at the right M1 (this is difficult to depict in the present still image but better seen with dynamic visualization of the blood flow during DSA). The neurovascular team opted for conservative treatment with double antiplatelet inhibition and slight augmentation of blood pressure levels, because of the high periprocedural risks of intracranial stenting and the lack of evidence for any benefit. However, 3 h later (**b, left**), his arm and leg weakness worsened, and he developed left-sided hemianopia as well as unilateral sensory and visual inattention (NIHSS 17). MR DWI confirmed a large left MCA infarction. Three months later (**b, middle and right**), the patient was able to walk unassisted despite spastic hemiparesis (NIHSS 6; mRS 2). Follow-up CT angiography showed that the right MCA was still slimmer than on the contralateral side although to lesser degree than during the acute stage. A large parenchymal defect was seen on CT

tive," progressing over 5–20 min to maximum severity, often followed by headache, nausea, and vomiting. Bear in mind that migraine-like headaches occur in certain rare stroke types, e.g., migrainous infarction, CADASIL, MELAS, and Susac's syndrome (Case 4.26).

- Functional (nonorganic) deficits. See Sect. 3.11.
- Headache with neurological deficits and CSF lymphocytosis (HaNDL), also termed pseudomigraine with pleocytosis. This is a rare and benign condition with migraine-like headache

attacks with transient neurological deficits and aseptic CSF pleocytosis, which affects primarily younger patients (15–40 years of age) and more commonly males. These attacks may reoccur several times, but lasting deficits are not part of this syndrome. Obviously, it is a diagnosis of exclusion. Postinfectious autoimmune leptomeningeal vasculitis has been suggested to cause HaNDL, but this remains to be proven.

- Structural brain lesions, e.g., brain tumors, chronic subdural hemorrhage, and sinus venous thrombosis, can occasionally present with symptoms of acute onset.

- Hypoglycemia may lead to transient focal symptoms, and when associated with long-standing diabetes, vegetative symptoms such as hunger and sweating may be lacking.
- Otogenic vertigo is usually not difficult to differentiate from vertigo due to a brainstem infarction because in the latter, there are almost always signs and symptoms related to the CNs and sensorimotor pathways. However, vertigo due to a cerebellar stroke can sometimes be hard to distinguish from otogenic vertigo, and careful analysis of eye movements is mandatory. Consult Chap. 3 for the "three-step oculomotor bedside examination."
- Mononeuropathies, HNPP, for instance, may lead to repeated episodes of weakness and sensory symptoms in the extremities.
- MS, e.g., brainstem plaques can sometimes lead to paroxysmal features, as outlined earlier.
- Transient global amnesia, if a reliable witness report is available, TGA should not be difficult to distinguish from acute aphasia.
- Fluctuating bulbar symptoms due to MG may occasionally be confused with stroke.

4.11.6 Hemorrhagic Stroke

It is not possible to distinguish between ischemic and hemorrhagic stroke by clinical means, which is why every patient with a suspicion of a cerebrovascular event should be investigated using neuroimaging without delay. As a rule, though, acute severe arterial hypertension, confusion, a history of anticoagulation, nausea, vomiting, and headache are more often associated with hemorrhagic than with ischemic stroke.

Most cases of *non-traumatic intracerebral hemorrhage* are believed to be due to:

- Uncontrolled hypertension and small vessel disease of the deep perforators. These bleedings typically occur with decreasing frequency in the putamen, thalamus, cerebellum, pons, and caudate nucleus ("typical ICH").

Less common causes of intracranial hemorrhage ("atypical ICH") include:

- Vascular malformations (AVM, cavernous malformation, dural AV fistula, aneurysms, moyamoya syndrome)
- Other vasculopathies, e.g., cerebral amyloid angiopathy (Cases 4.17 and 4.28), CADASIL (Case 4.20), vasculitis, infectious aneurysms, and intracranial artery dissection
- Intracranial venous thrombosis
- Primary or secondary brain tumors
- Hemostatic disorders (anticoagulation, antiplatelet therapy, congenital and acquired coagulation defects)

4.11.7 Subarachnoid Hemorrhage

Subarachnoid hemorrhage (SAH) may be due to rupture of an aneurysm or occur without an underlying aneurysm.

Aneurysms may present as follows:

- "Classical" saccular or berry aneurysms at the Circle of Willis. They are acquired lesions, responsible for roughly 80% of all non-traumatic SAH. Up to 2% of the general population has an unruptured intracranial saccular aneurysm, and multiple aneurysms may be found in 20–30% of these people. Women are three times more likely to have an aneurysm as compared to men. The vast majority of aneurysms (80–90%) occur in the anterior circulation. Apart from female sex, risk factors for intracranial saccular aneurysms include increasing age, cigarette smoking, hypertension, predisposing genetic conditions (autosomal dominant polycystic kidney syndrome, among others), and a family history with at least two first-degree relatives having an intracranial aneurysm. The risk of rupture depends on the size of the aneurysm (the larger, the higher the risk) and its location (posterior circulation aneurysms are more likely to rupture than anterior circulation aneurysms).
- Vertebrobasilar dolichoectasia. These are fusiform aneurysms affecting the posterior

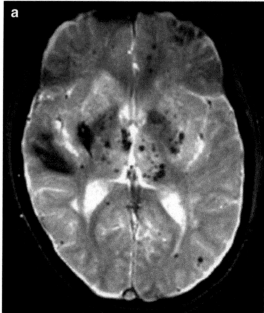

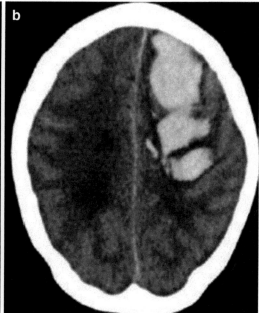

Case 4.28 Cerebral amyloid angiopathy. A 63-year-old female with a history of well-treated hypertension complained of spells of word-finding difficulty in the previous 6 months and slight forgetfulness. Routine neurological examination was normal, but neuropsychological assessment was not performed. MRI with gradient-echo sequences showed multiple microbleeds in both hemispheres (**a**). Moderate white matter hyperintense signal changes were evident on T2-weighted images (not shown). Three months later she was admitted with acute right-sided hemiplegia and decreased consciousness. CT of the brain showed an atypical lobar hemorrhage (as opposed to the "typical" deep hemispheric hemorrhages associated with uncontrolled arterial hypertension; **b**). Subsequent angiography revealed no vascular malformation, consistent with a diagnosis of probable CAA

circulation. They are associated with chronic hypertension and tend to increase with time in length and diameter. They may lead to sudden onset of brainstem deficits because of bleeding, ischemia (due to compromised microcirculation), and mass effect.

• Mycotic aneurysms associated with myxoma or endocarditis. In contrast to saccular aneurysms at the Circle of Willis (see above), these aneurysms tend to affect distal artery branches. They develop due to vessel wall damage secondary to local inflammation caused by embolic material. The bleeding risk is high.

• Extracranial pseudoaneurysms following ICA dissection. These are relatively benign lesions, which can be managed conservatively.

The differential diagnosis of non-aneurysmal subarachnoidal bleeding includes "angiogram-positive" and "angiogram-negative" subarachnoidal bleeding.

• Angiogram-positive subarachnoidal bleeding (non-aneurysmal)
  – Cerebral arteriovenous malformations (AVM)
  – Intracranial dural arteriovenous fistulas
  – Primary and secondary CNS vasculitis
  – Intracranial artery dissections
  – Cerebral venous thrombosis
  – Reversible cerebral vasoconstriction syndrome (RCVS)

• Angiogram-negative subarachnoidal bleeding
  – Cerebral amyloid angiopathy (CAA)
  – Perimesencephalic bleeding from the perimesencephalic venous plexus (which has an excellent prognosis)
  – Spinal bleeding sources
  – Abuse of sympathomimetics and stimulants such as cocaine and amphetamine
  – Sickle cell disease
  – Pituitary apoplexy
  – Tumors
  – Coagulation disorders

Of note, atraumatic, non-aneurysmal sub-arachnoidal bleeding localized on the brain convexities is typically due to CAA in the elderly (>60 years), whereas in younger patients it is often due to RCVS (Kumar et al. 2010).

4.12 The Differential Diagnosis of Demyelinating Disorders

4.12.1 Multiple Sclerosis

The great majority of patients with a demyelinating disease of the CNS will have MS.

According to the 2013 revisions of the International Advisory Committee on Clinical Trials of MS, the following MS phenotypes (i.e., disease courses) are distinguished:

- Relapsing disease
  - Clinically isolated syndrome (CIS). CIS is the first clinical presentation of a disease that is likely to manifest itself as MS in the future, but does not yet fulfill the criteria of dissemination in time. It is now accepted as an element of the MS phenotype spectrum. In addition, the revised McDonald MS diagnostic criteria allow some patients with a single clinical episode to be diagnosed with MS based on the single scan criterion for dissemination in time and space, thereby reducing the number of cases categorized as CIS.
  - Relapsing-remitting. This type is the most common phenotype (85% of all cases) and typically affects patients in their 20s or 30s.
- Progressive disease
  - Secondary progressive. In the majority of patients, MS becomes secondary progressive after 10–15 years.
  - Primary progressive. Roughly 10% of MS patients have primary progressive MS; usually these patients become symptomatic in their 40s and typically present with increasing leg stiffness and gait ataxia.

Both relapsing and progressive disease may be active or inactive as determined by clinical relapses and/or MRI activity (contrast-enhancing lesions; new or unequivocally enlarging T2 lesions assessed at least annually). The other important modifier besides activity is the presence or absence of disease progression (i.e., decline of neurological function, as assessed by at least annually clinical evaluation). Thus, perhaps somewhat counterintuitively, also primary progressive MS can be active or inactive and with or without progression. (Inactive primary progressive MS without progression would be labeled as "stable disease.")

The hallmark of relapsing-remitting MS is dissemination of neurological signs and symptoms in time and space. Clinically definite MS is defined as two or more attacks (time criterion) with two or more objective clinical symptoms (space criterion). Attacks are defined as "patient-reported symptoms or objectively observed signs typical of an acute inflammatory demyelinating event in the CNS, current or historical, with duration of at least 24 h, in the absence of fever or infection" (Polman et al. 2011). The Uhthoff's phenomenon is a common cause of pseudo-attacks in patients with MS. This phenomenon is due to temporary slowing of nerve conduction within a chronic plaque due to increased body temperature (e.g., because of a urinary tract infection, physical exercise, or hot weather), leading to worsening or reoccurrence of neurological deficits. When body temperature normalizes, nerve conduction recovers and the symptoms end.

Now that treatment options have become available, it is important to diagnose patients early because treatment may be associated with neuroprotection. The McDonald criteria have been established for this purpose, among others. These criteria enable the evaluation of patients presenting with a first demyelinating attack (e.g., optic neuritis, transverse myelitis, brainstem syndrome), including those with CIS. Instead of waiting for a second relapse to occur, an MRI may allow the clinician to document dissemination in space and time. Consequently, these patients can be diagnosed as having MS, and early treatment can be started.

Roughly 10% of all MS patients have a rather benign natural disease course. Positive prognostic factors include female gender, sensory symptoms at onset, low lesion load on T_2-weighted MRI, full recovery after first attack, low attack frequency in the first 2 years, and longtime interval between first and second attack. However, the severity and activity of the disease can change unpredictably, and therefore labels such as "benign" (and to a lesser degree "malignant") should be used very cautiously.

If the patient's presentation fulfills the McDonald criteria and no other diagnosis offers a better explanation, the diagnosis is MS. If the criteria are not completely met but suspicion is substantial, the diagnosis is *possible* MS. In addition, the McDonald criteria address the diagnosis of primary progressive MS.

Table 4.3 shows the McDonald criteria as revised in 2010 (Polman et al. 2011). McDonald criteria for MR are as follows.

Dissemination in space can be demonstrated by ≥1 T2 lesion (of note, contrast enhancement is not required) in at least two out of four areas in the CNS:

- Periventricular
- Juxtacortical
- Infratentorial
- Spinal cord[11]

Dissemination in time can be documented by:

[11] If the patient has a brainstem or spinal cord syndrome, the symptomatic lesions are excluded from the criteria and do not contribute to the lesion count.

Table 4.3   The revised McDonald criteria

Clinical presentation	Additional data needed
≥2 or more attacks; objective clinical evidence of ≥2 lesions	Not needed, if no better explanation than MS
≥2 or more attacks; objective clinical evidence of 1 lesion	Dissemination in space, demonstrated by:
	≥1 T2 lesion in at least 2 of 4 MS-typical regions of the CNS (periventricular, juxtacortical, infratentorial, or spinal cord) *or*
	Await further clinical attack implicating a different site
1 attack; objective clinical evidence of ≥2 lesions	Dissemination in time, demonstrated by:
	Simultaneous presence of asymptomatic gadolinium-enhancing and nonenhancing lesions at any time *or*
	A new T2 and/or gadolinium-enhancing lesion(s) on follow-up MRI, irrespective of its timing with reference to a baseline scan *or*
	Await a second clinical attack
1 attack; objective clinical evidence of 1 lesion (i.e., CIS)	Dissemination in time *and* space, demonstrated by:
	Dissemination in space:
	≥1 T2 lesion in at least 2 of 4 MS-typical regions of the CNS (periventricular, juxtacortical, infratentorial, or spinal cord) *or*
	Await a second clinical attack implicating a different CNS site
	Dissemination in time:
	Simultaneous presence of asymptomatic gadolinium-enhancing and nonenhancing lesions at any time *or*
	A new T2 and/or gadolinium-enhancing lesion(s) on follow-up MRI, irrespective of its timing with reference to a baseline scan *or*
	Await a second clinical attack
Insidious neurological progression suggestive of MS (this is primary progressive MS)	One year of disease progression (retrospectively or prospectively determined) *and* two of the following:
	1. Evidence for dissemination in space in the brain based on ≥1 T2 lesions in the MS-characteristic regions (periventricular, juxtacortical, or infratentorial)
	2. Evidence for dissemination in space in the spinal cord based on ≥2 T2 lesions in the cord
	3. Positive CSF[a]

Adapted from Polman et al. (2011)
MS multiple sclerosis, *MRI* magnetic resonance imaging, *CSF* cerebrospinal fluid
[a]Positive CSF findings include oligoclonal bands and increased IgG index

- A new T2 and/or gadolinium-enhancing lesion(s) on follow-up MRI, as compared to the initial MRI, irrespective of the timing of the baseline scan
- Simultaneous presence of asymptomatic gadolinium-enhancing and nonenhancing lesions at any time (Case 4.29)

Of note, incidental imaging findings suggestive of inflammatory demyelination in the absence of clinical signs or symptoms are termed *radiologically isolated syndrome* (RIS). RIS is not considered an MS subtype; however, there is a significant risk of developing MS in the future. This risk increases with gadolinium-enhancing lesions, asymptomatic spinal cord lesions, and signs of CSF inflammation.

The deficits of patients with MS are commonly assessed using the Kurtzke Functional System (FS) (Table 4.4) and graded according to the Kurtzke Expanded Disability Status Scale (EDSS) (Table 4.5). The EDSS quantifies disability in eight FSs (pyramidal, cerebellar, brainstem, sensory, bowel and bladder, visual, cerebral, and others) and allows the neurologist to assign a functional system score in each of these.

4.12.2 Other Forms of Demyelinating Disease and Related Conditions

If the clinical symptoms and signs are compatible with a demyelinating disease and it is not MS, the *differential diagnosis* is extensive (as outlined further below and shown in Fig. 4.8). There are nonetheless three rather common clinical scenarios:

- Hereditary conditions, such as one of the spinocerebellar ataxias (SCA), should be suspected if the MRI and CSF (cells, protein, IgG index, and oligoclonal bands) are normal despite severe ataxia and corticospinal tract signs.
- Although high CSF cell counts are occasionally seen with MS, a CSF pleocytosis exceed-

ing 30–50 cells should lead to examinations for infectious, malignant, and other autoimmune diseases.
- A history of extensive longitudinal myelitis (≥3 vertebral segments) is suspicious of neuromyelitis optica (NMO).

The following is a far from complete list of differential diagnoses to MS:

- Autoimmune diseases (typically not postinfectious)
  - NMO; Devic's disease. Myelitis is usually longitudinally extensive, expanding over three or more vertebral segments as revealed by MRI. The myelitis may be severe and lead to nervous tissue necrosis. With involvement of the cervical cord, respiratory failure is life-threatening. In recent years, though, it has become evident that myelitis can be mild and reversible. NMO is much more frequent in women than in men. The diagnosis of NMO requires a history of optic neuritis and myelitis as well as two out of the three following:
    Continuous spinal cord MRI lesion extending over three vertebral segments
    Brain MRI not meeting diagnostic criteria for MS
    NMO-IgG seropositive (NMO antibodies; these are antibodies against the water channel protein aquaporin 4)
  Of note, NMO antibody titers can be negative in some periods during the course of the disease and positive at other times; thus, it is useful to send for new antibody titers if the clinical suspicion of NMO is high (Case 4.30).

  - NMO spectrum disorders are those that do not fulfill the diagnostic criteria for NMO but are nevertheless associated with NMO antibodies. For instance, roughly half of all cases of longitudinally extensive myelitis (expanding over three or more vertebral segments) are associated with NMO antibodies, irrespective of optic neuritis. NMO antibodies may also induce a

Case 4.29 Multiple sclerosis. A 34-year-old female was diagnosed with the relapsing-remitting type of multiple sclerosis. Her MRI revealed classical periventricular, juxtacortical, and infratentorial lesions. Axial T2-weighted MR (**a, b**) and sagittal FLAIR (**c**) showed Dawson fingers, elongated periventricular white matter lesions arranged at right angles along medullary veins. Neuroimaging also revealed black holes (sagittal T1-weighted MRI; **d**) and a gadolinium-enhancing lesion (with a typical C-shaped appearance; axial contrast-enhanced T1-weighted MRI; **e**)

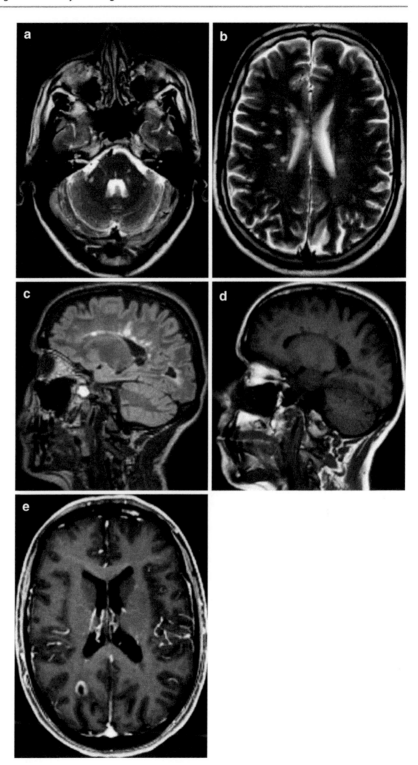

Table 4.4 Kurtzke Functional Systems Scores (Kurtzke 1983)

Pyramidal functions

0—Normal

1—Abnormal signs without disability

2—Minimal disability

3—Mild to moderate paraparesis or hemiparesis (detectable weakness but most function sustained for short periods, fatigue a problem); severe monoparesis (almost no function)

4—Marked paraparesis or hemiparesis (function is difficult), moderate quadriparesis (function is decreased but can be sustained for short periods), or monoplegia

5—Paraplegia, hemiplegia, or marked quadriparesis

6—Quadriplegia

9—Unknown

Cerebellar functions

0—Normal

1—Abnormal signs without disability

2—Mild ataxia (tremor or clumsy movements easily seen, minor interference with function)

3—Moderate truncal or limb ataxia (tremor or clumsy movements interfere with function in all spheres)

4—Severe ataxia in all limbs (most function is very difficult)

5—Unable to perform coordinated movements due to ataxia

9—Unknown

Brainstem functions

0—Normal

1—Signs only

2—Moderate nystagmus or other mild disability

3—Severe nystagmus, marked extraocular weakness, or moderate disability of other cranial nerves

4—Marked dysarthria or other marked disability

5—Inability to swallow or speak

9—Unknown

Sensory function

0—Normal

1—Vibration or figure-writing decrease only in one or two limbs

2—Mild decrease in touch or pain or position sense and/or moderate decrease in vibration in one or two limbs or vibratory decrease alone in three or four limbs

3—Moderate decrease in touch or pain or position sense and/or essentially lost vibration in one or two limbs or mild decrease in touch or pain and/or moderate decrease in all proprioceptive tests in three or four limbs

4—Marked decrease in touch or pain or loss of proprioception, alone or combined, in one or two limbs, or moderate decrease in touch or pain and/or severe proprioceptive decrease in more than two limbs

5—Loss (essentially) of sensation in one or two limbs or moderate decrease in touch or pain and/or loss of proprioception for most of the body below the head

6—Sensation essentially lost below the head

9—Unknown

Bowel and bladder function

0—Normal

1—Mild urinary hesitance, urgency, or retention

2—Moderate hesitance, urgency, retention of bowel or bladder, or rare urinary incontinence (intermittent self-catheterization, manual compression to evacuate bladder, or finger evacuation of stool)

3—Frequent urinary incontinence

4—In need of almost constant catheterization (and constant use of measures to evacuate stool)

5—Loss of bladder function

6—Loss of bowel and bladder function

9—Unknown

Visual function
0—Normal
1—Scotoma with visual acuity (corrected) better than 20/30
2—Worse eye with scotoma with maximal visual acuity (corrected) of 20/30.20/59
3—Worse eye with large scotoma, or moderate decrease in fields, but with maximal visual acuity (corrected) of 20/60.20/99
4—Worse eye with marked decrease of fields and maximal visual acuity (corrected) of 20/100.20/200; grade 3 plus maximal acuity of better eye of 20/60 or less
5—Worse eye with maximal visual acuity (corrected) less than 20/200; grade 4 plus maximal acuity of better eye of 20/60 or less
6—Grade 5 plus maximal visual acuity of better eye of 20/60 or less
9—Unknown
Cerebral (or mental) functions
0—Normal
1—Mood alteration only (does not affect EDSS score)
2—Mild decrease in mentation
3—Moderate decrease in mentation
4—Marked decrease in mentation (chronic brain syndrome—moderate)
5—Dementia or chronic brain syndrome—severe or incompetent
9—Unknown

Table 4.5 Kurtzke Expanded Disability Status Scale (EDSS)

0.0	Normal Neurological Exam
1.0	No disability, minimal signs in 1 FS
1.5	No disability, minimal signs in 2 of 7 FS
2.0	Minimal disability in 1 of 7 FS
2.5	Minimal disability in 2 FS
3.0	Moderate disability in 1 FS or mild disability in 3–4 FS, though fully ambulatory
3.5	Fully ambulatory but with moderate disability in 1 FS and mild disability in 1 or 2 FS, or moderate disability in 2 FS, or mild disability in 5 FS
4.0	Fully ambulatory without aid, up and about 12 h a day despite relatively severe disability, able to walk without aid 500 m
4.5	Fully ambulatory without aid, up and about much of day, able to work a full day, may otherwise have some limitations of full activity, or require minimal assistance. Relatively severe disability. Able to walk without aid 300 m
5.0	Ambulatory without aid for about 200 m; disability impairs full daily activities
5.5	Ambulatory for 100 m; disability precludes full daily activities
6.0	Intermittent or unilateral constant assistance (cane, crutch, or brace) required to walk 100 m with or without resting
6.5	Constant bilateral support (cane, crutch, or braces) required to walk 20 m without resting
7.0	Unable to walk beyond 5 m even with aid, essentially restricted to wheelchair; wheels self, transfers alone; active in wheelchair about 12 h a day
7.5	Unable to take more than a few steps; restricted to wheelchair; may need aid to transfer; wheels self, but may require motorized chair for full day's activities
8.0	Essentially restricted to bed, chair, or wheelchair but may be out of bed much of day; retains self-care functions, generally effective use of arms
8.5	Essentially restricted to bed much of day, some effective use of arms, retains some self-care functions
9.0	Helpless bed patient; can communicate and eat
9.5	Unable to communicate effectively or eat/swallow
10.0	Death due to MS

Adapted from Kurtzke (1983)
EDSS steps 1.0–4.5 refer to people with MS who are fully ambulatory. EDSS steps 5.0–9.5 are defined by the impairment to ambulation
FS functional system

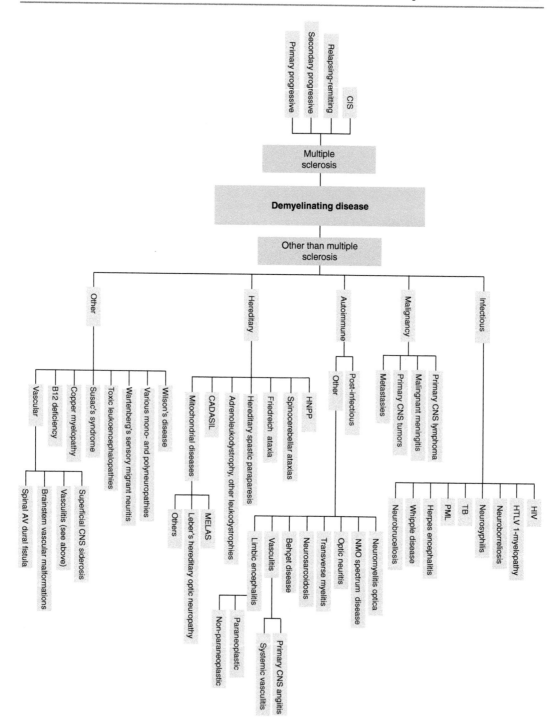

Fig. 4.8 Differential diagnosis of multiple sclerosis and other demyelinating diseases

condition of intractable nausea and vomiting due to involvement of the circumventricular organs.

– In analogy, demyelination previously associated with SLE, antiphospholipid syndrome, and other autoimmune diseases is increasingly being recognized as being due to NMO antibodies. Patients with NMO may have a variety of nonpathogenic antibodies that previously have been believed to represent markers of other autoimmune diseases.

– Tumefactive MS behaves clinically and radiologically like a mass lesion. Despite its name, this condition also appears to be associated with NMO antibodies.

– Transverse myelitis of presumed autoimmune origin, expanding over less than three vertebral segments, or those cases not associated with NMO antibodies (some of which occur with anti-MOG).

– Behçet disease (Case 4.31).

– Limbic and brainstem encephalitis.

– Neurosarcoidosis (Case 5.7).

– Optic neuritis, not progressing to MS.

– Vasculitis, either as part of a systemic disease or isolated to the CNS.

• Autoimmune diseases (typically, but not always, postinfectious)

– ADEM (more often seen in children)

– Acute necrotizing hemorrhagic leukoencephalitis (similar to ADEM, but more severe)

– GBS, including GBS variants

• Hereditary diseases

– Spinocerebellar ataxias

– Leukodystrophies, e.g., adrenomyeloneuropathy in men (and female carriers of the X-linked ABCD1 mutation who, if not asymptomatic, typically develop a mild myelopathy in their fourties)

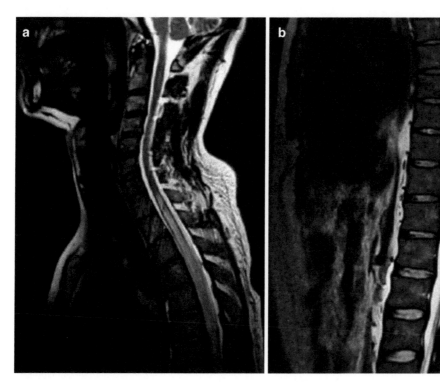

Case 4.30 Neuromyelitis optica. A 35-year-old female had painful vision loss of the right eye. She recovered following treatment with IV methylprednisolone. Four months later, the patient had an episode of tingling in both legs and slight urinary hesitancy but did not seek medical care. Two months later, the patient developed a spastic tetraplegia over the course of 5 days. T2-weighted MRI of the spinal cord showed an extensive longitudinally central lesion (**a, b**). MRI of the brain was normal. Of note, CSF analysis showed a polymorphonuclear pleocytosis (50 cells) and no oligoclonal bands. Although the first analysis for antibodies against aquaporin 4 antigen came out negative, the second analysis a few weeks later was positive. The patient was diagnosed with NMO. She regained the ability to walk following treatment with plasmapheresis and high-dose methylprednisolone, although slight spasticity remained. She was subsequently put on long-term immunomodulatory treatment to prevent further relapses

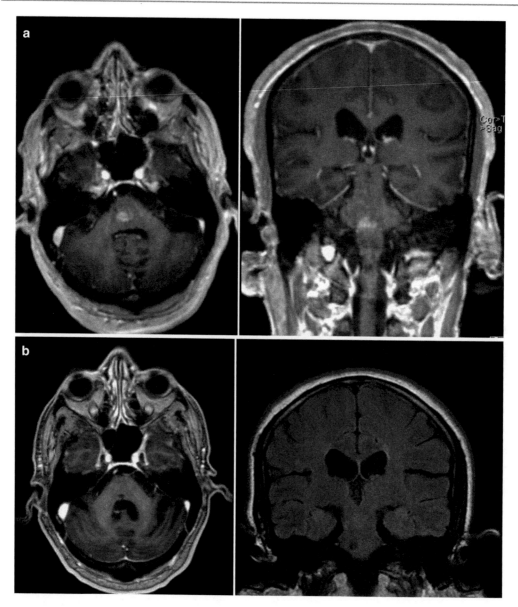

Case 4.31 Neuro-Behçet. A 59-year-old male from Morocco had been diagnosed with Behçet disease more than 30 years prior when he suffered from urogenital ulcers, uveitis, arthralgia, and skin changes (erythema nodosum). He had been hospitalized several times because of neurological deficits. On admission, examination showed cerebellar ataxia, diplopia because of right-sided abducens nerve palsy, a left-sided hemiparesis, and bulbar deficits including dysarthria and dysphagia. He had diffi-culty controlling tears and laughter. MRI revealed a contrast-enhancing lesion in the lower pons (**a**, **b**, T1 weighted following gadolinium). Following high-dose steroids and azathioprine, his condition improved. At fol-low-up a few months later, he was ambulatory with a walking cane, had safe swallowing, and emotional incon-tinence had completely resolved. Double vision was treated with eye muscle surgery. MRI contrast enhance-ment was no longer evident, but there was a small lacunar lesion compatible with neuronal loss due to infarction (**c**, axial T1 weighted with gadolinium; **d**, coronal FLAIR). Neuro-Behçet often has a relapsing-remitting course, although it typically becomes progressive without aggres-sive immunosuppression, much resembling the clinical course of MS. The most common manifestation of Neuro-Behçet is parenchymal involvement of the brainstem; the second most common is non-parenchymal Neuro-Behçet with involvement of large venous dural sinuses leading to isolated cerebral venous sinus thrombosis and intracranial hypertension. It is more common along the Silk Route, especially within the Mediterranean region and the Middle East. Virtually all patients with Neuro-Behçet also have systemic evidence of the disease, most commonly recurrent aphthous ulcers in the mouth. Onset is most fre-quent during the third or fourth decade of life. Behçet dis-ease affects males and females equally, although the disease tends to be more severe in males

- Cerebral autosomal dominant arteriopathy with subcortical infarcts and leukoencephalopathy (CADASIL)
- Friedreich's ataxia
- Hereditary spastic paraparesis (HSP)
- HNPP
- LHON
- Mitochondrial disorders
- Infectious diseases
  - HIV
  - HTLV-1-associated myelopathy

- PML
- Viral meningoencephalitis, e.g., tick-borne encephalitis (TBE), HSV-1 (rarely HSV-2)
- Neuroborreliosis
- Neurobrucellosis
- Neurocysticercosis
- Neurosyphilis
- Tuberculosis
- Whipple's disease
- *Listeria monocytogenes* (Case 4.32)

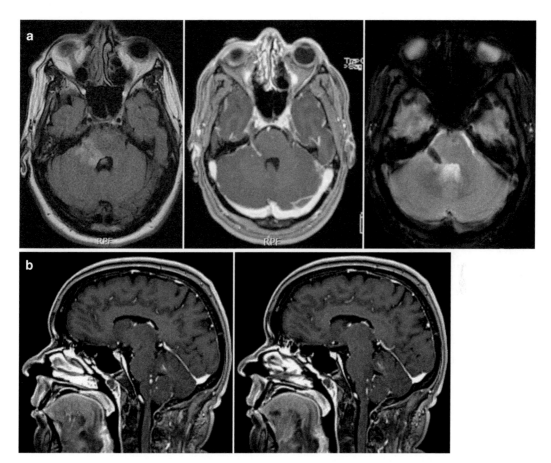

Case 4.32 Rhombenencephalitis due to *Listeria monocytogenes*. *Listeria monocytogenes* is associated with rhombencephalitis, but the exact mechanisms by which the pathogen invades the brainstem remain poorly understood. A 42-year-old female was admitted with serologically proven *Listeria monocytogenes* septicemia. Prior to any other neurological symptoms, she complained of hypoesthesia and a tingling sensation in the ipsilateral half of the face, consistent with sensory trigeminal nerve dysfunction on that side. T2-weighted and contrast-enhanced T1-weighted MRI revealed a cerebellopontine abscess, including involvement of the trigeminal nerve root, as well as selective contrast enhancement of the sensory trigeminal tract in the pons and medulla oblongata (**a, b**). This is in line with earlier data from animal experiments, showing that Listeria monocytogenes is capable of retrograde intra-axonal migration along cranial nerves and may induce rhombencephalitis in rodents after inoculation of bacteria into the facial musculature. Thus, in a subset of patients with rhombencephalitis, *Listeria monocytogenes* enters the cerebellopontine angle via the trigeminal nerve, invading the brainstem along the sensory trigeminal nuclei

- Malignancies
  - Primary CNS lymphoma
  - Malignant meningitis (meningeal carcinomatosis)
  - Other primary and secondary CNS neoplasms
- Others
  - Arnold-Chiari malformation
  - Superficial CNS siderosis
  - Brainstem vascular malformations
  - Vitamin B12 deficiency

- Copper deficiency myelopathy
- Small vessel disease and other cerebrovascular disease
- Spinal arteriovenous (AV) dural fistula and other spinal vascular malformations
- Susac's syndrome (Case 4.21)
- Toxic demyelination, e.g., due to heroin inhalation ("chasing the dragon"), cocaine leukoencephalopathy (Case 4.33), carbon monoxide (CO)-induced leukoencephalopathy

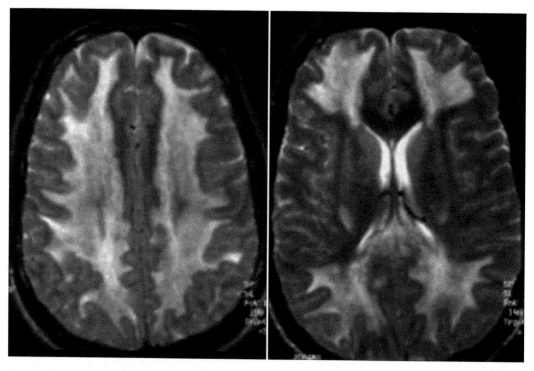

Case 4.33 Toxic leukoencephalopathy due to cocaine. A 21-year-old man had recurrent episodes of depression. He was found breathing, but deeply comatose in a hotel room with injection marks in the left cubital vein. A syringe and a farewell letter were beside him, and 14 empty packages with tracks of white powder, later identified as cocaine, were found close by. On admission, he was unresponsive and intubated with intact brainstem reflexes. There was bilateral hyperreflexia and moderately increased muscle tone, but normal plantar reflexes. Urine toxicology screening was positive only for cocaine. MRI of the brain on day 21 showed diffuse symmetrical WM changes in the cerebrum with hyperintense signal on the T_2-weighted images and preservation of U-fibers (**a**, **b**). Brainstem and cerebellum appeared normal. No con-trast enhancement was observed. Magnetic resonance angiography was unremarkable. Twenty-four days after admission, the patient died of pneumonia without having regained consciousness. Autopsy revealed severe leukoencephalopathy with pronounced demyelination, lipid-loaded macrophages, and liquefying of the central cerebral WM. Toxic leukoencephalopathy has been described with intravenous and inhalative consumption of cocaine, heroin, and other drugs of misuse. Whereas the clinical picture varies extensively, the radiological and histological findings are quite characteristic. Typically, T_2-weighted MRI shows diffuse bihemispheric WM lesions, often with preservation of U-fibers such as in this case (Adapted with permission from Kondziella et al. (2007a, b))

- Various mononeuropathies and polyneuropathies
- Wartenberg's migrant sensory neuritis
- Wilson's disease
- PRES

4.13   The Differential Diagnosis of Infectious Diseases

Infective agents may reach the CNS by several mechanisms, the first three of the following five being common (Fig. 4.9):

- Direct inoculation into the brain tissue (e.g., brain surgery, trauma).
- Per continuitatem (e.g., brain abscess secondary to a middle ear infection).
- Hematogenic spread (e.g., due to endocarditis).[12]
- Some viruses are neuroinvasive and reach neuronal cell bodies retrogradely via axons (e.g., rabies, HSV).
- Transmissible spongiform encephalopathies, or prion diseases, are exceptional in many ways. They are due to infectious proteins (prions) and can occur sporadically or may be familial or acquired (e.g., direct inoculation, orally).

The growing number of patients with immunosuppression because of cancer treatment, organ transplantation, HIV, or drug abuse contributes to the rising incidence of opportunistic infections. In addition, exotic infectious diseases are encountered with increasing frequency in Western societies due to immigration and intercontinental travel. The vast majority of conditions with infectious (and noninfectious) CSF inflammation managed by neurologists are associated with a lymphocytic CSF pleocytosis (as opposed to a neutrophil CSF pleocytosis, seen in bacterial meningitis and usually managed by infectious disease specialists). The list of human pathogens is huge, and many pathogens can affect the nervous system in many different ways. The most practical approach to the differential diagnosis of neuroinfectious diseases is therefore to list them according to the responsible microorganisms (e.g., viruses, bacteria, fungi, parasites) and to associate each of them with one or two characteristic features.

4.13.1   Viral Infections

- Virus, including:
  - Retrovirus
    HIV can infect nearly every part of the nervous system, from the muscle cell to cortical neurons. Neurological symptoms in HIV patients may be due to the virus itself, seroconversion (self-limiting aseptic meningitis), opportunistic infections, the side effects of antiviral therapy, and the immune reconstitution inflammatory syndrome (IRIS), a paradoxical reaction to HIV infection associated with reconstitution of the immune system following the start of highly active antiviral therapy (HAART). However, since the advent of HAART, the incidence of neurological disorders due to HIV has dramatically decreased, and they are almost always seen in HIV patients with low CD4+ counts (Case 4.34).
    Human T-lymphotropic virus type 1 (HTLV-1) is common in tropical regions, including Africa and the Caribbean, and leads to a chronic progressive myelopathy, hence the name tropical spastic paraparesis.
  - Herpes virus
    HSV-1 leads to classic herpes simplex encephalitis, the most common form of non-epidemic encephalitis in adults in

---

[12]Brain abscess is most commonly due to hematogenous spread. Less frequently, it occurs as a complication of sinusitis, otitis, mastoiditis, or penetrating trauma. Brain abscess may be caused by a single agent but can also be polymicrobial. Headache, fever, and focal neurologic signs are the classic triad of a brain abscess. However, most patients do not present with the complete triad, and the presentation is typically that of an intracerebral mass lesion with subacute onset. Intraventricular rupture of the abscess leads to ventriculitis and rapid deterioration.

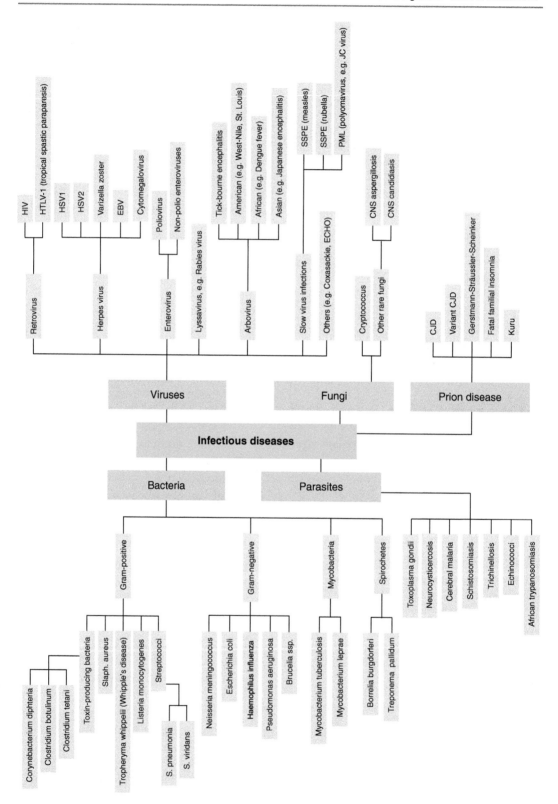

Fig. 4.9 Differential diagnosis of infectious diseases

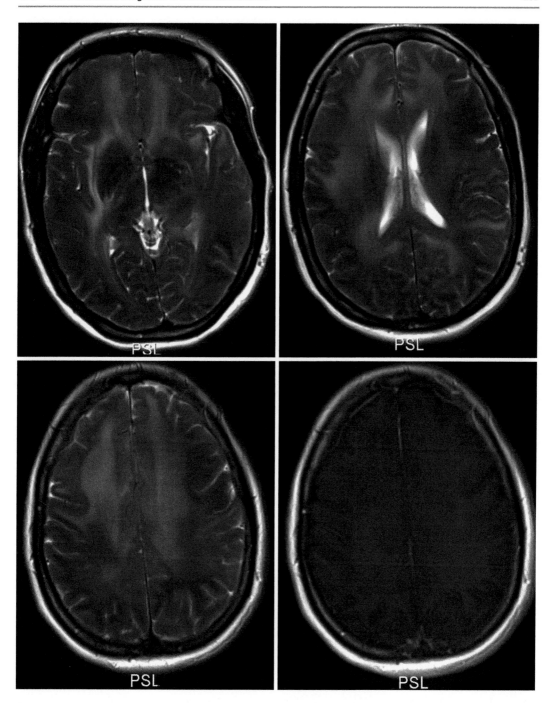

Case 4.34 HIV encephalitis. A 37-year-old HIV-positive woman stopped antiviral medication against advice from her physician, because she considered herself to be cured after intake of traditional herbal medicine. Four months later, she developed headache and bizarre behavior. There were no focal neurological deficits. MRI showed a pronounced leukoencephalopathy with sparing of U-fibers (axial T2 weighted, **upper row and lower row, left**) and no contrast enhancement (**lower row, right**). Lumbar puncture revealed a lymphocytic CSF pleocytosis (110 cells, 0.9 g protein). Tests for relevant opportunistic infections and sexually transmitted diseases other than HIV were negative. CSF flow cytometry and microscopy did not show evidence of lymphoma. However, her HIV viral copy load was much higher in CSF (1100 copies/ml) than in the blood (<50 copies/ml). When retroviral medication was reestablished, both her clinical condition and leukoencephalopathy on MRI improved, confirming the diagnosis of HIV encephalitis

the Western world (95%). Onset is usually within 1–5 days. Unspecific prodromal symptoms are followed by fever, confusion, headache, personality changes, altered consciousness, and focal neurological deficits related to the temporal lobes such as focal and secondarily generalized seizures, aphasia, and hemiparesis. Unfortunately, it is not uncommon that aphasic and hemiparetic patients presenting to the emergency room are misdiagnosed as suffering from ischemic stroke when the initial CT scan shows temporal lobe hypodensity (see Case 4.1). In the immunocompromised patient, herpes simplex encephalitis can take an atypical course with less prodromal symptoms and focal deficits, as well as more extensive cerebral involvement on MRI and occasionally a lack of CSF pleocytosis due to the host's ineffective immune response. Without immediate antiviral therapy, herpes simplex encephalitis is devastating and usually fatal, and therefore, it is essential not to wait for results from CSF analysis but to start aciclovir treatment right away. It is important to note that although polymerase chain reaction (PCR) amplification assays for the detection of HSV DNA in the CSF have high sensitivity and specificity in the first few days, false-negative results occur thereafter. Similarly, intrathecal synthesis of HSV-specific antibodies occurs in almost all patients but not usually until 3–10 days after the onset of symptoms, and therefore, false-negative results are possible in the beginning. It follows that it is mandatory to order both CSF PCR and antibody titer analyses.

HSV-2 is associated with mild relapsing-remitting meningitis (Mollaret's meningitis) and may lead to acute bladder palsy due to infection of the cauda equina and conus medullaris, as outlined in Chap. 2. Herpes simplex encephalitis, in contrast, is only rarely caused by HSV-2.

VZV leads typically to chicken pox in children and to shingles in adults after reactivation of the dormant virus in the sensory ganglia. VZV may also lead to myelitis and encephalitis, and in a patient with a peripheral facial nerve palsy and unusual pain, check for the typical erythematous rash in the ear canal, the tongue, and/or hard palate (herpes zoster oticus; Ramsay Hunt syndrome type II). Occasionally, VZV infections can occur without a rash (zoster sine herpete). Further, facial zoster in the elderly may lead to ipsilateral stroke a few days to weeks following the first signs of the painful rash.

Epstein-Barr virus causes infectious mononucleosis and has been implicated in several diseases such Hodgkin's lymphoma, nasopharyngeal carcinoma, and MS.

Cytomegalovirus usually leads to a mild aseptic meningitis but may have a much more aggressive course in the immunocompromised.

– Enterovirus

Enteroviruses are the most common agents associated with aseptic meningitis.

Poliovirus leads to poliomyelitis (and decades later, the post-polio syndrome may arise). Other enteroviruses such as *Coxsackie* and *ECHO virus* also have a predilection for the anterior horns cells and may lead to a similar form of acute anterior poliomyelitis.

– Arbovirus (= arthropod-borne viruses)

TBE is on the rise in Europe. In most cases, the symptoms of TBE develop in two distinct stages. Roughly 25% of people develop flu-like symptoms 2–28 days after a tick bite. Most patients make a full recovery within a week. The second stage, characterized by a meningoencephalitis, occurs a few days to weeks later.

Aggressive *arboviruses* are found in the Americas (e.g., East/West/ Venezuelan equine encephalitis, West Nile encephalitis, St. Louis encephalitis, tick-borne paralysis), Asia (Japanese encephalitis), and Africa (dengue fever, which has spread to other tropical regions around the globe).

– Lyssavirus

Rabies virus. Invariably fatal, rabies accounts for over 50,000 deaths annually according to the WHO, mostly in Africa and Asia. Bats are the most common vector in North America and dogs the most important vector globally. Depending on the distance the virus must travel to reach the CNS, the incubation period is usually a few months, following which the patient develops malaise, fever, and headache, then motor agitation, decreased consciousness, and the classic symptom of hydrophobia, which is due to reflexive spasms of the respiratory and pharyngeal muscles when attempting to swallow liquids—later, even the sound of running waters triggers these spasms. Finally, the patient becomes lethargic and eventually comatose. Death is usually due to respiratory insufficiency.

– Slow virus infections are not a family for themselves, but their distinct clinical course makes it practical for the neurologist to group them together:

Subacute sclerosing panencephalitis (SSPE) due to the *measles virus* usually affects children.

Rubella virus may lead to a disease similar to SSPE.

JC virus is a polyomavirus and the main agent behind PML. PML is usually seen in immunocompromised patients such as those with HIV, chemotherapy, organ transplantation or a history of sarcoidosis. It can be the initial AIDS-defining illness in up to 25% of patients. Of practical concern for MS patients is the possibility of developing PML with natalizumab treatment. JC virus affects oligodendrocytes and leads to large areas of multifocal demyelination. Although PML occasionally starts rather acutely, in the majority of cases, it evolves over days to months. The velocity of neurologic decline usually accelerates during the disease. Apart from hemiparesis and other focal signs, cognitive functions may be affected as well, e.g., PML may lead to dysphasia, cortical blindness, and alterations of personality. Seizures have been reported in up to 20% of cases. MRI shows characteristic conflating white matter involvement ("spilled milk" on FLAIR and T_2-weighted MRI) with cortical sparing (Case 4.9). The CSF cell count is usually normal (or only slightly increased). Cerebral involvement is more frequent than brainstem involvement. Contrast enhancement is only very rarely seen, but interestingly, in AIDS patients this is a favorable prognostic sign. The diagnosis of PML is based on the history, the typical neuroradiological appearance, and the finding of JC virus DNA in the CSF using PCR. Brain biopsy is rarely needed. If left untreated, PML leads to severe disability and finally death. The prognosis is poorer with a severe degree of immunosuppression, a high viral load, and involvement of critical locations (such as the brainstem). However, one needs to be aware that antiretroviral therapy in HIV patients or discontinuing natalizumab in patients with multiple sclerosis may lead to the development of IRIS, presenting with a paradoxical worsening of neurological deficits and possibly death.

4.13.2 Bacterial Infections

• Bacteria
  – Gram-positive bacteria and bacilli
    Staphylococcus usually leads to acute bacterial meningitis and/or cerebritis with subsequent abscess formation (Case 4.35).

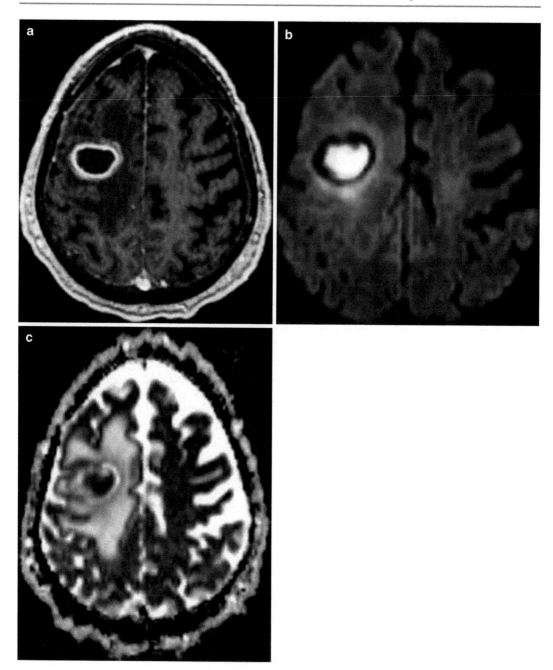

Case 4.35 Diffusion-weighted MRI in the assessment of brain abscesses. A 67-year-old male received chemotherapy for a plasmacytoma. The patient complained of an increasingly severe headache over the previous 7 days. He had fever and a left-sided hemiparesis. Contrast-enhanced T1-weighted MRI (**a**) showed a lesion in the right MCA territory, including perilesional edema and a ringlike contrast-enhancing periphery. MR DWI (**b**) showed hyperintense and ADC sequences (**c**) hypointense signal within the lesion, the characteristic MRI appearance of a cerebral abscess

Streptococcus pneumoniae also leads to acute bacterial meningitis.

Streptococcus viridans is often encountered with low-virulent infective endocarditis and foreign body infections.

Corynebacterium diphtheriae produces a toxin that causes diphtheria. Bilateral lower CN palsies including facial diplegia are typical, as are sore throat, swollen neck, and pseudomembranes on the tonsils.

Clostridium tetani produces tetanospamin, which is responsible for tetanus and usually acquired because of wound infections under poor sanitary conditions. Tetanus is rare in developed countries but common worldwide, probably killing half a million adults every year. The toxin is produced in the wound, binds to peripheral motor nerve terminals, and enters the spinal cord or brainstem via retrograde axonal transport. Depending on the site of spore inoculation, the incubation period varies from a few days to several weeks. In the generalized form, excessive excitation of spinal and bulbar motor neurons leads to sustained rigidity of the masseter muscles (trismus), the face (risus sardonicus), and the back (opisthotonus), as well as spasms of the laryngopharynx (e.g., triggered by simply looking at water and food). This form is always fatal without intensive medical care. The local form leads to stiffness near the injury and has a better prognosis.

Clostridium botulinum produces the most poisonous toxin of all and causes botulism which can be food-borne (canned food), neonatal (acquired during delivery under poor sanitary conditions), or associated with wounds (e.g., skin popping, the subcutaneous application of heroin by drug addicts). (See Case 2.1.)

Listeria monocytogenes is a significant cause of meningitis and meningoencephalitis in neonates, pregnant women, the immunocompromised, and the elderly. Ingestion of soft cheese and unpasteurized milk products is a typical cause, but *Listeria* has also been isolated from raw meat, vegetables, and seafood. CNS listeriosis preferentially involves the brainstem and the meninges. The case fatality rate exceeds that of salmonella infections (see Case 4.32).

Tropheryma whippelii is usually classified as a gram-positive *Actinobacteria*, although it may be gram-negative as well. It causes Whipple's disease, predominantly seen in middle-aged and elderly men with weight loss, progressive dementia, ataxia, and oculomotor disturbances. Oculomasticatory myorhythmia is pathognomonic for Whipple's disease but relatively seldom. *Tropheryma whippelii* is notoriously difficult to detect. Jejunum biopsy and CSF examination may be negative despite combined PCR analysis and microscopic evaluation, and often the last resort is brain biopsy.

– Gram-negative bacteria and bacilli

Neisseria meningococcus (together with *Streptococcus pneumoniae*) leads the list of community-acquired bacterial meningitis.

Haemophilus influenzae, previously the leading cause of bacterial meningitis in children under 5 years of age, is no longer common thanks to widespread vaccination.

Escherichia coli causes postsurgical infections and neonatal meningitis, usually associated with poor hygienic conditions.

Pseudomonas aeruginosa is a common hospital-acquired infection because it thrives in wet surroundings and on most surfaces, including medical equipment and catheters. *Pseudomonas aeruginosa* is the classic cause of otitis externa maligna (also called necrotizing external otitis). This life-threatening skull base infection is characterized by the following triad: (A) an elderly diabetic or otherwise immunocompromised patient presenting with (B) persistent headache, otalgia, and auditory discharge, usually after water irrigation for cerumen impaction, (C) complicated by multiple CN palsies. Due to its close proximity to the external acoustic meatus and the stylomastoid foramen, the facial nerve is the CN primarily involved (Case 4.36).

Brucella spp. is usually associated with unsterilized milk or meat from infected cattle; it may therefore lead to brucellosis (Malta fever) in, e.g., veterinarians and farmers. Neurobrucellosis is a differential diagnosis to Whipple's disease.

– Mycobacteria

Mycobacterium tuberculosis may cause meningovascular inflammation leading to ischemic infarction, basal meningitis with affection of multiple lower CNs, brain tuberculoma that behaves like a mass lesion, obstructive and communicating hydrocephalus, spondylitis, spinal abscess, and transverse myelitis (see Case 2.8).

Mycobacterium leprae and *Mycobacterium lepromatosis* give rise to leprosy, a granulomatous disease of the peripheral nerves, the upper respiratory tract, and the skin. Lesions of the latter are characterized by hypopigmented anesthetic areas.

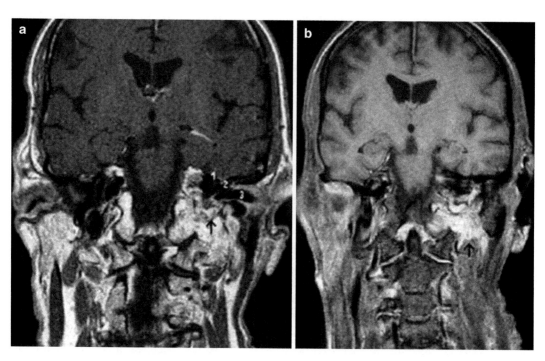

Case 4.36 Cranial neuropathy due to malignant external otitis. A 68-year-old male with poorly regulated diabetes mellitus consulted an otolaryngologist because of left ear deafness. After irrigation for cerumen impaction, hearing returned to normal. A week later he developed constant left-sided headache and painful drainage of a yellowish smelly fluid from the left ear. One month later, the patient noticed hypesthesia on the left side of his face. Two months later, he developed slurred speech and hoarseness. The month after he had difficulties with swallowing. Neurological examination revealed impairment of the left CN V, VIII, IX, X, and XII. T1-weighted MRI with gadolinium contrast showed the inner (*1*), middle (*2*), and external ear (*3*) as well as a subtemporal infectious process (**a**; *black arrow*), which extended caudally, causing massive soft tissue inflammation and bone erosion of the occipital condyle and mastoid (**b**; *black arrow*). Culture from a mastoid biopsy revealed *Pseudomonas aeruginosa*. The patient received 8 weeks of ciprofloxacin treatment and made an uneventful recovery (adapted with permission from Kondziella and Skagervik (2007))

- Spirochetes (in fact, also gram-negative bacteria)

  Borrelia burgdorferi is the agent in Lyme disease, the most common tick-borne disease in the Northern Hemisphere. Tick bites are acquired during outdoor activities in the warmer months of the year, which is why most patients present from June to November. Early localized infection leads to the characteristic circular, outwardly expanding rash called erythema chronicum migrans, but not all patients notice such a rash or having been bitten by a tick. Patients with neurological signs typically come to medical attention during early (second stage) neuroborreliosis. The most common manifestation is a painful lymphocytic meningoradiculitis (Bannwarth's syndrome), which either presents as an isolated radicular pain syndrome or together with muscle weakness. Characteristically, the patient complains about radiculopathic pain with attacks during the night, which clearly distinguishes it from radiculopathic pain due to degenerative spine disease. Peripheral facial palsy, often bilateral in adults, is another common syndrome. Involvement of the CNS, such as myelitis, is rare in early neuroborreliosis. If left untreated, 5–10% of patients suffer a chronic course of the disease, including chronic lymphocytic meningitis or third-stage encephalomyelitis. Monosymptomatic chronic headache due to pachymeningitis is another manifestation. Chronic Lyme disease is typically accompanied by vegetative signs, including general fatigue and malaise as well as unintended weight loss. Late disseminated infection may lead to cognitive symptoms, including dementia. CSF findings include high protein, lymphocytic pleocytosis, and Borrelia burgdorferi-specific intrathecal antibody synthesis, but despite clear CSF inflammation, meningeal signs are rare. The diagnosis of neuroborreliosis is based on the typical clinical presentation, CSF inflammatory changes and B. burgdorferi-specific intrathecal antibody production.

  Treponema pallidum leads to neurosyphilis. In the early stages, there is either asymptomatic meningitis or symptomatic meningovascular inflammation that may cause cerebral infarction. The late forms of neurosyphilis include tabes dorsalis with severe sensory ataxia due to destruction of the posterior columns[13] and dementia, traditionally known as general paresis. Another syndrome of tertiary syphilis is the Argyll Robertson phenomenon that denotes pupillary dysfunction with light-near dissociation. (This pupillary dysfunction has been memorized by generations of students using the mnemonic "a prostitute accommodates but does not react." However, Adie's tonic pupil is nowadays a more common cause for pupillary dysfunction with light-near dissociation.) Although neurosyphilis is rare nowadays, it is again on the rise. Since syphilis is treatable, it is mandatory to order a Venereal Disease Research Laboratory (VDRL) test in patients with a chronic CSF lymphocytosis.

4.13.3 Infections Due to Parasites, Fungi, and Prions

- Parasites
  - Neurocysticercosis is not only the most common parasitic infestation of the CNS, but it may also be one of the most frequent causes of epilepsy worldwide. It is caused by ingestion of eggs or larvae from *Taenia solium* in undercooked pork or from contaminated food or water. Brain cysticerci, usually multiple, develop in the brain after an incubation period of several months to years. Other manifestations than epilepsy

---

[13]Moritz Romberg (1795–1873, German neurologist) invented the eponymous test for the screening of sensory ataxia in large numbers of recruits to detect those unsuited for the army because of tabes dorsalis.

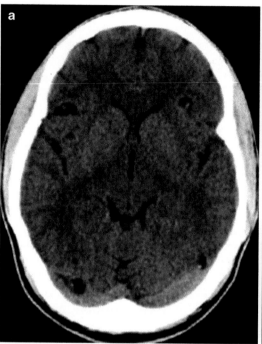

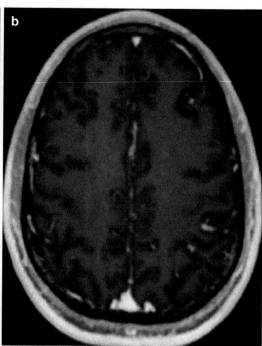

Case 4.37 Neurocysticercosis. A 23-year-old male exchange student from rural Latin America presented with headache and focal seizures evolving to bilateral convulsive seizures. His general physical and neurologic exam was normal. A CT and T1-weighted contrast-enhanced MRI demonstrated multiple cysticerci, consistent with a diagnosis of neurocysticercosis (**a, b**). A lumbar puncture revealed slightly elevated opening pressure and mild CSF pleocytosis. A serum cysticercosis enzyme-linked immunoelectrotransfer blot assay was positive. The patient was treated with albendazole and corticosteroids for 2 weeks as well as antiepileptic drugs. Two years later, neuroimaging showed a declining number of calcified cysts, and his epilepsy was well controlled

include obstructive hydrocephalus and focal neurological deficits (Case 4.37).

- *Toxoplasma gondii* is a parasitic protozoan for which the cat is the definite host. It is usually asymptomatic, but toxoplasma may be reactivated with immunosuppression. Toxoplasmosis is the most common opportunistic infection in patients with HIV. De novo infection in pregnancy may have catastrophic consequences for mother and fetus. Toxoplasmosis leads to various focal deficits, seizures, encephalopathy, and retinopathy.

- Cerebral malaria due to *Plasmodium falciparum* should be suspected in every traveler returning from endemic countries and presenting with neurological symptoms of unknown origin. Although cerebral malaria is often fatal and the course severe, outcome can be strikingly good (Case 4.38).

- Schistosomiasis (or bilharziosis) is infection with flukes (small parasitic worms) after contact with water from rivers and lakes contaminated by freshwater snails. *Schistosoma* (*S.*) *mansoni* and *S. haematobium* characteristically lead to granulomatous disease of the spinal cord with flaccid paraplegia and bladder palsy, whereas *S. japonicum* may evoke granulomatous disease of the brain.

- Ingested larvae from *Trichinella* can cause symptomatic or asymptomatic trichinosis. Affection of the CNS is rare but usually fatal.

- *Echinococcus granulosus* and *Echinococcus multilocularis*, for which dogs, respectively, foxes, are the definite hosts, may lead to hydatid cysts in the human brain and increased ICP, focal deficits, and seizures.

- African trypanosomiasis produces the classic sleeping sickness with characteristic lymphadenopathy at the back of the neck (Winterbottom's sign), followed later by confusion, sleep cycle disturbance, and, if left untreated, coma and death.

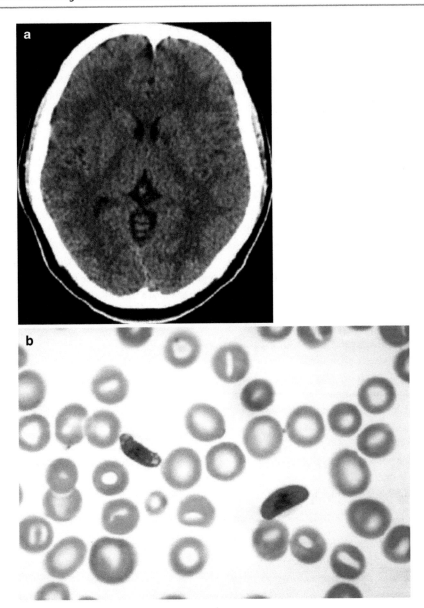

Case 4.38 Cerebral malaria. A 31-year-old male sailor was found unresponsive in his cabin. On admission to the emergency room, he had a fever (40.4 °C). The patient was awake, but not responding; there was occasional eye contact, but he did not talk or follow any commands. There was meningism, generalized hypertonia, and intermittent opisthotonus; tendon reflexes were brisk and plantar responses extensor. Following the bedside examination, he developed a generalized tonic-clonic seizure without evident focal onset. According to witnesses, 6 h prior to admission, the patient had complained of feeling unwell but had appeared otherwise normal. He had been treated with antibiotics for an unspecified infection 14 days earlier. During the last 3 months, his crew had traveled to various ports in Eastern and Western Africa. A CT of the brain was normal (**a**). A lumbar puncture revealed a slightly increased opening pressure (28 cm H$_2$O) but normal cells and protein. Screening for illicit drugs was negative. Routine blood tests, including arterial gases, showed slight microcytic anemia and metabolic acidosis and significantly increased C-reactive protein and leukocytosis. Examination of a thick blood film under light microscopy revealed macrogametocytes of the parasite *Plasmodium falciparum* (**b**). Artemisinin-based combination therapy for cerebral malaria was initiated. The patient regained consciousness 2 days later. On follow-up 3 months later, he was back at work but complained of slight cognitive sequelae regarding concentration and short-term memory

- Fungi
  - Cryptococcosis due to *Cryptococcus neoformans* is a defining opportunistic infection for AIDS and the most frequent fungal meningitis in these patients.
  - CNS infection with other fungi such as candida and aspergillus is very unusual and only seen in the immunocompromised.
- Prion diseases (known as transmissible spongiform encephalopathies) include:
  - Creutzfeldt-Jakob disease (CJD) may be sporadic, familial, or iatrogenic. It is a common cause of rapidly progressive dementia. Ataxia, myoclonus, and enhanced startle as well as various focal deficits are commonly seen. Death is inevitable and usually occurs within 6 months. For further information, see Sect. 4.4.
  - The new variant form of Creutzfeldt-Jakob disease (vCJD; first described in 1996) typically leads to prominent neuropsychiatric symptoms. It affects people at a much earlier age (median age 28) than classic CJD and has a somewhat more protracted cause (12–18 months). Most cases of vCJD are from the UK.
  - Kuru is another classic prion disease, now history. It occurred in Papua New Guinea and was transmitted among members of the Fore tribe because of cannibalistic funeral practices.
  - Gerstmann-Sträussler-Scheinker disease, one of the familial prion diseases.
  - Fatal familial insomnia, another familial prion disease.

4.14 The Differential Diagnosis of Malignancy, Including Paraneoplastic Conditions

Malignancy may affect the nervous system in several ways (Fig. 4.10):

- Primary CNS tumors and secondary malignancies (metastasis)
- Paraneoplastic syndromes
- Side effects of cancer treatment

- Radiotherapy, e.g., radiation plexopathy and leukoencephalopathy
- Chemotherapy, e.g., peripheral neuropathy and toxic leukoencephalopathy
- Surgery, e.g., focal neurological deficits following neurosurgery

4.14.1 Primary Tumors of the CNS and PNS and Secondary Malignancies

Primary brain tumors may be histologically benign or malignant. However, due to their mass effect causing brain tissue shifts, even histologically benign tumors can be fatal. The common primary brain tumors are listed here according to their cellular origin.

- Glial cells
  - Astrocytes, astrocytoma grades I–IV. Astrocytomas grades I and II may be curable (e.g., pilocytic astrocytoma in children). Grade III tumors progress after several years into astrocytoma grade IV. The latter is identical with glioblastoma multiforme, which may arise de novo or, as stated, from a low-grade astrocytoma. Astrocytomas are the most common primary malignant brain tumors. Of note, brainstem glioma in adults has a rather unique presentation (see Case 2.6). In contrast to supratentorial gliomas (and brainstem gliomas in children), the course of glioma in the brainstem tends to be prolonged. When these patients present to the neurologist, they usually have surprisingly few clinical symptoms despite extensive tumor infiltration as seen on MRI. Another malignant condition that may have a rather unusual presentation is gliomatosis cerebri (Case 4.39).
  - Oligodendrocytes, oligodendroglioma. These usually have a somewhat better prognosis than astrocytoma but tend to become increasingly more malignant as well. CT of the brain typically shows a calcified process.

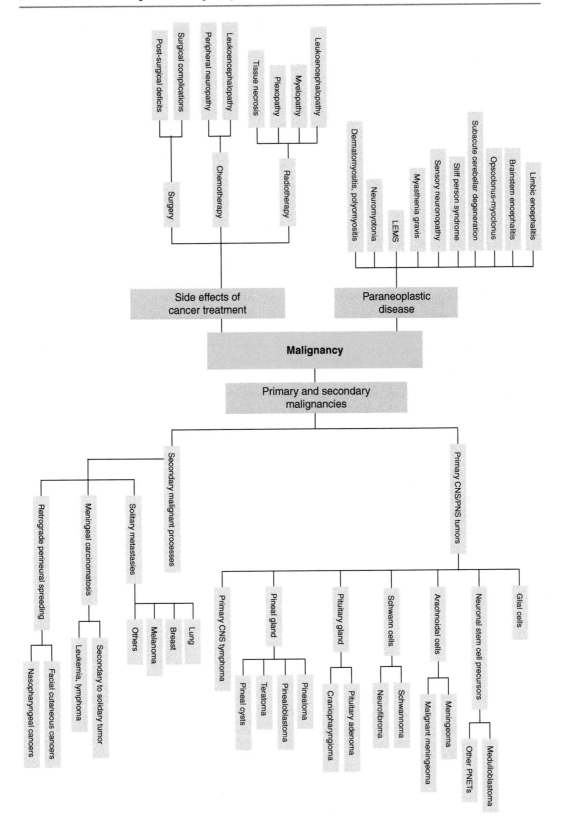

Fig. 4.10 Differential diagnosis of malignancy and paraneoplastic disorders

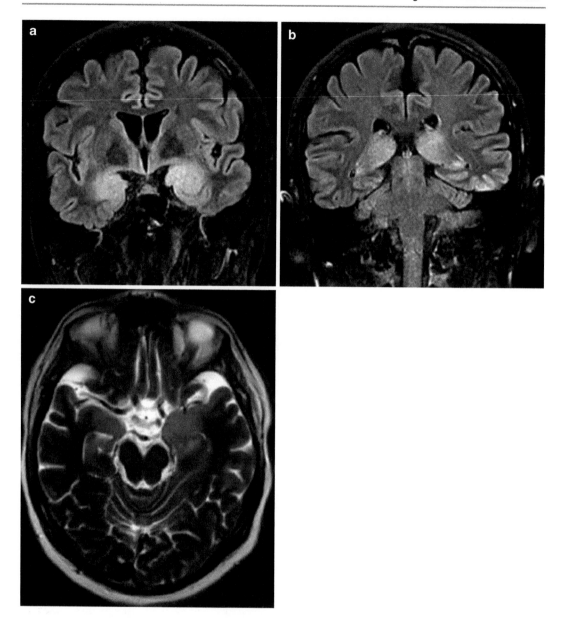

Case 4.39 Gliomatosis cerebri. A 45-year-old female was referred with a working diagnosis of limbic encephalitis because of a history of short-term memory deficits and temporal lobe epilepsy as well as an MRI showing bilateral edematous mesial temporal lobes. However, upon admission, the patient stated that her symptoms had started gradually more than 3 years ago with only slight progression. The time course was rather unusual for autoimmune limbic encephalitis. In addition, on FLAIR (**a, b**) and T2-weighted MRI (**c**), signal changes were relatively widespread, involving the entire hippocampal formation and the posterior thalamus on both sides, and follow-up MRI 3 months later showed unchanged abnormalities. There was no contrast enhancement after gadolinium injection. Extensive diagnostic procedures for autoimmune limbic encephalitis, systemic malignancy, and infectious agents were negative. Following a brain biopsy, the patient was diagnosed with a low-grade astrocytoma (gliomatosis cerebri, WHO grade II)

- Ependyma, ependymoma. The common location of intracranial ependymoma is the fourth ventricle. In adults, it also occurs at spinal locations.
- Neurons. Limited neurogenesis in the adult human brain is restricted to certain areas such as the hippocampus and the subventricular zone. Thus, since neurons do not proliferate, there are no neuronal tumors other than those that derive from neuronal stem cell precursors. These are the primitive neuroectodermal tumors (PNET), the most common being medulloblastoma. The tumors have a strong tendency to metastasize within the CNS (e.g., spinal drop metastases). Neuroblastoma is another tumor that derives from the neural crest; it is a neuroendocrinal tumor and one of the most common extracranial solid cancers in childhood.
- Arachnoidal cells, meningioma. This is the most common benign tumor of the CNS; more malignant and much rarer varieties include atypical (grade II) and anaplastic (grade III) meningiomas.
- Schwann cells, schwannoma, and neurofibroma. Schwann cells are for the PNS what oligodendrocytes are for the CNS; they produce myelin. Schwannoma may be associated with any cranial (CN III–CN XII) or spinal nerve, but vestibular schwannoma is most common. (These tumors are often but incorrectly called acoustic neurinoma.) Bilateral vestibular schwannoma is pathognomonic for neurofibromatosis type II. Neurofibromas arise also from Schwann cells, but in contrast to schwannomas, they incorporate other types of cells and structural elements as well. Plexiform neurofibromas, which may sometimes undergo malignant transformation, are the hallmark of neurofibromatosis type I.
- Pineal gland. Pineal gland tumors include, e.g., pinealomas, pineoblastomas, pineal cysts, and astrocytomas. Also germ cell tumors (either germinomatous or nongerminomatous) frequently arise in proximity of the pineal gland. All these tumors may present with acute or subacute hydrocephalus, gait disturbances, and midbrain signs such as the Parinaud's syndrome (see Chap. 2).
- Pituitary gland, pituitary adenoma, and craniopharyngioma
  - Pituitary adenomas account for approximately 10% of all intracranial neoplasms. They may manifest with bitemporal hemianopia and hormonal disturbances (e.g., Cushing syndrome, acromegaly, galactorrhea, sexual dysfunction). Pituitary apoplexy may lead to sudden headache, diplopia (due to CN III compression), and coma. Postpartum pituitary necrosis due to infarction of or hemorrhage into a pituitary adenoma during delivery is called Sheehan syndrome.
  - Another tumor of the parasellar region, craniopharyngioma tends to reoccur after surgery despite being histologically benign. Craniopharyngiomas present with visual field defects and diencephalic disturbances and may lead to obstructive hydrocephalus (Case 4.40).
- Primary CNS lymphoma. This non-Hodgkin's lymphoma is confined to the CNS. The etiology of cerebral lymphoma in the immunocompetent patient is unknown. In immunosuppressed patients, particularly those with AIDS or transplant recipients, Epstein-Barr virus seems to play an etiologic role. In recent decades, the frequency of primary CNS lymphoma has been increasing in both immunocompetent and immunosuppressed patients. Following corticosteroid therapy, CNS lymphomas typically decrease in size or may even disappear on brain imaging (only to recur after some time; this is the ghost tumor phenomenon), which is why imaging and brain biopsy of presumed lymphomatous tumors are best performed before steroids are given (Case 4.41).

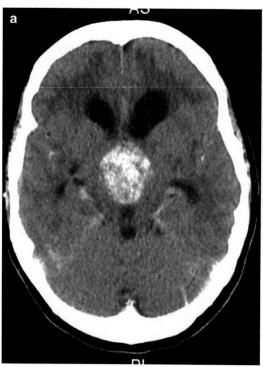

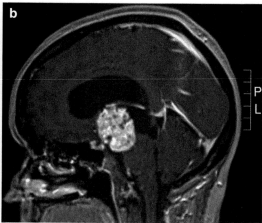

Case 4.40 Craniopharyngeoma and obstructive hydro-cephalus. A 53-year-old female with an unremarkable medical history was brought to the neurologist by her husband. He complained that his wife had difficulties with balance and gait; she was constantly tired and fell asleep several times during the day. In addition, she was slow-cerebrated and had memory difficulties, and she had become incontinent for urine. Symptoms had started 3 months prior and were progressive. Although the patient confirmed the history, she seemed unconcerned. Examination revealed bilateral extensor plantar reflexes, increased muscle tone in the legs, as well as cognitive deficits and a broad-based shuffling gate. The clinical history (gait ataxia, urine incontinence, and cognitive decline) was consistent with a hydrocephalus, most likely obstructive because of the recent onset. Contrast-enhanced CT (axial, **a**) and MRI (sagittal, **b**) showed an enhancing well-demarcated tumor obstructing the third ventricle and leading to ventricular dilatation. Following resection of the tumor, the patient's condition was normalized except for mild urinary urge. Histology revealed a papillary cra-niopharyngioma (WHO grade 1)

Secondary malignancies may affect the nervous system as follows:

- Single or multiple metastases. Brain metasta-ses are much more common than primary brain tumors. Data on the ratio of primary vs. secondary brain tumors are very inconsistent in the literature, though. This is due to the fact that some authors refer to neurosurgical data, while others refer to autopsy studies. Obviously, brain metastases are more common in the latter.
  - Lung cancer, breast cancer, and malignant melanoma (in this order) are the most com-mon primaries and account for two-thirds of all brain metastases.
  - All neoplasms, including leukemia and systemic lymphoma, are theoretically capable of metastasizing to the brain.
  - In 10% of cases, the primary cancer remains unknown despite extensive inves-tigations. At autopsy, the most commonly found primary tumor is lung cancer.
  - Metastases may of course also affect the spinal cord, plexus, and peripheral nerves. For plexus infiltration of lung cancer, the so-called Pancoast tumor, see Case 2.3.

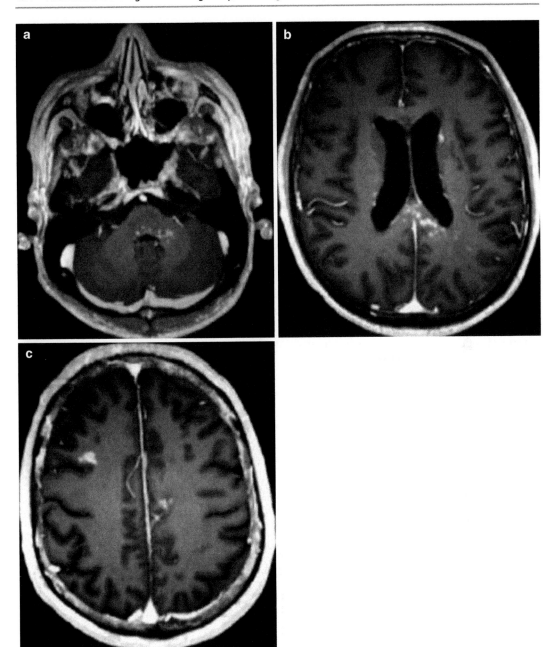

Case 4.41 Primary CNS lymphoma. A 65-year-old male presented with a focal seizure starting in the left half of his face and evolving into bilateral convulsions. He had a 2-month history of short episodes of twitching of the left corner of the mouth as well as gait ataxia and dysarthria. Examination further revealed saccadic pursuit, hyperre- flexia in all extremities, and bilateral extensive plantar reflexes. T1-weighted MRI showed contrast-enhancing lesions in the brainstem (**a**), the corpus callosum (**b**), and the right frontal lobe (**c**). Following a brain biopsy, the patient was diagnosed as having a primary CNS lymphoma

- Meningeal carcinomatosis. This is the spread of malignant cells into the lepto-meninges. Frequent symptoms include multiple and successive CN palsies, weakness in the extremities because of polyradiculopathy, back pain, headache, and mental changes. The most common causes are, in decreasing frequency, breast cancer, leukemia, systemic lymphoma, lung cancer, CNS tumors (e.g., medulloblastoma, glioblastoma), and malignant melanoma. The median survival is 6 months despite aggressive treatment.
- Retrograde perineural spreading of cutaneous (e.g., squamous cell carcinoma, basalioma) or mucosal (e.g., nasopharyngeal cancer) tumors. These tumors are a much rarer cause of secondary malignancy affecting the nervous system The typical history is of a (initially successfully) treated cancer in the skin or nasopharynx, until pain and numbness evolve many years later in the ipsilateral half of the face due to the spread of tumor cells into the trigeminal nerve, followed after weeks or months of ipsilateral abducens, oculomotor, facial, and other CN palsies. Typically, the diagnosis is delayed because many physicians are unfamiliar with the disease, and without thin-sliced contrast-enhanced MRI sequences, the perineuronal tumor infiltration is easily overlooked. Invasion of the brainstem will eventually lead to bulbar and sensorimotor symptoms and, ultimately, death.

4.14.2 Paraneoplastic Conditions

Paraneoplastic neurological syndromes result from damage to organs or tissues remote from the site of the primary malignancy or metastases. The pathogenesis is immune-mediated and due to cross-reaction against antigens shared by the tumor and cells in the CNS or PNS. Paraneoplastic neurological diseases are often related to intracellular antineuronal antibodies (as compared to synaptic/surface antigens, which are more commonly detected in non-paraneoplastic conditions). Various cancers are associated with paraneoplastic syndromes, the most common being SCLC, cancer of the breasts, testicles, and ovaries, and teratoma. The number of known antibodies is increasing steadily. It is no longer practical to learn them all by heart, and it does not seem useful either. Instead, it is advisable to know the most significant paraneoplastic syndromes and a few associated antibodies and to consult up-to-date literature in case of doubt. Listed from central to peripheral, the following syndromes are often (but not always) paraneoplastic conditions:

- Limbic encephalitis (e.g., SCLC, breast, ovaries, testicles, teratoma; anti-Yo, anti-Hu, anti-VGKC, anti-NMDA receptors, and many more; for a detailed account, see Sect. 4.5).
- Multifocal encephalomyelitis (SCLC, various others; anti-Ri, anti-Hu, anti-amphiphysin).
- Opsoclonus-myoclonus (lung, breast, testicles, others; anti-Yo, anti-Ri, anti-Hu, anti-amphiphysin; see Chap. 2).
- Brainstem encephalitis (testicles, lung, others; anti-Ma1, anti-Ma2) (Case 4.42).
- Subacute cerebellar degeneration (e.g., SCLC, breast, ovaries, testicles, teratoma, Hodgkin's lymphoma; anti-Yo, anti-Ri, anti-Hu, anti-amphiphysin, anti-VGKC).
- Stiff person syndrome (breast, lung, others; anti-amphiphysin, anti-GAD).
- Sensory neuronopathy (SCLC, plasma cell dyscrasias, others; anti-Hu, anti-amphiphysin, anti-CV2). Subacute sensory neuronopathy and neuropathies with anti-Hu or anti-CV2 antibodies are definite paraneoplastic disorders. Possible paraneoplastic neuropathies are heterogeneous.
- Neuromyotonia (also termed Isaac's syndrome; thymoma, SCLC; anti-VGKC).

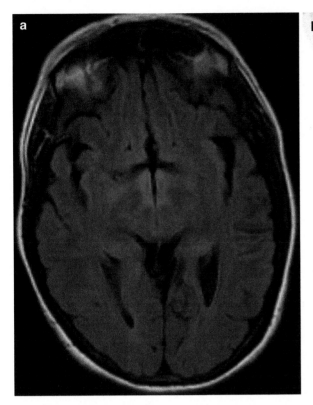

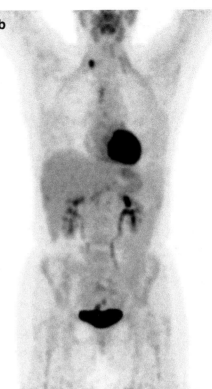

Case 4.42 Anti-Ma2-associated paraneoplastic brainstem encephalitis. A 56-year-old woman, previously healthy, developed double vision. A few days later, she noticed weakness in her legs and arms and slurred speech. Her relatives stated that she appeared slightly confused. Within 6 weeks, she was admitted to the intensive care unit because of tetraplegia and shortness of breath requiring artificial respiratory support and a tracheostomy. Horizontal eye movements were preserved, but there was complete vertical gaze palsy. She was awake and generally drowsy although she could communicate using preserved horizontal eye movements and neck flexion. Despite her fulminant brainstem syndrome, the only abnormality on MRI was a midline FLAIR hyperintensity at the level of the mesencephalon (**a**, left; but no contrast enhancement; this was confirmed by a second MRI a few weeks later), and lumbar puncture revealed a very minor lymphocytic CSF pleocytosis (9 cells, normal protein).

However, whole-body PET/CT showed a suspicious neck lymphadenopathy on the right side (**a**, right). Histology revealed adenocarcinoma; despite extensive diagnostic procedures, the primary malignancy was not found. When CSF analysis revealed a strongly positive IgG anti-Ma2 antibody titer, she was diagnosed as having anti-Ma2-associated paraneoplastic brainstem encephalitis. Despite treatment with IV steroids, plasma exchange, and chemotherapy, she died 3 months after onset of double vision. Autopsy confirmed inflammatory changes in the brainstem, thalamus, and basal ganglia, confirming the clinical diagnosis. Anti-Ma2-associated encephalitis is a rare paraneoplastic neurological syndrome that gives rise to a typical clinical picture of progressive diencephalic and brainstem dysfunction. Although MRI and CSF abnormalities can be very subtle, as shown here, the prognosis is usually poor

- LEMS (SCLC; voltage-gated calcium channel antibodies (anti-VGCC)).
- MG (thymoma; anti-acetylcholine receptor (AChR), anti-MuSK).
- Dermatomyositis and polymyositis (ovaries, GI, breast, lung). Dermatomyositis is more often paraneoplastic than polymyositis.

4.15   The Differential Diagnosis of Movement Disorders

Movement disorders can be divided into:

- Hypokinetic-rigid disorders, commonly referred to as parkinsonism

- Hyperkinetic disorders, often associated with normal or decreased muscle tone (chorea, choreoathetosis, hemiballism, myoclonus, tics), but not always (dystonia)

4.15.1 Hypokinetic Movement Disorders (Parkinsonism)

Parkinsonism is defined as bradykinesia in combination with at least one of the following signs: muscular rigidity, a pill-rolling rest tremor, and postural instability. Parkinsonism can be due to (Fig. 4.11):

- PD. See Chap. 2 (basal ganglia) for the discussion of the clinical features of Parkinson's disease. PD is most often idiopathic. It is rarely familial, dominant (PARK1, PARK4, PARK8), or recessive (PARK2, PARK6, PARK7). The diagnosis of PD is best achieved using this three-step approach:
  - First, it is necessary to verify that the patient has parkinsonism (i.e., bradykinesia, with at least one of the following: muscular rigidity, 4–6 Hz rest tremor, postural instability).
  - Second, it must be confirmed that the patient does not meet exclusion criteria, suggesting atypical parkinsonism (Babinski sign, early and severe autonomic dysfunction, early and severe dementia, oculogyric crises, supranuclear gaze palsy, strictly unilateral symptoms after 3 years, cerebellar signs) or symptomatic parkinsonism (history of repeated strokes with stepwise progression, repeated head trauma, encephalitis, neuroleptic treatment at onset, presence of tumor, or hydrocephalus).
  - Third, look for supportive prospective positive criteria for Parkinson's disease, including unilateral onset, presence of 4–6 Hz rest tremor, symptom progression, persistent asymmetry, excellent levodopa response, levodopa response of more than 5 years, severe levodopa-induced chorea, and prolonged clinical course of ≥10 years.

- Atypical parkinsonism (sporadic). At least in the beginning, atypical parkinsonism is often misdiagnosed as PD. Red flags that parkinsonism is not due to PD include, e.g., poor levodopa response, symmetrical symptoms at onset, strictly unilateral symptoms after 3 years, wheelchair dependency, severe and early autonomic failure (e.g., orthostatic hypotension, erectile dysfunction, urinary incontinence, diarrhea at night), oculomotor palsies, unprovoked falls, early cognitive deficits, cerebellar signs, and the Babinski sign. Also, a history of antipsychotic drug treatment, repeated head trauma or stroke, definite infectious encephalitis, and familiar disposition with more than one affected relative suggest another disorder than PD.
  - PSP is characterized by parkinsonism associated with supranuclear ophthalmoplegia, usually starting with slowing of vertical gaze saccades (only downgaze impairment is specific). The patient develops a characteristic starring gaze with square wave jerks and a striking lack of spontaneous blinking. Early and frequent unprovoked falls due to postural instability are another diagnostic clue. Also, neck dystonia (sometimes with classic posteroflexion), axial rigidity, pseudobulbar palsy (e.g., increased facial reflexes, spastic dysarthria, dysphagia), as well as behavioral impairment of the frontotemporal type (e.g., motor recklessness, frontal disinhibition, dementia) are typical signs (Case 4.43).
  - MSA. The hallmark of MSA is parkinsonism with early and severe autonomic dysfunction, including orthostatic hypotension, urinary retention and/or urgency incontinence, erectile dysfunction, coldness and grayish discoloration of the hands, and Raynaud's phenomenon. Inspiratory stridor (initially nocturnal, later throughout the day), severe dysphonia, and dysarthria are also characteristic features. Indeed, in advanced cases, inspiratory stridor may allow for instant diagnosis. Apnea periods may occur often, but not exclusively, during sleep. (Rarely, the disease may even

Fig. 4.11 Differential diagnosis of parkinsonism

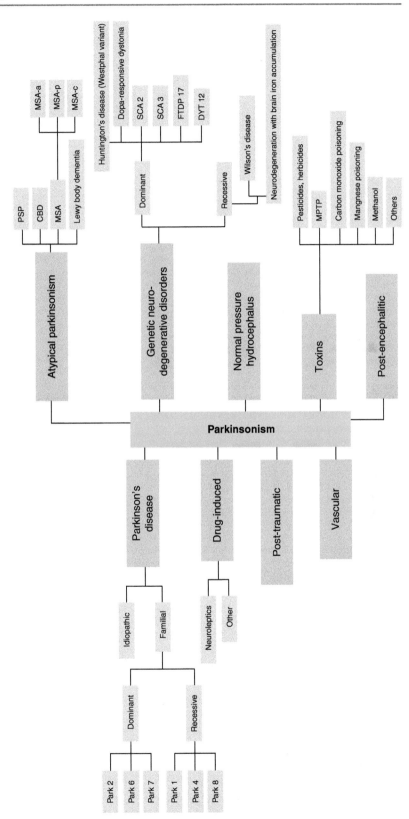

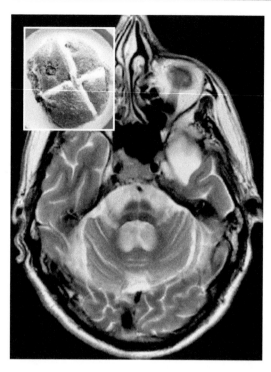

Case 4.43 Multisystem atrophy. A 63-year-old female had a 10-year history of unusually vivid dreams, including dream enactment behavior, consistent with a diagnosis of REM sleep behavior disorder. Five years later she developed autonomic symptoms, including urinary urgency, orthostatic hypotension, and diarrhea. About 4 years ago, she developed gait difficulties and dysarthria. Soon thereafter, she could no longer walk and needed a wheel chair ("wheel chair sign"). She developed neck dystonia of the antecollis type, left upper extremity rigidity, and rest tremor, as well as inspiratory stridor and severe dysphonia. Treatment with L-dopa had no effect. Her MRI showed atrophy of the medulla, pons, cerebellum, and middle cerebellar peduncles with a cross-shaped T2 signal hyperintensity within the pons ("hot cross bun sign"). She was diagnosed with MSA-p as the parkinsonian features were most prominent

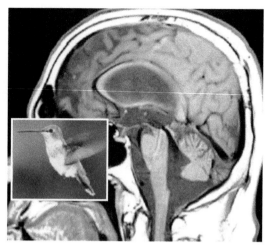

Case 4.44 Progressive supranuclear palsy. A 63-year-old female complained of double vision and several episodes of unexpected falling. A detailed history revealed that she also had abnormally vivid night dreams, consistent with a diagnosis of REM sleep behavior disorder. Examination revealed abnormal oculomotor function, including square wave jerks, hypometric saccades with slowing, particularly in the downward direction, a staring facial expression, axial rigidity, a wide-based gait ataxia, and retropulsation. During the following 4 years, her speech turned nonfluent, and she developed severe dysphagia, bradykinesia, and urinary incontinence, as well as disturbances of cognition and personality. T1-weighted sagittal MRI showed marked atrophy of the mesencephalon ("hummingbird sign"), corroborating the clinical diagnosis of PSP

start with respiratory insufficiency as the predominant symptom.) Early postural instability is common. Neck dystonia, if present, is usually of the antecollis type. Camptocormia (forward flexion of the trunk) and the Pisa syndrome (lateroflexion of the trunk) may also occur. Myoclonic jerks of the fingers can be seen. In contrast to PSP, overt dementia is not a typical feature in MSA patients, but dysexecutive behavioral symptoms and psychomotor slowing may occur. MSA leads to death within 5–10 years. REM sleep behavior disorder is common and can precede the onset of other symptoms by several years. MSA is divided into three entities, according to the most prominent accompanying features:

MSA with predominantly autonomic features (MSA-a, historically known as Shy-Drager syndrome)

MSA with predominantly cerebellar features (MSA-c, olivopontocerebellar atrophy)

MSA with predominantly parkinsonian features (MSA-p, striatonigral degeneration) (Case 4.44)

– CBD. This is a rare form of FTD that, in contrast to PSP and MSA, is associated with strikingly asymmetric motor features, as well as language impairment. The most characteristic complaint is of one arm becoming increasingly useless (alien limb phenomenon), whereas the other arm appears completely normal. Examination reveals asymmetric rigidity, akinesia, and dystonia, as well as cognitive deficits, mainly consisting of unilateral/asymmetric apraxia, astereognosis, and impaired graphesthesia, in addition to aphasia. Myoclonus may also be seen. Although gait apraxia can occur, balance is typically preserved. However, CBD is a neuropathological diagnosis; similar clinical features (i.e., the corticobasal syndrome) can also occur with PSP and other neurodegenerative diseases (Armstrong et al. 2013).

– DLB. This has been discussed in Sect. 4.4.

• Hereditary disorders with parkinsonism (other than familial PD):

– Dominant

HD. Juvenile onset of an akinetic-rigid syndrome with fast progression is suggestive of the so-called Westphal variant of HD.

Dopa-responsive dystonia (hereditary progressive dystonia with diurnal fluctuation, also known as Segawa disease or DYT5 dystonia; dominantly inherited with incomplete penetrance). These are usually young patients with asymmetric and fluctuating dystonia of the lower limbs (and less often true parkinsonism) that tends to be worse in the afternoon and evening. As the name suggests, patients respond very well to low doses of levodopa.

Spinocerebellar ataxia type 2 (SCA2).

Spinocerebellar ataxia type 3 (SCA3).

FTD with parkinsonism related to chromosome 17 (FTDP 17).

Rapid onset dystonia-parkinsonism (DYT12).

– Recessive

Wilson's disease (hepatolenticular degeneration). In this disease copper accumulates particularly in the brain and liver. Characteristic features of Wilson's disease include neuropsychiatric features, parkinsonism and other extrapyramidal movement disorders, liver failure, as well as the Kayser-Fleischer cornea ring (the

detection of which may require slit-lamp examination). All patients below 50 years of age with a movement disorder of unknown origin should be screened for Wilson's disease by checking S-ceruloplasmin and urinary copper secretion.

Pantothenate kinase-associated neurodegeneration, also termed NBIA, is formerly known as Hallervorden-Spatz syndrome.[14]

– Uncertain

Parkinson-dementia-ALS complex of Guam

• Secondary parkinsonism:

– Drug-induced parkinsonism

Parkinsonism associated with antipsychotic treatment. This is usually due to first-generation antipsychotics, including phenothiazines and butyrophenones, and usually presents with marked akinesia and rigidity but relatively little tremor. Orofacial dyskinesias may develop with chronic treatment.

Neuroleptic malignant syndrome is due to acutely decreased dopaminergic activity in the brain because of neuroleptic treatment, leading within days to weeks to severe rigidity, fever, decreased consciousness, autonomic dysfunction with labile blood pressure, and tachycardia as well as increased creatine kinase levels. If untreated, neuroleptic malignant syndrome is often fatal due to rhabdomyolysis and secondary renal and multiorgan failure.

Neuroleptic malignant-like syndrome is seen in Parkinson patients with sudden withdrawal of dopaminergic medication. The symptoms, treatment, and

---

[14]In the Third Reich, German pathologists Julius Hallervorden (1882–1965) and Hugo Spatz (1888–1969) collaborated with the Nazi regime and collected the brains of several hundred NS-euthanasia victims. Based on material from "euthanized" patients, Hallervorden published 12 papers after World War II (several of which are listed in MEDLINE) (Kondziella 2009).

potentially fatal outcome are similar to true neuroleptic malignant syndrome.

A few other drugs have been associated with parkinsonism, e.g., amiodarone and metoclopramide.

- Parkinsonism associated with toxins

MPTP-induced parkinsonism. In the 1970s MPTP was abused by a group of young people in California; MPTP is now the most common animal model of PD.

CO poisoning. CO, alone or in combination with smoke intoxication, is one of the major causes of poisoning injury and death worldwide. CO intoxication is often overlooked because CO is an odorless gas and induces various non-specific symptoms (headache, fatigue, nausea, and concentration difficulties). The brain and heart are particularly vulnerable to CO, and consequently, high-dose exposure may lead to myocardial ischemia, cardiac arrhythmia, and to neurological disturbances, including coma, seizures, and focal neurological signs. Carboxyhemoglobin (COHb) levels at the time of arrival in the emergency department can be normal again—therefore, a high level of suspicion is necessary. Two distinct clinical syndromes may occur after acute CO poisoning: a condition of chronic, persistent neurological deficits and the interval form of CO poisoning. The latter may occur in 15–40% of survivors following acute CO poisoning. In patients with the interval form of CO poisoning, neurological impairment occurs, for poorly understood reasons, days to weeks after a lucid period. In both syndromes, deficits usually include motor and neuropsychiatric symptoms; the patients can be totally mute, unresponsive, and bedridden with parkinsonian features. MRI typically shows pallidum infarcts, and cortical and white matter may be affected as well. Following hyperbaric oxygen therapy long-term outcome is sometimes sur-prisingly good despite severe initial neurological deficits (Case 4.45).

Manganese poisoning.

Other toxins, e.g., methanol, carbon disulfide, thallium, pesticides, and herbicides.

- Posttraumatic parkinsonism

Rarely seen after an isolated trauma that per definition must lead to a demonstrable, persistent structural brain injury.

Pugilistic parkinsonism results from the cumulative effects of numerous concussions to which boxers are subject, Muhammad Ali being the most prominent example. It is often associated with dementia (dementia pugilistica or punch-drunk syndrome).

- Postencephalitic parkinsonism. The best example is encephalitis lethargica, which occurred in the 1920s (von Economo encephalitis); cases of the non-Economo type (e.g., after Japanese encephalitis, post-streptococcal) may appear months or years following infectious encephalitis. An autoimmune reaction with antineuronal antibodies (e.g., anti-basal ganglia antibodies) is now believed to be the cause. Parkinsonism may also occur with ongoing CNS infection such as CJD. However, CJD should not be difficult to diagnose due to severe and rapidly progressive ataxia, myoclonus, and dementia.

- Vascular parkinsonism used to be a common but probably often incorrectly diagnosis. The disorder has numerous other names, including arteriosclerotic parkinsonism, lower-body parkinsonism, senile gait, and vascular pseudo-parkinsonism. Elderly patients present with a primary gait difficulty that includes parkinsonian features such as festination and altered postural reflexes. In addition, other features such as apraxia or cerebellar symptoms, including a wide-based ataxic gait, may occur. (This is rather different from the shuffling gait seen in PD.) Of note, tremor is often lacking and the upper extremities can be normal (hence the term lower-body

Case 4.45 Carbon monoxide poisoning (interval form).
A 40-year-old female with depression was found unconscious but breathing in a garage in her car with the engine running. The blood COHb level was 25%. Five sessions of hyperbaric oxygen therapy were administered. The patient regained consciousness 2 days after admission. A week later she was discharged without neurological deficits. However, after 3 weeks, she developed odd behavior, followed 2 days later by akinetic mutism, generalized muscular rigidity, and double incontinence. Coronal FLAIR and an axial T2-weighted MR of the brain showed widespread white matter signal change (*upper and middle rows*). The patient was diagnosed with the interval form of CO poisoning. Another cycle of hyperbaric oxygen therapy was initiated. Four months later the patient complained of moderate difficulties with memory and concentration but was independent in her daily activities (mRS 2). MRI revealed normalization of white matter signal changes but also subtle enlargement of the cerebral sulci, suggesting mild cerebral atrophy (*lower row*)

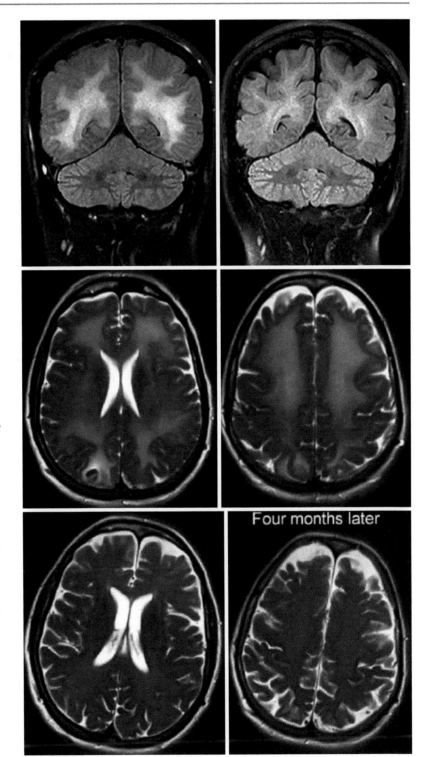

parkinsonism). Vascular parkinsonism is usually a chronic, stepwise progressing condition. On MRI and CT, white matter abnormalities are typically seen. This is consistent with the perception that vascular parkinsonism is more a disorder of white matter than of the basal ganglia. However, the basis of this gait abnormality is not entirely clear.

- The gait disturbance of vascular parkinsonism must be distinguished from the gait apraxia of NPH.

4.15.2 Hyperkinetic Movement Disorders

As stated above, hyperkinetic disorders include chorea, choreoathetosis, hemiballism, myoclonus, tics (all associated with normal or decreased muscle tone), and dystonia (associated with increased muscle tone) (Fig. 4.12).

The differential diagnosis of *chorea* and *choreoathetosis* include:

- Genetic disorders
  - HD. This autosomal dominant disease is associated with mutation of the Huntingtin gene on chromosome 4, which leads to neuropsychiatric symptoms and chorea and, ultimately, death. HD is a cytosine, adenine, guanine (CAG) triplet repeat disorder, and therefore, anticipation may occur.[15]
  - Benign hereditary chorea.
  - Neuroacanthocytosis. Acanthocytosis denotes spiked red blood cells and is associated with several inherited neurological disorders. Neuroacanthocytosis refers to autosomal recessive chorea-acanthocytosis and X-linked McLeod syndrome, but other movement disorders are associated with

erythrocyte acanthocytosis as well, e.g., HD-like 2 disorder and pantothenate kinase-associated neurodegeneration (NBIA, formerly known as Hallervorden-Spatz disease). Phenomenologically, there is significant overlap between these syndromes. Genetic testing is available.

- Dentatorubral-pallidoluysian atrophy (DRPLA). This is another autosomal dominant CAG repeat disorder with spinocerebellar degeneration and is characterized by juvenile onset (<20 years), early adult onset (20–40 years), or late adult onset (>40 years) of ataxia, choreoathetosis, dementia, seizures, and myoclonus.
- Wilson's disease. (See above.)
- Drug-induced chorea
  - Neuroleptics
  - Oral contraceptives
  - Phenytoin
  - Excessive L-dopa and dopamine agonists
  - Cocaine, amphetamine, and other central stimulants
  - Levothyroxine
- Postinfectious chorea
  - Sydenham chorea, also called chorea minor and usually seen in children after streptococcal infections, is rare nowadays.
- Chorea secondary to systemic disease
  - Thyrotoxicosis. This may be spontaneous, iatrogenic, or due to abuse of levothyroxine (in order to lose weight).
  - Antiphospholipid antibody syndrome/lupus erythematosus.
  - Polycythemia vera.
  - Paraneoplastic disease.
  - HIV/AIDS.
  - Hyperglycemia. Nonketotic, hyperglycemic chorea-ballism is a not-fully-understood disorder of sudden onset, typically occurring in elderly patients with poorly controlled diabetes. The movement disorder disappears with insulin therapy and symptomatic treatment with neuroleptics. It has been suggested that a reversible ischemic-hyperglycemic injury to the basal ganglia is responsible for this peculiar phenomenon.

---

[15] Anticipation is a phenomenon characterized by increasingly severe symptoms and earlier outbreak in the subsequent generation due to accumulation of CAG repeats. In Huntington's disease, this is mainly the case if the disease is transmitted by the father.

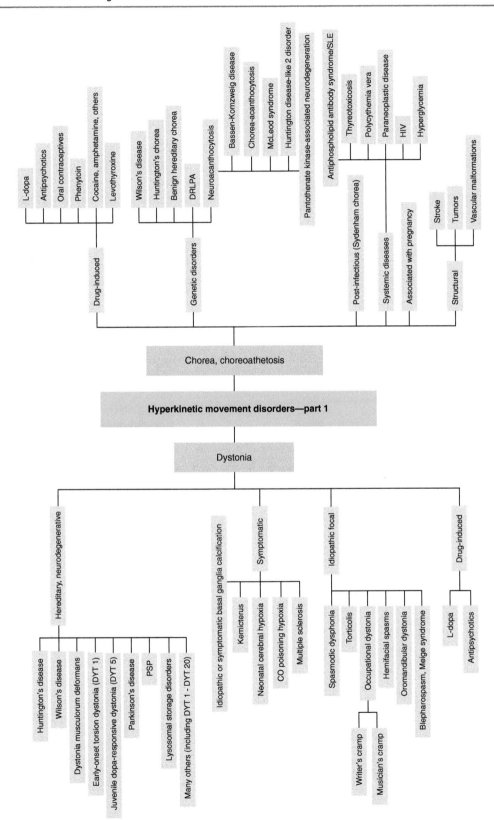

Fig. 4.12 (**a**) Differential diagnosis of hyperkinetic movement disorders I. (**b**) Differential diagnosis of hyperkinetic movement disorders II

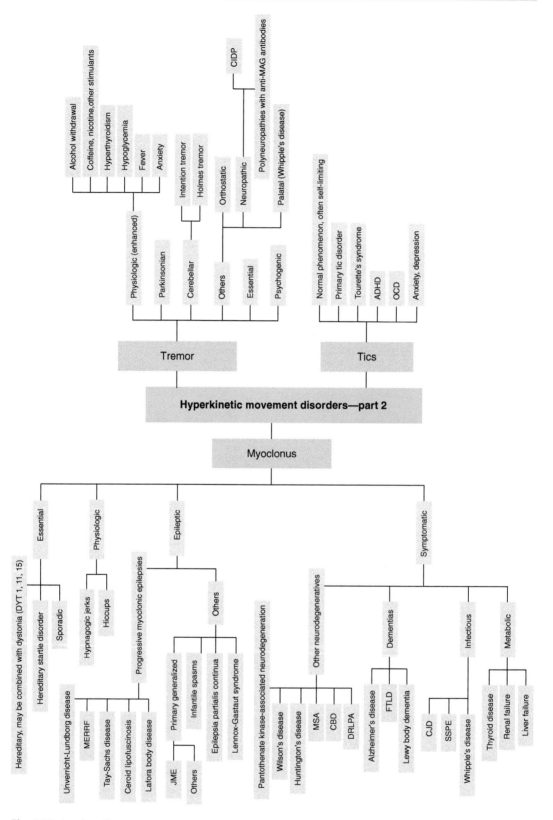

Fig. 4.12 (continued)

- Chorea in pregnancy
  - Chorea gravidarum usually resolves by itself after delivery.
- Structural brain lesions such as stroke, brain tumors, and vascular malformations may occasionally lead to hemichorea.

Hemiballism usually occurs in the elderly and is of acute onset, almost always due to infarction of the contralateral subthalamic nucleus.

Akathisia denotes an inner restlessness and the inability of the patient to sit still. It is usually associated with neuroleptic drug treatment, seldom with SSRI use or withdrawal, and it may occasionally be seen in PD as well.

Dystonia is focal, segmental, multifocal, hemidystonia, or generalized. It can further be divided according to etiology (primary vs secondary), age at onset (congenital, early or late childhood, teenage years, early or late adulthood), course of the disease (progressive or nonprogressive), concomitant medical or neurological disorders (present or absent), and whether it is constant, periodic, action-induced and/or task specific. The differential diagnosis includes:

- Hereditary and degenerative diseases with dystonia
  - HD.
  - Wilson's disease.
  - Dystonia musculorum deformans.
  - Juvenile dopa-responsive dystonia (Segawa disease). Classic L-dopa-responsive dystonia is characterized by the triad of dystonia, diurnal fluctuation of signs, and dramatic response to low-dose L-dopa therapy. There are cases of children incorrectly diagnosed with cerebral palsy who responded dramatically to L-dopa. Thus, a clinical trial with L-dopa (e.g., 200 mg tid for 2 months) is mandatory, if in doubt.
  - Dystonia associated with PD.
  - PSP.
  - More than 30 DYT mutations have been described so far (e.g., early-onset torsion dystonia (DYT1)), and more mutations are constantly added. See the Online Mendelian

Inheritance in Man database for recent updates (http://omim.org/).
  - Various metabolic diseases, e.g., lysosomal storage diseases.
  - Many other rare syndromes, e.g., idiopathic basal ganglia calcifications, which may occur as a sporadic disease or may be inherited as an autosomal dominant disorder (Fahr disease).
- Drug-induced dystonia
  - Neuroleptics
  - Excessive L-dopa and dopamine agonists
- Symptomatic (secondary) dystonia
  - Cerebral hypoxia in neonates (Vogt-Vogt syndrome).
  - Kernicterus.
  - Acquired hepatocerebral degeneration.
  - Basal ganglia calcification due to hypo−/hyperparathyroidism and pseudohypoparathyroidism. When neuroimaging shows bilateral subcortical calcifications in the brain, serum calcium and parathormone levels should be checked.
  - Idiopathic basal ganglia calcification (sporadic variant); however, non-symptomatic basal ganglia calcification as a benign, incidental radiological finding is much more common.
  - Carbon monoxide poisoning.
  - Methanol poisoning.
  - MS (occasionally).
  - HIV/AIDS.
- Idiopathic focal dystonias
  - Writer's cramp, musician's cramp, and other occupational dystonias
  - Blepharospasm and Meige syndrome
  - Torticollis
  - Hemifacial spasm
  - Oromandibular dystonia
  - Spasmodic dysphonia

Myoclonus is sudden and brief shock-like involuntary movements due to muscular contraction (positive myoclonus) or inhibition (negative myoclonus, e.g., asterixis seen in liver and kidney failure and other metabolic disturbances). Like dystonia, it can be focal, multifocal, segmental, and generalized.

Myoclonus has multiple causes and may arise from several sites in the nervous system.

The anatomic origin of myoclonus can be:

- Cortical (e.g., myoclonus associated with AD, CJD, and epilepsy; postanoxic myoclonus)
- Subcortical (basal ganglia, brainstem)
- Spinal (e.g., associated with transverse myelitis, spinal cord tumors)
- Peripheral (e.g., hemifacial spasms)

The etiology of myoclonus may be:

- Physiologic
  - Myoclonic jerks when falling asleep
  - Hiccups
- Essential
  - Autosomal dominant; may be combined with dystonia (DYT11)
  - Hereditary exaggerated startle syndrome
  - Sporadic
- Epileptic
  - Progressive myoclonic epilepsies. Most of these are untreatable and ultimately fatal syndromes.
    ○ Lafora body disease
    ○ Ceroid lipofuscinosis (Batten disease, Kufs disease)
    ○ Unverricht-Lundborg disease
    ○ GM2 gangliosidosis (Tay-Sachs disease; includes dementia and blindness; usually affects Ashkenazi Jews)
    ○ Mitochondrial disease (myoclonic epilepsy with ragged red fibers (MERRF))
  - Other epilepsies with myoclonus
    ○ Primary generalized
      - JME
      - JAE with myoclonus
      - Photosensitive epileptic myoclonus
    ○ Focal epilepsies
      - Epilepsia partialis continua
    ○ Infantile spasms
    ○ Lennox-Gastaut syndrome
- Symptomatic
  - Neurodegenerative disorders
    ○ AD
    ○ DLB
    ○ FTD

○ Wilson's disease
○ Huntington's disease
○ NBIA (formerly known as Hallervorden-Spatz disease)
○ Multiple system atrophy
○ CBD
○ DRPLA
- Infectious
  ○ CJD
  ○ SSPE
  ○ HIV
  ○ Whipple's disease (e.g., oculomasticatory myorhythmia)
  ○ Other infections with cortical or subcortical irritation
- Metabolic-toxic-hypoxic
  ○ Thyroid disease.
  ○ Liver failure.
  ○ Renal failure.
  ○ Electrolyte disturbances.
  ○ Hyperglycemia.
  ○ Posthypoxic. Coma with generalized myoclonus after hypoxic-ischemic brain injury, such as after cardiac arrest, suggests a very poor prognosis. (In contrast, action myoclonus developing a few days or weeks after the event, termed Lance-Adams syndrome, may still be associated with favorable cognitive recovery.)
  ○ Drug-induced. Many CNS drugs may potentially induce myoclonus, e.g., selective serotonin reuptake inhibitors (SSRIs), antiparkinson medications, neuroleptics, lithium, AED, and benzodiazepines. Also, antibiotics such as quinolones and anesthetic agents, including propofol, can provoke myoclonus.
  ○ Serotonergic syndrome. SSRI alone or in combination with other antidepressants and serotonergic medication (e.g., tramadol) can lead to serotonergic syndrome. This is due to excessive serotonergic activity and is characterized by mental changes (confusion, agitation, and decreased consciousness), myoclonus, tremor, and autonomic dysfunction (fever, tachycardia, diarrhea, sweating, shivering). In contrast to neuroleptic malignant syndrome, it develops very

rapidly within hours to days and rigidity is less common. Rhabdomyolysis, metabolic acidosis, and secondary organ failure, however, occur in both syndromes and can be potentially fatal. Mild serotonergic syndrome is usually quickly reversible when the offending medication is discontinued.

– Autoimmune, non-paraneoplastic
  ○ Post-infectious opsoclonus-myoclonus-ataxia syndrome (see Sect. 4.13)
  ○ Hashimoto's encephalitis (steroid-responsive encephalopathy with thyroid antibodies)
– Autoimmune, paraneoplastic
  ○ Opsoclonus-myoclonus-ataxia syndrome (see Sect. 4.13)
  ○ Brainstem encephalitis
– Structural
  ○ Trauma
  ○ Stroke
  ○ Vascular malformations

Tremor includes:

• Physiologic tremor usually has a postural component, e.g., the amplitude increases when the arms are elevated and stretched out. This type of tremor can become more pronounced with:
  – Alcohol withdrawal
  – Hyperthyroidism
  – Hypoglycemia
  – Various medications, e.g., valproate, antidepressants, sympathomimetics, and lithium
  – Caffeine, nicotine, and illicit drugs
  – Fever
  – Anxiety
• Essential tremor is often autosomal dominant; there are no other neurological deficits, and the tremor characteristically diminishes with slight amounts of alcohol. The tremor has a resting and postural component. The hands are most often involved but head, tongue, legs, and trunk may also be affected. Head tremor is of the yes-yes or no-no type. Essential tremor can also involve the vocal cords, leading to voice tremor.
• Parkinsonian. This is the typical asymmetric 4–6 Hz rest tremor (pill-rolling tremor) that occurs in PD.

• Cerebellar tremor:
  – Intention tremor, the classic cerebellar tremor, is absent in rest and occurs with purposeful movements. The amplitude increases at the end of the movement, e.g., when the finger reaches the target.
  – Holmes' tremor (rubral tremor) occurs with lesions of the brainstem, cerebellum, and thalamus leading to interruption of the cerebellorubrothalamic pathway. It is a tremor of low frequency, usually below 4.5 Hz. Holmes' tremor is a tripartite tremor; thus, it has rest, intention, and postural components. Ataxia, ophthalmoplegia, and bradykinesia are associated features.
• Dystonic tremor. This type of tremor affects a body part that also displays clear dystonic features, e.g., tremulous torticollis. (Some authorities argue that this definition is too narrow.) Dystonic tremor in a limb may develop prior to overt dystonia.
• Orthostatic tremor. A typical patient with orthostatic tremor is a middle-aged woman who reports unsteadiness while standing, which is relieved by walking and sitting. This unusual complaint (balance problems while standing, but not while walking) is often misdiagnosed as hysterical, especially so because formal neurological examination tends to be normal. EMG reveals a high-frequency tremor of 12–16 Hz in the thighs. (The tremor is too high in frequency to be seen, but it can be felt. Listening with the stethoscope over the skin of the thighs may occasionally reveal a sound that resembles the noise of a helicopter.)
• Neuropathic tremor. Chronic demyelinating and paraproteinemic polyneuropathies, particularly CIDP or those associated with IgM antibodies to MAG (anti-MAG antibodies), can cause a disabling postural and action tremor that, if severe, may occur in the resting position as well. The degree of the tremor is not necessarily correlated with the degree of the neuropathy.
• Palatal tremor (earlier termed palatal myoclonus) is a rhythmic contraction of the soft palate (1–2 Hz). It may be essential or secondary due

to brainstem or cerebellar disease. The palatal contractions impart a repetitive audible click that usually ceases during sleep if the tremor is essential, but not if it is symptomatic. Symptomatic palatal tremor is due to a lesion that disrupts the connections between the red nucleus and inferior olivary nucleus in the brainstem and the dentate nucleus in the cerebellum. Symptomatic palatal tremor may occur with Wilson's disease, brainstem stroke, tumor, or inflammation. Also, Whipple's disease may produce a similar phenomenon, and in addition it often involves oculomasticatory myorhythmia, which is pathognomonic for this disease.
- Psychogenic tremor has been discussed previously together with the examination of the functional patient in Chap. 3.

Tics can be defined as unintentional, sudden, fast, nonrhythmic, and stereotyped movements or sounds with a pathognomonic premonitory urge, which steadily increases if the tics are voluntarily suppressed, until the patient no longer can hold them back. They may occur as:

- A normal temporary phenomenon, especially in children
- Primary tic disorder
- Part of other disorders, including:
  - Tourette's syndrome
  - Obsessive compulsive disorder (OCD)
  - Attention deficit hyperactivity disorder (ADHD)
  - Anxiety and depression

4.16 The Differential Diagnosis of Ataxia

The origin of ataxia can be (Fig. 4.13):

- Cerebellar
- Sensory
- Vestibular

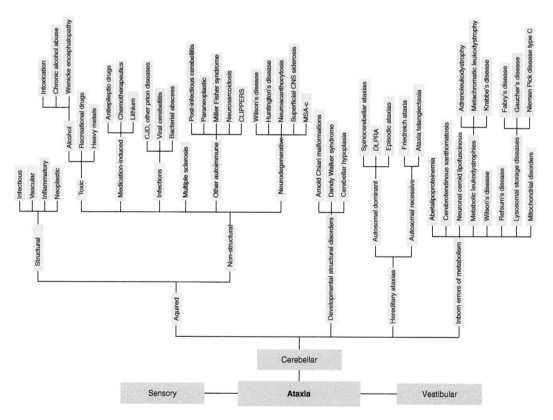

Fig. 4.13 Differential diagnosis of ataxia

How to differentiate clinically between these three types of ataxia has been covered earlier. Please refer to Chaps. 2 and 3 and the relevant parts on cerebellar, oculomotor, vestibular, and dorsal column function.

The differential diagnosis of *cerebellar ataxia* includes:

- Acquired diseases
  - Cerebellar mass lesions
    - Cerebellar mass lesions of vascular, infectious, inflammatory, and malignant etiology
  - Nonstructural
    - Toxic substances (e.g., alcohol, recreational drugs, heavy metals).
    - Various medications (e.g., valproate and other AEDs, chemotherapeutics, lithium, metronidazole).
    - MS and other demyelinating diseases.
    - Viral, bacterial, and prion infections.
    - Postinfectious viral cerebellitis (usually seen in children and young adults).
    - Miller-Fisher syndrome (variant of GBS).
    - Subacute cerebellar degeneration (paraneoplastic).
    - Superficial CNS siderosis. This is due to chronic subarachnoidal hemorrhage leading to hemosiderin deposits in the subpial layers of the brain and spinal cord many years or even decades after CNS trauma, neurosurgery, and other injury, but in roughly 30% of patients, no cause is identified. Superficial CNS siderosis presents with a characteristic triad of sensorineural deafness, cerebral ataxia, and various sensorimotor deficits. Identification of the bleeding source and stopping it are the only definitive therapy and may halt otherwise relentless progression, which, however, is only rarely possible. In patients with this disorder who do not have a history of trauma or surgery, the most common bleeding source is spinal, e.g., dural ectasias. High-

quality MRI of the brain and spine is mandatory (Case 4.46).
    - Chronic lymphocytic inflammation with pontine perivascular enhancement responsive to steroids (CLIPPERS) is a CNS inflammatory disease responsive to immunosuppressive therapy. Subacute onset over weeks of diplopia, nystagmus, and ataxia is typical. MRI shows a typical picture with patchy spotlike gadolinium enhancement in a salt-and-pepper-like appearance in the pons, midbrain, and cerebellum. The thalamus, white cerebral matter, and the spine may be involved as well but usually to a lesser degree. Brain biopsies show diffuse perivascular infiltration by small mature lymphocytes. Of note, other inflammatory diseases such as sarcoidosis, neuroinfections, and CNS lymphoma have to be excluded. Early treatment with steroids leads to rapid clinical improvement and marked resolution of MRI lesions. If treatment is delayed, however, subsequent development of generalized cerebral and cerebellar atrophy may be associated with long-term neurological deficits (Case 4.47).
  - Heat stroke, if severe, may lead to bilateral cerebellar infarcts.
  - Neurodegenerative disorders (e.g., MSA-c, Huntington's disease, Wilson's disease, neuroacanthocytosis).
- Developmental structural diseases of the posterior cranial fossa
  - Dandy-Walker syndrome
  - Arnold-Chiari malformations
  - Cerebellar hypoplasia syndromes
- Hereditary ataxias. These are dominant or recessive hereditary diseases with ataxia being the dominant feature. (Various other hereditary diseases with inborn errors of metabolism may lead to ataxia; that, however, is not necessarily the dominant symptom; see below.)
  - Autosomal dominant, e.g.:
    - SCA. Currently around 30 different forms of SCA have been identified, and

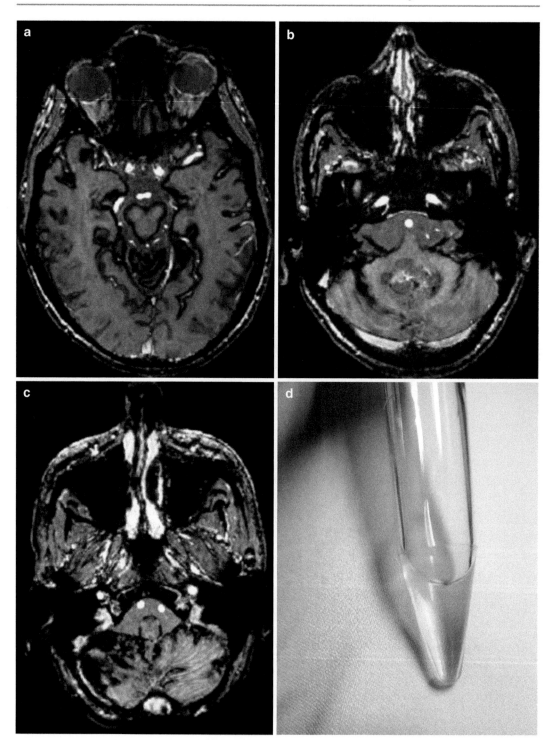

Case 4.46 Superficial CNS siderosis. A 35-year-old male presented with a 5-year history of slowly progressive gait ataxia, bilateral sensory hearing loss, spastic paresis of both legs, dysarthria, and urge incontinence. He had been treated surgically for a medulloblastoma more than 20 years previously. MRI of the brain showed excessive leptomeningeal hemosiderin deposits around the midbrain (**a**), in the basal cerebral sulci, around CN VIII (**b**), and the cerebellum (**c**). CSF showed xanthochromia, which did not clear with successive tubes. Spectrophotometric measurement revealed bilirubin, consistent with chronic subarachnoidal bleeding (**d**). Superficial CNS siderosis was diagnosed. Although the chronic subarachnoidal bleeding most likely was associated with the previous neurosurgical procedure, no bleeding source was found that could have been subject to surgical repair

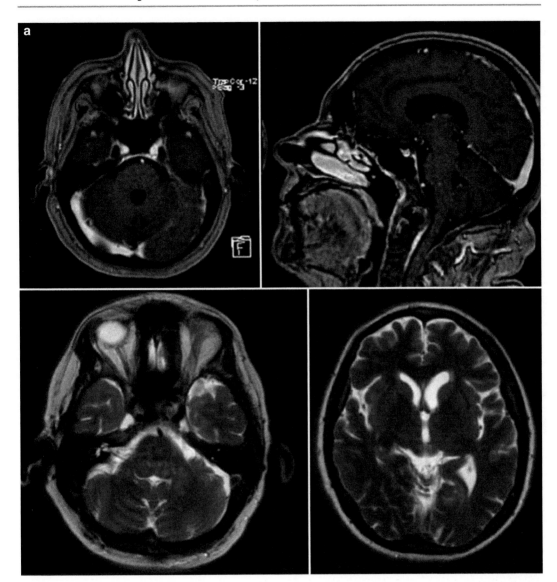

Case 4.47 Chronic Lymphocytic Inflammation with Pontine Perivascular Enhancement Responsive to Steroids (CLIPPERS). A 58-year-old woman had a 4-week history of subacute gait ataxia, dysarthria, and paresthesia of the face, hands, and feet. She recovered but had four relapses during the follow-up period from 2007 to 2013. Coronal gadolinium-enhancing T1-weighted MRI showed typical spotlike, enhancing perivascular lesions in the pons (**a**, upper row, left) and the medulla (**a**, upper row, right). Serial MRI showed progressive cortical cerebral and cerebellar atrophy (**a**, middle row, 2007; lower row, 2013; T2 weighted). On tissue biopsy from the cerebellum accumulation of CD3+ T cells and CD68+, microglia/macrophages was noted (**b**, 50×). Repeated CSF analysis showed mild lymphocytosis but no oligoclonal bands. In 2013, the patient was severely dysarthric, moderately cog-

nitively impaired, wheel-chair bound, and had mild involuntary movements of tongue and hands consistent with chorea (modified ranking scale 4). CLIPPERS is an inflammatory CNS disorder characterized by (1) subacute onset of cerebellar and brainstem symptoms, (2) peripontine contrast-enhancing perivascular lesions with a "salt-and-pepper" appearance on MRI, and (3) angiocentric, predominantly T-lymphocytic infiltration as revealed by brain biopsy. Inflammatory diseases including neuroinfections, CNS lymphoma, and neurosarcoidosis must be excluded. Potentially severe neurological deficits and progressive parenchymal atrophy (as seen here on follow-up MRI) may suggest neurodegenerative features, which emphasizes the need for early immunomodulatory treatment (adapted with permission from Kerrn-Jespersen et al. (2014))

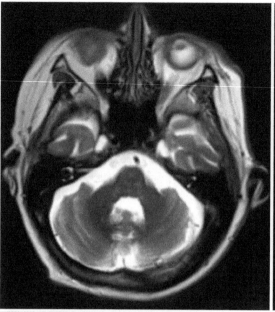
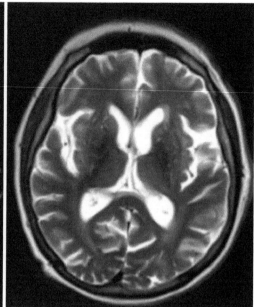

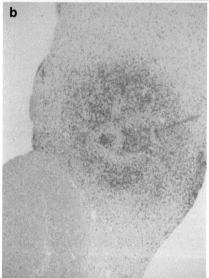

Case 4.47 (continued)

probably many more will be discovered in the future. Some of the more common ones include SCA-1 (neuropathy, pyramidal signs), SCA-2 (dementia, neuropathy, slow saccades), SCA-3 (amyotrophy, neuropathy, parkinsonism, pyramidal signs), SCA-6 (pure cerebellar ataxia), and SCA-7 (blindness due to pigmentary retinopathy, deafness).

• DRPLA (chorea, dementia, myoclonus, seizures).

• Episodic ataxia 1–7.

– Autosomal recessive, e.g.:

• Friedreich's ataxia is the most common autosomal recessive ataxia. It is characterized by cerebellar ataxia, corticospinal tract signs, and dorsal column dysfunction (leading to deep areflexia combined with Babinski sign). Many patients develop pes cavus, dysarthria, and cardiomyopathy. According to Harding's essential diagnostic criteria for Friedreich's ataxia (Harding 1981),

Friedreich's ataxia is very likely when symptoms have been present for less than 5 years, and:

- – Onset of symptoms occurs before 25 years of age.
- – Progressive ataxia affects all limbs and gait.
- – Knee and ankle tendon reflexes are absent.
- – Babinski sign is present.
- – Motor nerve conduction velocity is greater than 40 m/s in the upper extremity with small or absent sensory responses.

- Ataxia-telangiectasia and other disorders of DNA repair. In ataxia-telangiectasia, slowly progressive cerebellar ataxia is associated with characteristic telangiectasia of the skin and conjunctiva, choreoathetosis, susceptibility to sinopulmonary infections, and increased incidence of lymphoreticular and other malignancies.
  - – X-linked, e.g., fragile X-associated ataxia/tremor syndrome (FXATS) (see Sect. 5.7)
- Various inborn errors of metabolism lead to ataxia as *one* of many different symptoms. These disorders are too many and too rare to name but a few:
  - – Abetalipoproteinemia (mental retardation, neuropathy, retinitis pigmentosa, steatorrhea).
  - – Cerebrotendinous xanthomatosis (atherosclerosis, cataracts, dementia, xanthomas). This autosomal recessively inherited disorder leads to deposition of cholestanol in the brain and other tissues. It is typically characterized by progressive cerebellar ataxia developing in the second or third decade of life and tendinous or tuberous xanthomas, e.g., xanthomas of the Achilles tendons are very characteristic. Also, bilateral cataracts during childhood or adolescence and chronic diarrhea in infancy are strong clues to the diagnosis. Various other features such as premature atherosclerosis and learning disabilities may occur as well. Although very rare, it is easily diagnosed using plasma cholestenol, and it should not be overlooked because it is one of the few inborn errors of metabolism that are amenable to specific treatment.
  - – Neuronal ceroid lipofuscinosis (blindness, myoclonic seizures, psychomotor retardation). There are several subtypes, which are grouped according to age at onset (e.g., Batten disease in juveniles, Kufs disease in adults).
  - – Refsum disease leads to a characteristic triad of polyneuropathy, deafness, and visual deficits (retinitis pigmentosa with night blindness, visual field deficits, hypersensitivity to light, and cataracts). Other important symptoms include skeletal dysplasia, skin changes such as ichthyosis, as well as cardiac arrhythmias. Refsum disease is equivalent to HSM III.
  - – Wilson's disease (movement disorder, bulbar dysfunction, hepatic disease, Kayser-Fleischer rings, neuropsychiatric symptoms).
  - – Various leukodystrophies, including:
    - • Adrenoleukodystrophy (faulty peroxisomal fatty acid beta oxidation results in the accumulation of very-long-chain fatty acids in body tissues; Addison disease, CNS leukodystrophy, myelopathy) (Case 4.48)
    - • Krabbe disease (globoid cell leukodystrophy associated with dysfunctional metabolism of sphingolipids; late-onset form with blindness, neuropathy, spasticity)
    - • Metachromatic leukodystrophy (caused by a deficiency of the enzyme arylsulfatase A; peripheral neuropathy, spasticity, visual impairment)
  - – Various lysosomal storage diseases, such as:
    - • Fabry disease (angiokeratoma, cardiomyopathy, cerebrovascular disease, dysarthria, painful crises, renal failure)
    - • Gaucher type 3 (gaze palsy, myoclonus, seizures)
    - • Niemann-Pick type C (brainstem symptoms, dementia, hepatosplenomegaly, psychosis, spasticity, supranuclear palsy)
  - – Mitochondrial disorders
    - • Kearns-Sayre syndrome (KSS), (external ophthalmoplegia, retinopathy)
    - • MELAS
    - • MERRF
    - • Neuropathy, ataxia, and retinitis pigmentosa (NARP)

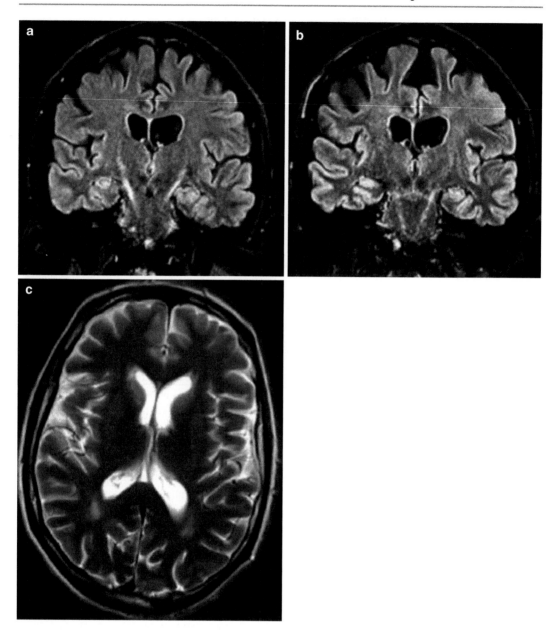

Case 4.48 Adult-onset adrenoleukodystrophy. A 47-year-old male was admitted with a 4-year history of increasingly spastic tetraparesis, dysarthria, and dysphagia. Plasma levels of very-long-chain fatty acids were elevated, and genetic testing for mutations of the *ABCD1* gene (which encodes for a peroxisomal membrane transporter protein) on the X chromosome confirmed the diagnosis of adult-onset adrenoleukodystrophy. MR FLAIR revealed signal change associated with the corticospinal tracts (**a, b**), and T2-weighted MRI showed hyperintense signal change related to the poles of the frontal and occipital horns (**c**). The patient had two sisters who were female carriers: one was asymptomatic and the other had a mild myelopathy (which had been incorrectly diagnosed as primary progressive MS)

4.17 The Differential Diagnosis of Gait Disorders

The differential diagnosis of gait disorders has been discussed in Sect. 3.6 ("Gait"). Consider also the sections on the differential diagnoses of ataxia, movement disorders, myelopathy, motor neuron disease, peripheral neuropathy, and myopathy in the present chapter. Gait disturbances may have orthopedic, vascular (intermittent claudication),

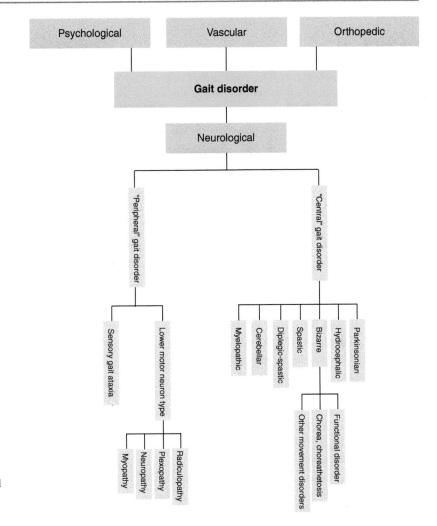

Fig. 4.14 Differential diagnosis of gait disturbance

psychological, or neurological causes, and in case of the latter, one can distinguish between gait ataxia of central and peripheral origin (Fig. 4.14).

4.18 The Differential Diagnosis of Cranial Nerve Deficits

CN deficits may be divided into:

- Deficits of isolated CNs. Chapter 2 discusses the differential diagnosis of isolated CN palsies.
- Deficits of multiple CNs *without* corticospinal and spinothalamic tract signs suggest that the lesion is near the skull base but outside of the brainstem. Differential diagnoses include, among others:

- Basilar meningitis/basilar meningeal inflammation as seen with tuberculosis, Lyme disease, and neurosarcoidosis.
- Meningeal carcinomatosis and lymphomatosis.
- GBS and its variants.
- Retrograde perineural spreading of skin and nasopharynx cancers has a protracted course and has been discussed together with the differential diagnosis of malignancy.
- Malignant external otitis due to *Pseudomonas aeruginosa* (see Case 4.36).
- Bear in mind that diphtheria, botulism, and MG, although neuromuscular junction diseases, may also lead to acute onset of bilateral facial weakness and oculomotor paresis.

- Deficits of multiple CNs *with* corticospinal and spinothalamic tract signs point toward a lesion that affects the brainstem. The differential diagnoses include the usual kinds of vascular, inflammatory, infectious, and malignant diseases.

4.19 The Differential Diagnosis of Myelopathy

Myelopathy may occur with lesions that are (Fig. 4.15):

- Extradural
  - Trauma.
  - Malignancy, e.g., spinal metastases.
  - Degenerative, e.g., spondylosis, spondylolisthesis, disc herniation. Myelopathy due to cervical canal stenosis is probably the most frequently observed myelopathy in general practice. (An important differential diagnosis to cervical spondylosis is ALS; see below. It is not uncommon that ALS patients are operated on for asymptomatic cervical degenerative disease before they receive the correct diagnosis.)
  - Infectious, e.g., spinal osteomyelitis and epidural abscess (Case 4.49).
  - Congenital spinal malformations, ranging from spina bifida occulta (typically diagnosed accidentally in patients with back pain examined by MRI of the lumbar spine) to meningomyelocele (resulting in congenital paraplegia and sphincter dysfunction).
- Intradural-extramedullar
  - Tumors, e.g., meningioma, schwannoma (rarely neurofibroma) of spinal nerve roots, and meningeal carcinomatosis.
  - Arachnoiditis, infectious or aseptic (e.g., following spinal subarachnoidal bleeding, CT myelography, and spinal radiation therapy).
  - Spinal dural AV fistula. The typical patient is an elderly man with stepwise progressive gait ataxia, resulting after a few months in the inability to walk and stand upright. Sagittal T2-weighted MRI of the spine reveals enlarged and tortuous veins on the dorsal aspect of the spinal cord (Case 4.50).
- Intramedullar
  - Primary malignancies, e.g., astrocytoma and ependymoma.
  - Secondary malignancies, e.g., lung, breast, and prostate cancer. Intramedullar metastases are much rarer than spinal bone metastases (see Case 2.5).
  - Spinal cord syrinx, enlargement of the central canal (syringomyelia), or cysts secondary to trauma, tumors, and infections.
  - Transverse noninfectious myelitis. Idiopathic.
    MS.
    NMO (including NMO spectrum disease).
    Other autoimmune disorders, such as systemic lupus erythematosus, have been associated with myelitis, but most of these cases are probably caused by NMO or anti-MOG antibodies.
  - Infectious.
    HTLV-1-associated myelopathy (tropical spastic paraparesis).
    Poliovirus and other *Enteroviruses.*
    HIV
    Schistosomiasis.
    Bacterial abscess (usually per continuitatem from extramedullar abscess).
    Tertiary syphilis (tabes dorsalis).
  - Metabolic.
    Vitamin B12 deficiency.
    Copper deficiency myelopathy (or myeloneuropathy) leads to dysfunction of the dorsal columns (impairment of proprioception and vibration) as well as corticospinal tracts. It is usually due to a GI malabsorption (e.g., after gastric surgery) or excessive intake of zinc supplements. Clinically, it is indistinguishable from myelopathy due to vitamin B12 deficiency. Anemia and neutropenia may or may not be seen.

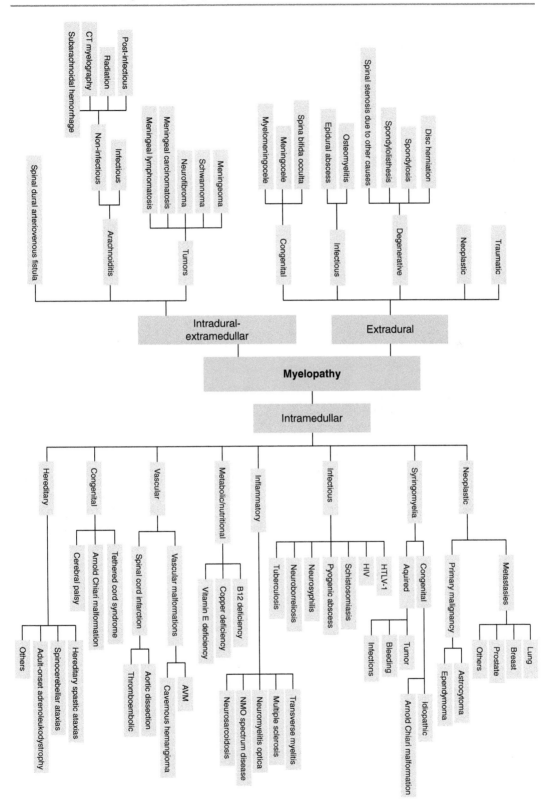

Fig. 4.15 Differential diagnosis of myelopathy

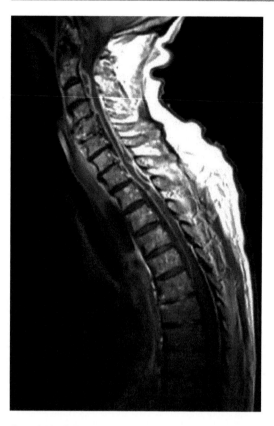

Case 4.49 Spinal epidural abscess. A 76-year-old female had surgical excision of a soft tissue abscess in the left leg. Ten days later she complained of fever and upper back pain. During the following 2 days, she became tetraplegic and developed urinary and fecal incontinence. Examination also revealed bilateral extensor plantar responses and a truncal sensory level. Contrast-enhanced MRI of the spinal cord showed a multilobulated cervico-thoracic epidural spinal abscess

An important differential diagnosis to B12 deficiency myelopathy, copper deficiency can be screened for by checking serum copper and ceruloplasmin levels and urinary copper excretion, which all are reduced.

Vitamin E deficiency due to malabsorption syndromes or rare disorders of fat metabolism.
– Vascular malformations.
AVM.
Cavernous hemangioma.

– Spinal cord infarction (typically because of occlusion of the anterior spinal artery, leading to the anterior cord syndrome). (See Sect. 2.4.3.)

Aortic dissection. Aortic imaging (CT or MRI) should be mandatory in any patient presenting with a suspicion of spinal cord infarction. Of note, the area of the aortic wall dissection can be very small and may be overlooked, if the images are not carefully reviewed.

Thrombotic/embolic

Fibrocartilaginous embolism. Spinal cord infarction due to embolization of nucleus pulposus material into the vascular circulation is a serious and very likely underdiagnosed cause of spinal cord infarction. Fibrocartilaginous material may prolapse under pressure into the cancellous bone of the vertebral body, thereby causing retrograde arterial embolization to several segments of the spinal cord, usually in the territory of the anterior spinal artery. This condition should be considered particularly in younger patients without cardiovascular risk factors who develop a subacute onset of paraplegia, a sensory level and sphincter disturbances following minor or moderate trauma associated with traffic or sport accidents, somersaults, handstands, Valsalva-like maneuvers, and so on. There is typically a very intense back or neck pain directly associated with the trauma, followed by progressive onset of a myelopathy (≤24 h). Particular attention should be paid to signs of disc protrusion and Schmorl's nodes at the level of the spinal cord ischemia on MRI. This condition is often misdiagnosed as an acute transverse myelitis. In contrast to thrombotic spinal cord ischemia, which typically is associated with substantial recovery, prognosis tends to be poor, and most

Case 4.50 Spinal arteriovenous dural fistula. A 56-year-old male developed stepwise progressive weakness in his legs and urinary retention during a 6-month period. Two weeks prior to admission, he experienced rapid deterioration and was no longer able to walk. On examination, there was normal power in the arms but spastic motor weakness in the legs, decreased sensation in the trunk and legs, and anal sphincter dysfunction. MR showed characteristic spinal cord edema and perimedullary dilated veins (**a**, **b**). Spinal angiography (not shown) confirmed the diagnosis of spinal AV dural fistula. Following repeated neurointerventional procedures with superselective embolization with a liquid embolic agent, the patient regained the ability to walk, although slight spasticity in the legs remained

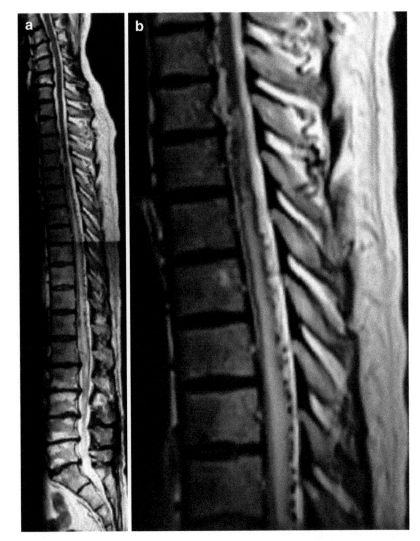

patients remain paraplegic. Fatal cases due to fibrocartilaginous embolism at the cervical level with subsequent cervical cord and brainstem infarctions are exceedingly rare but well described.

– Congenital, e.g.:
Tethered cord syndrome.
Arnold-Chiari malformations.
Cerebral palsy.

– Hereditary diseases.
Adrenoleukomyeloneuropathy, late-onset form of adrenoleukodystrophy, presenting with progressive myelopathy ± neuropathy in males; female carriers of the X-linked ABCD1 mutation sometimes develop a mild myelopathy in their fifth decade. (See Case 4.48.)

Other leukodystrophies of adult onset.

HSP, may be dominantly and recessively inherited; strictly myelopathic (pure forms of HSP) or in combination with other neurological deficits (complicated forms of HSP).

Spinocerebellar ataxias (SCA).

- An important but rare differential diagnosis of spastic paraparesis (with or without incontinence) is bilateral injury to the corticospinal tract within the frontal lobes, usually seen with a large falx meningioma or rupture of ACOM aneurysm.[16]

4.20   The Differential Diagnosis of Motor Neuron Disease

ALS is the most common (and dreaded) MND, but it is crucial to rule out ALS mimics such as cervical spondylosis or one of the other MNDs (Fig. 4.16).

4.20.1 Amyotrophic Lateral Sclerosis

Although it has become evident that ALS is a neurodegenerative process affecting many parts of the nervous system, the clinical hallmark of ALS is signs and symptoms referable to damage of the first and second motor neurons in different body regions. Importantly, sensory and autonomic (e.g., bladder) functions remain intact. Also, extraocular muscles are preserved. At first sight, cognitive function often seems undisturbed as well, although formal neuropsychological evaluation will reveal slight deficits in roughly every second patient, and a significant number of patients (15%) will fulfill the diagnostic criteria of FTD. Median survival in ALS patients is roughly 3 years. Ten percent may survive as much as 10 years and longer, and roughly as many have rapid progression with death arriving within a few months.

Variants of ALS include:

- Progressive bulbar palsy. This starts with prominent bulbar symptoms such as tongue atrophy, dysarthria, and dysphagia, whereas power in the extremities is relatively unaffected. These patients develop early weight

---

[16]With acute rupture of an ACoMA aneurysm, the paraparesis will be flaccid; only later does spasticity develop.

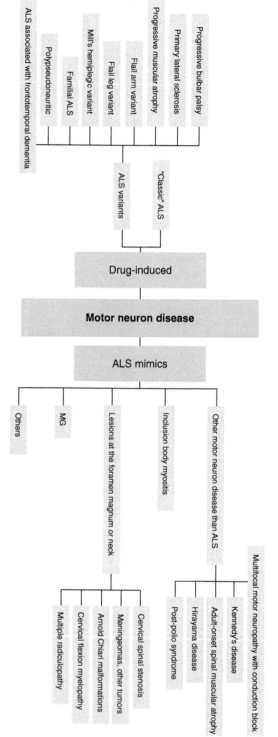

Fig. 4.16 Differential diagnosis of motor neuron disease

loss, aspiration pneumonia, and anarthria. Median survival is usually very short. Women are affected more frequently than men.

- Primary lateral sclerosis. In these patients damage is relatively restricted to the UMN, and progression tends to be rather slow.
- Progressive muscular atrophy is a poorly defined variant involving predominantly the second motor neurons.
- Flail arm variant. Flail arm syndrome occurs in up to 10% of patients and is characterized by relatively symmetrical proximal and distal bibrachial wasting with positive Babinski sign. Survival is somewhat longer than with classic ALS. Drop head can be another typical presentation with ALS.
- Mills hemiplegic variant. This ALS variant is a well-recognized but rare entity presenting with upper motor and LMN signs isolated to one side.
- Familial ALS is clinically indistinguishable from sporadic disease in individual cases. Between 5% and 10% of patients attending MND clinics have a history of a first-degree relative with MND. Median age of onset is about 3 years earlier than sporadic ALS. Several autosomal dominantly inherited adult-onset ALS genes have been reported so far, e.g., the *C9ORF72* gene (see below) and the copper-zinc superoxide dismutase (*SOD1*) gene on chromosome 21q22.1
- As stated above, ALS can be associated with progressive dementia, which is usually of the frontotemporal type and which has been termed the FTD-ALS syndrome. The relation between FTD and ALS has been underpinned by the finding that a hexanucleotide repeat expansion in a noncoding region of the *C9ORF72* gene causes both familial and sporadic forms of these two diseases.

4.20.2 Other Motor Neuron Diseases

The differential diagnosis of ALS is of utmost importance. Diagnostic red flags include:

- Lack of progression.
- Major fluctuations in function.
- Symptoms and signs confined to one part of the body.
- Limb weakness without wasting.
- Unusual and prominent sensory symptoms.
- Dysphagia preceding dysarthria (suggesting IBM).
- Significant bladder or bowel involvement.
- Fasciculations without weakness. The crucial features that differentiate benign fasciculations from those occurring in MND are lack of muscle atrophy and weakness, as well as repetitive switching of one muscle fiber at a time (as compared to widespread switching involving several parts of the body simultaneously).

Careful consideration of the following entities ensures very high diagnostic accuracy.

- Lesions at the level of the foramen magnum and cervical spine:
  - The most common cause of misdiagnosis is probably degenerative cervical spine disease. Spondylotic myelopathy and radiculopathy may lead to LMN signs in the upper limbs and to UMN signs in the lower limbs. Many patients with ALS have been operated on for asymptomatic cervical canal stenosis. Importantly, with cervical spinal stenosis, bulbar symptoms are missing and the jaw jerk is normal.
  - Tumors and other mass lesions at the foramen magnum and in the posterior fossa.
  - Arnold-Chiari malformation. If severe, downward displacement of the cerebellar vermis and medulla through the foramen magnum may lead to progressive bulbar symptoms. Similar to what is seen with other posterior fossa lesions, vertigo, ataxia, and long tract signs may occur.
  - Cervical flexion myelopathy. In a patient with brachial diplegia and electrophysiological signs of anterior horn cell disease,

cervical MRI is mandatory to rule out a cervical myelopathy. Occasionally, spinal cord compression can be temporary and may be overlooked with MRI in neutral position. It is essential to order MRI of the spine during neck flexion in patients with the man-in-the-barrel syndrome in whom a standard MRI shows no compressive myelopathy but a cervical process (e.g., an intradural or arachnoid cyst). Otherwise the opportunity for early diagnosis and surgical intervention might be missed (Case 4.51).

– Hirayama disease (juvenile muscular atrophy of the distal upper extremity). This disorder is also associated with intermittent spinal cord compression during neck flexion. This is a self-limiting, distal, brachial mono- or diplegia due to segmental anterior horn cell lesion, affecting young people. The typical teenage onset corresponds with juvenile growth spurt. Males are more frequently affected, and many of them participate in competitive sports or regular strenuous physical activity. Sensory symptoms are absent. Hirayama disease usually presents with unilateral weakness and severe atrophy of the intrinsic hand muscles. Atrophy and weakness spread to the

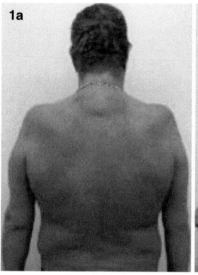
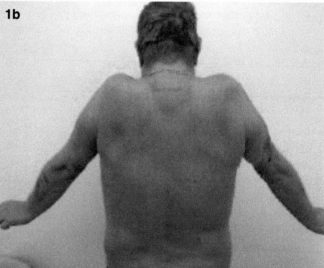

Case 4.51 Cervical flexion myelopathy. A 44-year-old male presented with a 7-year history of slowly progressive weakness of shoulder and proximal arm muscles. Nerve conduction studies and electromyography had indicated a segmental motor neuron disorder. Standard MRI of the spine had shown an intradural arachnoid cyst dorsal to the spinal cord (C5/Th2) without medullary compression. A diagnosis of the flail arm variant of ALS had been made. Due to lack of clinical progression during the last 3 years, the patient was referred for a second opinion. On examination, symmetric atrophy, severe paresis, and fasciculations of upper limb-girdle muscles were noted (**1a, b**). Biceps and brachioradialis reflexes were missing bilaterally. There were no signs of pyramidal tract or bulbar muscular dysfunction. Sensory examination was normal. MRI of the spinal cord in neutral position and during neck extension showed no compression of the spinal cord (**2a, b**). During neck flexion, however, the spinal cord was pressed against the posterior wall of the vertebral column because of an intradural cyst, leading to significant medullary deformation (**2c**). No intramedullar signal changes were seen, but the spinal cord was slightly atrophic at the level of the intradural cyst. Motor evoked potentials from upper and lower extremities were normal. It was concluded that intermittent medullary compression by the intradural cyst during neck flexion was causing chronic anterior horn cell damage. The patient was told that he did not have ALS but cervical flexion myelopathy associated with an intradural cyst. Since the benefit-to-risk ratio in this chronic, nonprogressing condition was considered to be low, surgical excision of the cyst was not performed

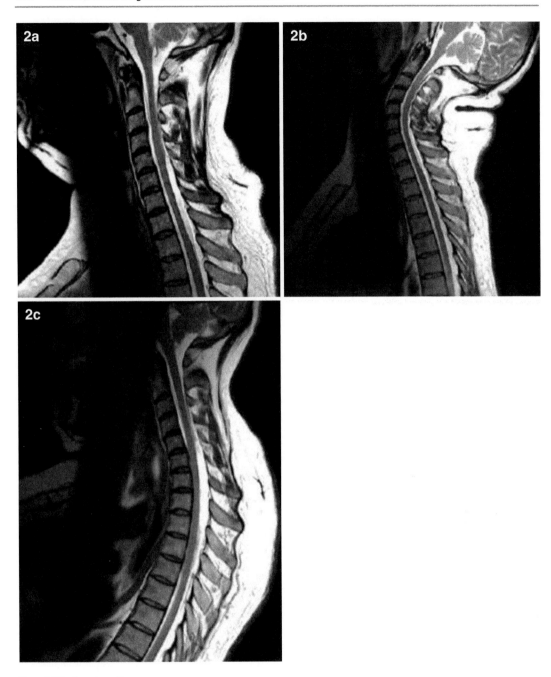

Case 4.51   (continued)

forearm flexors and extensors before reaching a plateau 1–2 years after symptom onset. The hallmark of this disease is anterior displacement of the cervical spinal cord against the vertebral bodies during neck flexion. MRI of the cervical spine may show compression of the cervical spinal cord by anterior displacement of the dura (only!) during neck flexion. Intermittent medullary compression is believed to induce chronic microvascular ischemia of the anterior horn cells, and disproportionate growth of the vertebral column and the dural sac may be the underlying structural cause of this phenomenon.

- MNDs that may simulate ALS include:
  - MMN typically affects arms more than legs and men more often than woman. As the name suggests, there are no sensory symptoms. Characteristically, there is little or no atrophy of the muscles despite considerable weakness. Careful electrophysiological examination will usually show multifocal motor conduction blocks at sites distinct from common entrapment or compression syndromes. More than half of all MMN patients have increased titers of IgM anti-GM1 gangliosides antibodies. First-line treatment is with intravenous immunoglobulin (IVIG), and many, if not all patients, have a favorable response.
  - Bulbospinal neuronopathy (Kennedy's disease) is a CAG trinucleotide repeat disorder with dysfunction of the androgen receptor gene. This disease is inherited in an X-linked fashion and thus affects men only. Typical symptoms are gynecomastia, infertility, and LMN symptoms with prominent fasciculations in the face, especially in the mentalis muscle. Prognosis is much better than with ALS, since the disease evolves slowly over many years.
  - Benign monomelic atrophy usually affects young people. Juvenile distal atrophy of the upper limb (Hirayama disease), as discussed above, belongs to this entity.
  - Spinal muscular atrophy (SMA). The current classification of SMAs is based on age of onset and rate of progression: SMA I (acute infantile, Werdnig-Hoffmann disease), SMA II (intermediate, chronic infantile, arrested), SMA III (chronic juvenile, Kugelberg-Welander disease), and SMA IV (adult onset). The last one should be considered as a differential diagnosis to ALS. Inheritance of SMA IV can be heterogeneous and can be mistaken for familial ALS. SMA IV most commonly presents with symmetric, proximal muscle weakness and atrophy and has a slow disease progression. Serum creatine kinase (CK) activity may be slightly elevated.
  - Poliomyelitis and post-polio syndrome. Poliomyelitis due to poliovirus is more or less eradicated in the Western world. Post-polio syndrome, however, is not unusual. Progressive muscular weakness and muscular pain in the affected limbs appear several decades after recovery from the original paralytic attack. A polio- and post-polio-like disorder may also occur with non-poliovirus, e.g., ECHO virus and Coxsackie virus.
- IBM is probably the most common inflammatory myopathy and is characterized by a very characteristic pattern of atrophy of the extremities (finger flexors and quadriceps muscles) and dysphagia. This is one of the more frequent ALS mimics. There is sometimes a "neurogenic" pattern on EMG, which may cause diagnostic uncertainty. A muscle biopsy will usually resolve the problem.
- As stated previously, ALS is a frequent diagnosis in a patient with a recent history of head dropping but other differential diagnoses comprise MG, isolated neck extensor myopathy (including radiation-induced myopathy), and MSA.
- Atypical parkinsonism, pseudobulbar paralysis due to bilateral damage of corticopontine tracts as seen with multiple lacunar strokes, hereditary spastic paraplegia, subacute combined degeneration of the spinal cord due to vitamin B12 or copper deficiency, MG, and myotonic dystrophy are usually easy to distinguish from ALS, but not always.

4.21 The Differential Diagnosis of Peripheral Nerve Disorders

The differential diagnosis of peripheral mono-neuropathies, plexus lesions, and spinal radiculopathies (including the cauda equina syndrome) as well as GBS and its variants has been discussed in Sect. 2.3. Here, a three-step approach to the differential diagnosis of polyneuropathy is presented.

In general, polyneuropathies are either predominantly axonal or demyelinating. The most common axonal polyneuropathies are due to diabetes and alcohol. Pharmaceutical drugs and chronic renal failure are also frequent causes of axonal polyneuropathies. Demyelinating polyneuropathies are much less frequent. They can be acute or chronic, and they may be hereditary, autoimmune-mediated, or occur in association with a monoclonal gammopathy. Importantly, most acquired demyelinating polyneuropathies (such as GBS, CIDP, and MMN) can be treated by IVIG and other forms of immuno-modulatory therapy. Compared to acquired demyelinating polyneuropathies, hereditary demyelinating neuropathies (including the various forms of CMT disease) usually have different clinical (e.g., foot deformities) and neurophysiological characteristics (non-focal, generalized demyelination).

The following algorithm allows systematic, stepwise evaluation of polyneuropathies. Preferably, every patient is investigated with blood test screening for the most common causes of polyneuropathy. If the routine investigation is negative, a targeted approach based on clinical and neurophysiological examination is recommended. Algorithms similar to the following one have been shown to reduce the number and cost of investigations for each patient without loss of diagnostic reliability (Vrancken et al. 2006).

4.21.1 Algorithm for Evaluation of Polyneuropathies

Polyneuropathies may be evaluated using the following approach (Fig. 4.17):

The first consultation is usually at primary care level. The history and examination should focus on whether an association can be established between the polyneuropathy and:

- Diabetes mellitus
- Alcohol
- A positive family history
- Neurotoxic medication
- Renal failure

If this is the case, more extensive investigation is usually only indicated if symptoms and signs are atypical or unexpectedly severe or if the course of the disease suggests another etiology.

The following blood tests are useful at this stage: fasting blood glucose, glycated hemoglobin (HbA1c), full blood count, liver function tests (perhaps combined with carbohydrate-deficient transferrin (CDT)), renal function tests (creatinine, blood urea nitrogen), C-reactive protein (CRP), erythrocyte sedimentation rate, serum protein electrophoresis, vitamin B12, folate, and thyroid function tests.

If fasting blood sugar or HbA1c levels are borderline, impaired glucose tolerance may be checked for by performing an oral glucose tolerance test. If there is a positive family history of polyneuropathy, genetic testing as suggested below can be considered. Despite careful testing, the cause of chronic polyneuropathy remains unknown in roughly 25% of cases. In an elderly patient with mild and stationary, mainly sensory symptoms, it is therefore reasonable to waive further investigation.

If the diagnostic process is to be continued, the next step is to refer the patient for nerve conduction studies (NCS). Neurophysiological evaluation is performed in order to answer the

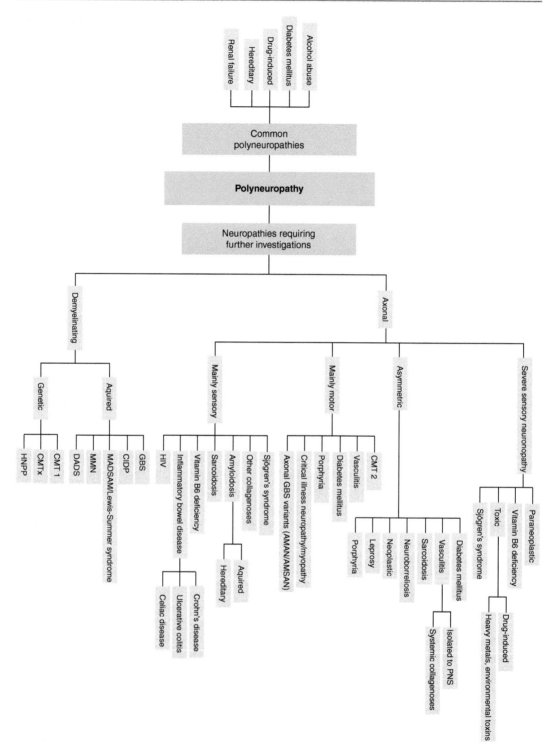

Fig. 4.17 Differential diagnosis of polyneuropathies

question: Is this a demyelinating or axonal neuropathy? The neurophysiological results and the clinical presentation are evaluated. The relevant clinical features include symptom manifestation and distribution (e.g., primarily sensory versus primarily motor symptoms; symmetrical versus asymmetrical), time course, risk factors, coexisting medical diagnosis, and the family history.

Based on the clinical and neurophysiological data, a working diagnosis is established in order to guide specific testing.

- Exclusively or mainly demyelinating neuropathies
  - Proximal and distal, symmetrical sensorimotor PNP

    ○ AIDP, classic GBS with rapid onset, CN defects, autonomic disturbances, and elevated CSF protein[17]
    ○ CIDP, e.g., elevated CSF protein
  - Asymmetric PNP
    ○ MMN; deficits are restricted to motor symptoms (no sensory symptoms!); there is relative lack of atrophy despite severe weakness, usually affecting the upper extremities first; IgM anti-GM1 antibodies are positive in up to 80%; CSF protein is normal or mildly elevated.
    ○ Multifocal acquired demyelinating sensory and motor neuropathy (MADSAM) or Lewis-Sumner syndrome is an asymmetric neuropathy initially affecting upper extremities with predominantly sensory or sensorimotor symptoms. Like other demyelinating neuropathies, it responds to treatment with IVIG.
  - Distal sensorimotor symptoms

    ○ Distal acquired demyelinating symmetric (DADS) polyneuropathy, paraprotein-associated demyelinating neuropathy, M-component, and anti-MAG
  - Chronically progressing distal symptoms, positive family history, and possible foot deformities
    ○ CMT (CMT1, CMT3, CMT4), CMTx (genetic testing: *PMP22*, *MPZ*, connexin)
  - Recurrent pressure palsies and positive family history
    ○ Hereditary neuropathy with liability to pressure palsies (HNPP; genetic testing: *PMP22* gene)
  - Slowly progressive, distal, symmetric, mainly sensory, and age > 50 years
    ○ Neuropathies associated with monoclonal gammopathies (due to either plasma cell dyscrasia or monoclonal gammopathy of unknown significance/MGUS) are associated with elevated CSF protein and EMG findings that may be mixed axonal demyelinating. Neuropathies with additional antibodies against MAG (anti-MAG) can be distinguished from CIDP using NCS showing disproportionate prolongation of distal motor latencies.
  - Although drug-induced polyneuropathies are almost always of the axonal type, polyneuropathy due to medication with amiodarone has demyelinating features.
- Exclusively or mainly axonal neuropathies
  - Severe sensory neuronopathy (leading to pronounced posterior column dysfunction and sensory ataxia)
    ○ Paraneoplastic (onconeuronal antibodies, lumbar puncture, screening for SCLC, and other malignancies using whole-body PET/CT)
    ○ Toxic substances
  - Drugs (e.g., cisplatin, chloroquine, dapsone, disulfiram, doxorubicin, ethambutol, gold, isoniazid, metronidazole, nitrofurantoin, nitrous oxide, nucleoside

---

[17]Important variant forms of GBS include pharyngeal-cervical-brachial paresis, oculopharyngeal weakness, pure sensory GBS, pure autonomic failure, ataxic GBS, and the Miller-Fisher syndrome.

analogue reverse transcriptase inhibitors, phenytoin, pyridoxine, thalidomide, vincristine)

- Heavy metals and industrial and environmental toxins (e.g., acrylamide, arsenic, carbon disulfide, lead, mercury, organic solvents, organophosphates, thallium)
- Sjögrens syndrome and other collagenoses (antinuclear antibody (ANA)/antineutrophil cytoplasmic antibodies (ANCA), other autoantibodies; Schirmer test; oral mucosa biopsy)
- Vitamin B6 deficiency or intoxication
• Asymmetric polyneuropathy
- Diabetes mellitus
- Vasculitis/collagenoses (antibodies, suralis biopsy)
- Neuroborreliosis (CSF)
- Sarcoidosis (CT thorax, serum angiotensin-converting enzyme, lymph node biopsy)
- Malignancy with infiltration of peripheral nerves (nerve biopsy, malignancy screening)
- Leprosy (skin biopsy)
- Porphyria (urine porphyrias)
• Mainly motor symptoms and subacute
- Axonal GBS variants (AMAN, AMSAN).
- Vasculitis.
- Diabetes mellitus.
- Porphyria (urine estimation of porphobilinogen; if necessary, further biochemical analysis of blood, urine, and stool).
- Critical illness polyneuropathy/myopathy (CIPM). This condition occurs in ICU patients with sepsis (or the systemic inflammatory response syndrome) and multiple organ failure. CIPM is a common neurological cause for delayed weaning from the ventilator. Of note, depressed tendon reflexes are not encountered in all of these patients. An important differential diagnosis to CIPM is prolonged neuromuscular blockade seen in patients with abnormal renal function who have been treated with non-depolarizing agents. CIPM requires prolonged and intensive neurorehabilitation, and patients may need 1–2 years to fully recover.

• Mainly motor symptoms, subacute progressive, positive family history
- CMT disease type 2 (genetic testing, but false negatives possible)
• Mainly sensory symptoms
- Sjögren syndrome (Sjögren syndrome type A and type B antibodies (SSA/SSB), lip biopsy, Schirmer test) and other collagenoses
- Sarcoidosis (CT thorax, lymph node biopsy)
- Amyloidosis due to plasma cell dyscrasia/myeloma (fat tissue biopsy, bone marrow biopsy)
- Vitamin B6 deficiency and intoxication
- Celiac disease (anti-transglutaminase antibodies; duodenal biopsy)
- Crohn's disease (colonoscopy)
- Ulcerative colitis (colonoscopy)
- Chronic obstructive lung disease (spirometry)
• Prominent involvement of small fibers, severe autonomic dysfunction, and autosomal dominant family history
- Transthyretin familial amyloid polyneuropathies (TTR-FAPs) usually manifest in the second to fourth decade with a length-dependent axonal neuropathy with prominent small fiber involvement (pain, sensory deficits) and dysautonomic features (e.g., postural hypotension, erectile dysfunction, diarrhea, weight loss), typically evolving to multiorgan systemic failure and death within 10 years. Diagnosis in patients who present as nonfamilial cases is often delayed.
• Of note, NCS are normal with *small fiber polyneuropathy*. A history of prominent pain and dysesthesias in the distal extremities in combination with normal tendon reflexes and posterior column function dur-

ing bedside examination suggests a small fiber polyneuropathy. Thermoregulatory sweat testings may be abnormal, and a skin biopsy may show a decreased amount of small nerve fibers. Of note, the discovery of *gain of function SCN9A mutations* related to sodium channels has been crucial to understand the mechanisms of painful conditions such as paroxysmal extreme pain disorder, which often were labeled as functional disorders due to the lack of objective clinical findings.

If in doubt, seek early advice from a neuromuscular specialist colleague. Rare diagnoses are numerous but rare indeed, e.g., Refsum disease, Fabry disease, or POEMS (polyneuropathy, organomegaly, endocrinopathy, M protein, and skin changes). The most often neglected cause of a peripheral neuropathy is genetic.

4.22   The Differential Diagnosis of Neuromuscular Junction Disorders

The differential diagnosis of neuromuscular junction disorders is easy at first sight—either it is MG or it is not (Fig. 4.18).

4.22.1 Myasthenia Gravis

The clinical features of ocular and generalized MG have been discussed in Chap. 2. Patients with generalized MG are usually acetylcholine receptor positive (>90%), but those with isolated ocular MG are often seronegative. A few patients have muscle-specific kinase (MuSK) antibodies (0–3%). When performing a tensilon test, use a syringe with tensilon and at least one or two with saline in order to "blind" the patient. Choose muscles and activities that can easily be tested and quantified, e.g., the time the patient can look up before ptosis occurs (Jolly's test) or lift the head from the bed or the

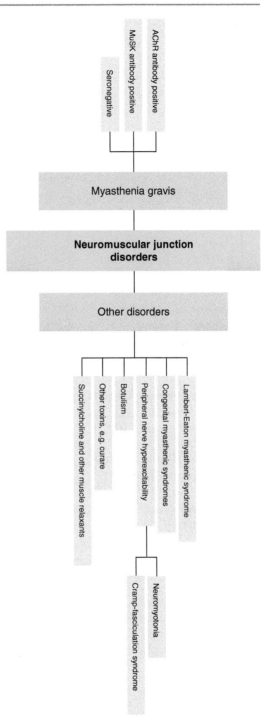

Fig. 4.18 Differential diagnosis of disorders of the neuromuscular junction

number of squats he can perform.[18] In case the patient has ptosis, ice-on-eyes is another useful bedside test.[19]

The differential diagnosis of myasthenic crisis (in patients with known and well-treated MG) includes:

- Exacerbation of myasthenic symptoms due to systemic infections
- Exacerbation of myasthenic symptoms due to certain medications
  - AED (e.g., phenytoin)
  - Antibiotics (e.g., aminoglycosides, sulfon-amide, tetracyclines)
  - Sedatives (e.g., barbiturates, benzodiazepines)
  - Others (e.g., opioids, neuroleptics)
- Cholinergic crisis (rarely seen with Mestinon® dosage ≤800 mg/day)
- Disorders unrelated to MG, e.g., acute cardiopulmonary disease (including pulmonary embolism), pneumonia, brainstem stroke, cervical myelitis, and organophosphate poisoning

4.22.2 Other Neuromuscular Junction Disorders

Neuromuscular junction disorders other than MG include (Fig. 4.18):

---

[18] To perform a tensilon test, start with 1 mL normal saline IV (placebo), and then use edrophonium IV (10 mg/mL; give 0.2 mL, if no adverse reactions give another 0.8 mL). Atropine 0.5 mg IV (antidote) must be available at the bedside. The tensilon test is used to:

- Verify the diagnosis of MG
- Evaluate treatment (increase of pyridostigmine dosage possible?), performed 2 h after last pyridostigmine dose
- Differentiate between myasthenic and cholinergic crisis (rarely necessary)

[19] To perform the ice-on-eyes test, fill a rubber glove with crushed ice, and place it over the patient's eyes for 2 min or less. If this is too cold, put a paper towel between the eyes and the glove. Coldness increases synaptic transmission and ameliorates the ptosis. This test is believed to have even higher specificity and sensitivity than the tensilon test and is not associated with cardiovascular complications but can only be performed in patients with ptosis.

- LEMS is caused by antibodies to the presynaptic VGCC leading to decreased release of acetylcholine. The majority of patients with paraneoplastic LEMS have a small cell carcinoma of the lung. An underlying malignance is ultimately found in roughly 50% of all LEMS cases (but it may take up to two to four years before the malignancy will have "declared itself"). Weakness in the upper and lower limbs is proximal and symmetrical. In contrast to myasthenia, bulbar and oculomotor symptoms are usually missing. Thirst, however, is a frequent complaint probably due to cross-reaction of antibodies with salivary glands. (Many LEMS patients carry a bottle of water with them wherever they go, a useful clinical sign.)
- Botulism due to *Clostridium botulinum* toxin often affects families or other groups that have shared contaminated food. Intravenous or subcutaneous abuse of heroine using contaminated syringes is another cause. Botulism may also occur in neonates following delivery under bad sanitary conditions. Bulbar symptoms (diplopia, ophthalmoplegia, dysarthria, dysphonia, dysphagia, and facial weakness) and pupillary dysfunction (loss of accommodation with blurred vision, fixed mydriasis) are common. Paralysis of the extremities develops over 1–3 days. Deep tendon reflexes are hypoactive or absent. Due to weakness of respiratory muscles, mechanical ventilation is usually necessary. Smooth muscle paralysis typically involves constipation, paralytic ileus, and urinary retention. Botulinum toxin is said to be the most toxic of all natural toxins (Case 2.1).
- Other toxins of the neuromuscular synapse include curare (the traditional South American arrow poison), tetrodotoxin (found in exotic fishes), and muscle relaxants such as succinylcholine.
- Congenital myasthenic syndromes (e.g., AChR deficiency, rapsyn deficiency, Dok-7 synaptopathy), usually present at birth or in childhood, but adult-onset cases are well described.

- Neuromyotonia (Isaacs' syndrome) and cramp-fasciculation syndrome are the two main disorders of acquired peripheral nerve hyperexcitability. Acquired neuromyotonia is a condition associated with muscle hyperactivity, resulting in muscle stiffness, cramps, myokymia, pseudomyotonia, and weakness. It may be associated with thymoma or autoimmune disorders. The diagnosis requires the presence of antibodies to the VGKC of the presynaptic nerve terminal.

4.23   The Differential Diagnosis of Myopathy

The general neurologist is likely to encounter the following myopathies at least a few times during his career:

- Myotonic dystrophy
- Drug-induced myopathies
- IBM
- Polymyositis and dermatomyositis
- Myopathy associated with thyroid dysfunction
- Limb-girdle muscular dystrophies
- FSH
- Mitochondrial disorders
- CIPM

All other myopathies are usually only seen in dedicated neuromuscular outpatient clinics or occasionally during grand rounds at tertiary level institutions.

Important hints from the history include:

- Age of clinical onset, e.g., DMD presents before the age of 6 and IBM in middle life.
- Family history (autosomal, X-linked, or mitochondrial (maternal) inheritance), including history of nonmuscular symptoms in family members, e.g., early-onset cataract and diabetes associated with myotonic dystrophy.
- Pulmonary (respiratory failure, e.g., Pompe's disease) and cardiac complications (cardiomyopathy, arrhythmias).

- Severe orofacial weakness, e.g., FSH.
- Limb-girdle muscle atrophy, e.g., limb-girdle muscular dystrophies and FSH.
- Medication. Drugs that have been associated with myopathy include alcohol, amiodarone, chloroquine, cimetidine, colchicine, corticosteroids, cyclosporine, d-penicillamine, glycyrrhizin (licorice), isoniazid, lithium, nifedipine, propofol, quetiapine, salbutamol, statins, vincristine, and zidovudine.
- Myopathies can be divided into acquired and genetic myopathies (Fig. 4.19).

4.23.1   Acquired Myopathies

- Idiopathic inflammatory myopathies.
  - IBM, as discussed in Sect. 4.19
  - Polymyositis
  - Dermatomyositis (usually paraneoplastic)
- Drug-induced myopathies. For a list of offending drugs, see above. Statin- and corticosteroid-induced myopathies are the most common drug-induced myopathies in clinical practice. The combination of cholesterol-lowering agents and steroids may lead to a particularly severe myopathy.
- CIPM. As explained earlier (Sect. 4.20), CIPM is a common neurological cause for delayed weaning from the ventilator in ICU patients with sepsis and multiple organ failure. Of note, while serum creatine kinase levels can be normal, myoglobin levels are typically markedly elevated.
- Infectious myositis.

4.23.2   Genetic Myopathies

See also Sect. 2.1.

- Muscular dystrophies
  - Myotonic dystrophy type 1
  - Myotonic dystrophy type 2 (proximal myotonic myopathy (PROMM))
  - DMD
  - Becker muscular dystrophies

for initial management of minimal, mild and moderate head injuries in adults: an evidence and consensus-based update. BMC Med. 2013;11:50–87.

Vrancken AF, Kalmijn S, Buskens E, et al. Feasibility and cost efficiency of a diagnostic guideline for chronic polyneuropathy: a prospective implementation study. J Neurol Neurosurg Psychiatry. 2006;77:397–401.

Waldemar G, Burns A, editors. Alzheimer's disease. London: Oxford University Press; 2009.

Waubant E, Weinshenker B, Wolinsky JS. Diagnostic criteria for multiple sclerosis: 2010 revisions to the McDonald criteria. Ann Neurol. 2011;69:292–302.

Wegener M, la Cour M, Milea D. Loss of sight and hearing and cognitive dysfunction—Susac's syndrome? Ugeskr Laeger. 2009;171:618–20.

World Health Organization. International Statistical Classification of Diseases and Related Health Problems, 10th revision, vol. 2. 2010 ed. www.who.int/classifications/icd/.

Wu CM, McLaughlin K, Lorenzetti DL, et al. Early risk of stroke after transient ischemic attack: a systematic review and meta-analysis. Arch Intern Med. 2007;167(22):2417–22.

Zhang S, Ma Y, Feng J. Clinicoradiological spectrum of reversible splenial lesion syndrome (RESLES) in adults: a retrospective study of a rare entity. Medicine. 2015;94:e512.

Zongo D, Ribéreau-Gayon R, Masson F, et al. S100-B protein as a screening tool for the easy assessment of minor head injury. Ann Emerg Med. 2012;59:209–18.

Ancillary Investigations

5

Abstract

The neurologist has a continuously expanding arsenal of ancillary investigations at hand. Good clinical skills are mandatory to put the patient on the right diagnostic track and to ensure correct interpretations of the results. Every investigation ordered should serve a specific purpose and help to answer a well-considered and well-formulated question. Close cooperation and, preferentially, personal communication with appropriate colleagues such as radiologists, neurophysiologists, and geneticists are mandatory. Given the book's focus on bedside skills, the following overview of neuroimaging, neurophysiology, ultrasound techniques, laboratory evaluations of blood and cerebrospinal fluid, genetic testing, and neuropsychological evaluation is short but covers many elementary technical and clinical facts relevant to the general neurologist. Clinical neurophysiology is discussed in somewhat greater detail, since it is the domain of the neurologist in many countries.

Keywords

Ancillary investigations • Autonomic nervous system testing • Cerebrospinal fluid • Computed tomography • Electroencephalography • Electromyography • Evoked potentials • Genetic testing • Lumbar puncture • Magnetic resonance imaging • Nerve conduction studies • Neuroimaging • Neuropsychological testing • Polysomnography • Positron emission tomography • Single photon emission computed tomography • Sleep studies • Ultrasound investigations

5.1 Neuroimaging

No other technological field is having a greater impact on clinical neurology than neuroimaging. The advent of MR angiography, MR diffusion-weighted imaging, and MR gradient-echo sequences, for instance, has made formerly unknown or exceptionally rare conditions rather commonplace, e.g., RCVS, PRES, superficial CNS siderosis, CLIPPERS, and mild encephalopathy with a reversible splenial lesion (MERS) (Case 5.1). A thorough review

© Springer International Publishing AG 2017
D. Kondziella, G. Waldemar, *Neurology at the Bedside*, DOI 10.1007/978-3-319-55991-9_5

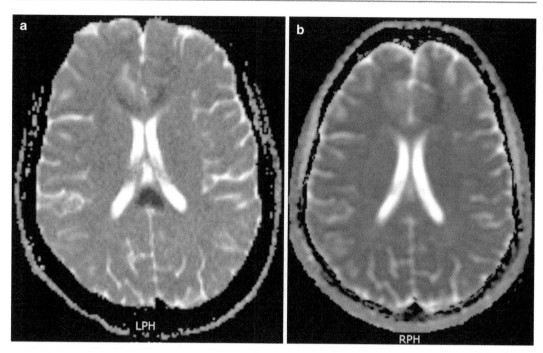

Case 5.1 Mild encephalopathy with a reversible splenial lesion (MERS). A 23-year-old male presented with subacute onset of headache, confusion, fever, and decreased consciousness. MRI showed a singular lesion in the splenium of the corpus callosum (**a**, ADC). CSF analysis was notable for a lymphocytic pleocytosis. His previous medical history was unremarkable, and he did not take any medication. Screening for infectious agents was positive for influenza A (PCR in nasopharyngeal swab). The patient made an uneventful recovery, and follow-up MRI a few weeks later was normal (**b**). Mild encephalitis/ encephalopathy with a reversible splenial lesion (MERS, also known as "reversible splenial lesion syndrome") is a clinico-radiological syndrome characterized by a transient mild encephalopathy and a singular, reversible lesion in the midline of the splenium of the corpus callosum on MRI. Occasionally, reversible lesions may also be seen outside of the splenium. MERS has been described in a variety of conditions, including neuroinfections (e.g., influenza, herpesviridae, and mycoplasma), antiepileptic drug withdrawal, hyponatremia, high-altitude cerebral edema, and cesarean section

of the available neuroimaging modalities is not possible here due to space limitations, but gathering adequate knowledge in this field is highly advisable. This is best achieved on a day-to-day basis in close cooperation with the neuroradiologist. Accurate referrals based on decent clinical observations and with a clearly stated question are mandatory to choosing the right neuroimaging modality and to interpreting the imaging data correctly. Moreover, scans should be looked at jointly with the neuroradiologist instead of relying on a written report. Attending the daily radiology conference (if available) should be mandatory. However, unexpected findings on MRI (and CT) are not uncommon, and therefore, examinations should not just be ordered "for the benefit of doubt" but should always serve a well-defined purpose (Cases 5.2 and 5.3).

5.1.1 Computer Tomography (CT)

CTs digitally reformat a large series of cross-sectional, two-dimensional X-ray images to allow visualization within a few minutes of the body anatomy, usually in axial sections. The spiral CT technique uses multiple roentgen-ray tubes that continually rotate in one direction, while the patient table moves forward at a constant speed.

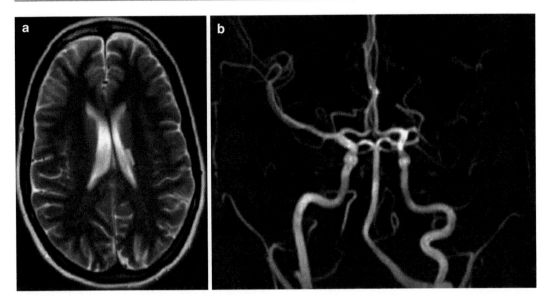

Case 5.2 Clinically silent middle cerebral artery occlusion. A 24-year-old male medical student volunteered to participate in the control group of a medical study and was examined by MRI. His previous medical history was unremarkable, and he was a nonsmoker. Surprisingly, T_2-weighted MRI showed a periventricular lacunar infarction (**a**), and MR angiography revealed a left-sided MCA occlusion and compensatory collateral vessels (**b**, moyamoya phenomenon). Extensive cerebrovascular follow-up was unremarkable. Following an in-depth discussion with the patient, he opted for prophylactic antithrombotic treatment with clopidogrel

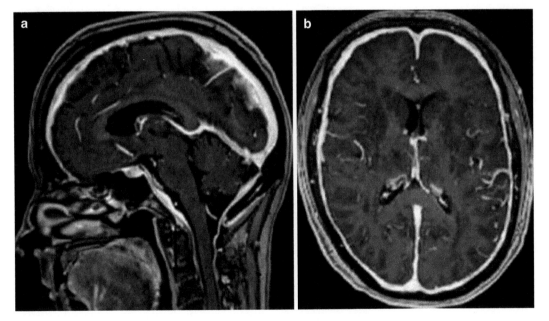

Case 5.3 Idiopathic hypertrophic pachymeningitis. A 58-year-old female consulted a neurologist for transient sensory symptoms, which he felt were unspecific. The neurological examination was normal. An MRI of the brain was ordered "for the benefit of doubt." T_1-weighted contrast-enhanced sequences showed thickened and enhancing dura mater, which was considered an incidental finding (**a, b**). A lumbar puncture revealed normal CSF opening pressure (16 cm H_2O), a mild lymphocytic pleocytosis (10 cells/ mm^3), and slightly increased protein (0.67 g/L). After extensive workup for possible autoimmune, infectious, and neoplastic disorders, as well as sarcoidosis, a diagnosis of idiopathic hypertrophic pachymeningitis was made. Follow-up MRI 1 year later showed unchanged dural inflammation. IgG4-related disease (which in the CNS frequently manifests as hypertrophic pachymeningitis) was considered, but a meningeal biopsy was not performed. The patient had no symptoms and refused further investigations

Compared to MR imaging, CT is more available, cheaper, and less time-consuming. Disadvantages include the lower resolution and the use of X-rays. One CT brain scan exposes the patient to a radiation of 1.5 mSv. The equivalent figures for chest X-ray and the annual average background exposure in Western Europe are 0.1 and 1–3 mSv, respectively (Case 5.4). Contrast medium can cause renal failure. Hydration therapy is important to prevent contrast-induced nephropathy. A creatinine level above 1.4 mg/dL puts the patient at risk. If contrast imaging is indispensable, four doses of 600 mg N-acetylcysteine (two the day of procedure, two the next day) and intravenous fluids can prevent

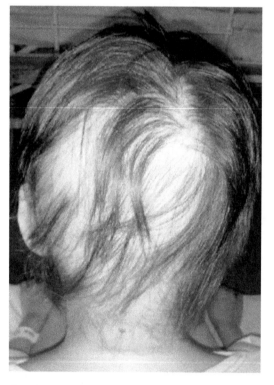

Case 5.4 Radiation toxicity. A 28-year-old female with CVST was treated with repeated endovascular interventions for extensive thrombosis of the deep central veins and declining consciousness despite IV heparin. The patient made a full neurological recovery. However, because of radiation toxicity associated with frequent CT-based neuroimaging and digital subtraction angiographies, she suffered from temporary hair loss

renal damage. Normal saline with bicarbonate, 154 mEq/L (1 h before and 6 h after the procedure at a rate of 3 mL/kg/h), is an alternative.

The Hounsfield scale, named after one of the inventers of CT, is a quantitative scale of tissue density. It ranges from −1000 to +1000 Hounsfield units (HU). Roughly, air has −1000 HU, fat −100, water 0, CSF 10, white matter 30, gray matter 40, muscle 40, blood 100, contrast medium 130, and bone ≥600. The more HU, the brighter the object; thus, on CT, air appears darker than fat and CSF, and gray matter appears lighter than white matter.

CT offers generally excellent imaging but is poor at demonstrating lesions that are small (<1 cm), that have a similar attenuation to that of the brain (e.g., MS plaques) or of the bone (particular if lesions are close to the skull base), and that are situated within the posterior fossa or spinal canal.

Although digital subtraction angiography is still the gold standard for imaging of the cerebral vasculature, CT angiography has become the first choice for most diagnostic procedures, since it is more widely available, faster, and noninvasive. In patients with ischemic cerebral infarction, it is important to order a computed tomography angiography (CTA) that includes the neck vessel and the aortic arch; otherwise, proximal stenoses and dissections of the carotid and vertebral arteries might be missed. CT venography can be used to evaluate for cerebral venous sinus thrombosis, but false-negative results may occur because of contrast enhancement of the thrombotic material falsely suggesting intact passage. MRI venography appears to be superior in this regard.

CT perfusion imaging is used to study CBF in acute ischemic stroke, vasospasm secondary to subarachnoidal hemorrhage, and brain trauma. In patients with suspected acute stroke, the site of vascular occlusion, infarct core, salvageable brain tissue, and collateral circulation can be assessed by a combination of non-contrast CT, CT perfusion, and CT angiography. It has been suggested that CT perfusion may help in decision making for thrombolysis when there is no certain time of symptom debut. CT perfusion protocols are difficult to standardize, however, and data evaluation is affected by a relatively low signal-to-noise ratio.

5.1.2 Positron Emission Tomography (PET)

PET measures emissions from radioactively labeled metabolically active chemicals that have been injected intravenously. The most commonly used PET tracer is fludeoxyglucose (^{18}F-FDG), a labeled form of glucose. FDG-PET, combined with CT of the brain, is useful in assessing metabolic activity (hyper- vs. hypometabolic) of various acquired brain diseases (e.g., brain tumors, CNS lymphoma, autoimmune limbic encephalitis), including neurodegenerative disorders (e.g., AD, FTD). Imaging of brain beta-amyloid with ^{11}C-PIB PET (or with ^{18}F labeled tracers) may be used to increase the certainty of a diagnosis of AD in unclear cases (Case 5.5).

5.1.3 Single Photon Emission Computed Tomography (SPECT)

SPECT is a nuclear medicine tomographic imaging technique using gamma rays. The most commonly used tracer is ^{99m}Tc-labeled HMPAO for studying regional CBF. Interictal and ictal SPECT may demonstrate CBF increase within epileptogenic foci and is used in the workup for epilepsy surgery. Like ^{18}F-FDG-PET, ^{99m}Tc-HMPAO SPECT can help differentiating between AD and other dementias. For instance, AD is most often associated with temporoparietal hypometabolism (hypoperfusion), and bvFTD is associated with symmetric bilateral frontal hypometabolism (hypoperfusion).

SPECT scanning using ioflupane (^{123}I FP-CIT), a presynaptic dopamine transporter marker, also known as dopamine transporter scanning (DAT scan), can help distinguish between essential tremor (normal DAT scan) and Parkinson's disease (reduced binding in striatum) (Case 5.6). A DAT scan may also help differentiate between DLB (reduced binding) and AD (normal). However, it cannot be used to distinguish between Parkinson's disease and atypical Parkinsonism (e.g., MSA and PSP/CBS).

5.1.4 Magnetic Resonance Imaging (MRI)

Unlike CT, MRI does not require ionizing radiation but uses a powerful magnetic field to align hydrogen atoms in the water of body tissues. Radio frequency fields are applied in order to systematically alter the alignment of the magnetization, causing the protons to produce a rotating magnetic field that is detected by the scanner. The signal can be manipulated by additional magnetic fields in order to gather the information to construct an image.

MRI is usually superior to CT for all clinical questions, with the possible exception for bony pathology. However, MRI is less available, more expensive, and more time-consuming. (Although not of the highest quality, a single-shot, fast spin echo sequence in an uncooperative unstable patient is usually free of artifacts and takes less than a minute for the entire brain.) Potential contraindications for MRI include claustrophobia, magnetic implants, and foreign bodies such as cardiac pacemakers, insulin pumps, and electrodes for deep brain stimulation (DBS). Nowadays, many devices are compatible with MRI but need to be readjusted after the procedure. If foreign bodies are suspected, e.g., eye splinters in a metalworker, perform a plain skull X-ray prior to MRI. Pregnancy is not a contraindication per se, but be restrictive with gadolinium contrast.

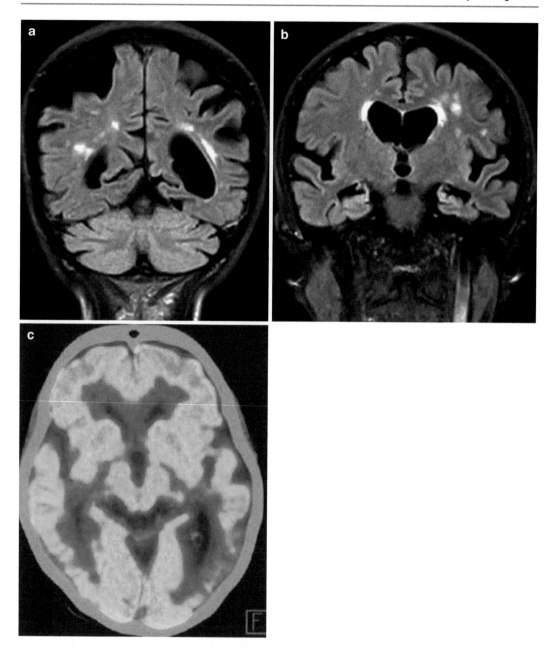

Case 5.5 Alzheimer's disease with atypical onset (posterior cortical atrophy). A 72-year-old retired primary school teacher, living alone without assistance, was referred for subjective word-finding difficulties with particular difficulties in retrieving names of places, persons, and concepts. Symptoms had been progressing over 1–2 years. There was no significant functional impairment and reasonable day-to-day memory. Her family confirmed that her performance in activities of daily living was normal. Neurological examination was unremarkable except for cognitive impairment. The MMSE score was 30/30. Neuropsychological examination revealed pronounced anomia, visuo-constructional deficits, simultanagnosia, optic ataxia, and mild impairment of word fluency, writing, and calculation (partial Balint's syndrome). Episodic and semantic memory, comprehension, judgment, abstraction, and insight were all unremarkable. MRI revealed pronounced bilateral superior temporoparietal atrophy (**a**, **b**) and FDG-PET bilateral posterior temporoparietal hypometabolism (**c**). Amyloid PET (^{11}C-PIB PET) was positive (*not shown*). Although the patient did not meet the formal criteria for dementia due to intact memory, she did meet criteria for AD dementia with atypical onset (posterior cortical atrophy). She was started on a cholinesterase inhibitor (PET images courtesy of Ian Law, Department of Clinical Physiology and Nuclear Medicine, Rigshospitalet, Copenhagen)

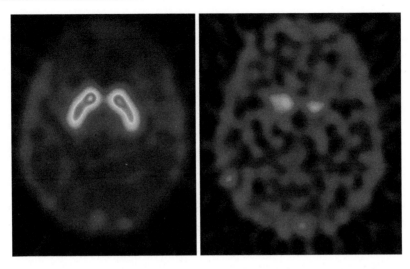

Case 5.6 Dopamine transporter (DAT) imaging in Parkinson's disease. DAT scan of a healthy volunteer (*left*) and a patient with Parkinson's disease (*right*) is depicted here. The patient was a 50-year-old man with a 3-year history of bradykinesia, rigidity, and a pill-rolling tremor worse on the right side. DAT scanning (following intravenous application of tracer [123I]-PE2I) showed asymmetry and reduced uptake in the striatum. L-dopa treatment was started with good clinical response (SPECT images courtesy of Gerda Krog Thomsen, Neurobiology Research Unit, Rigshospitalet, Copenhagen, Denmark (Adapted with permission from Kondziella (2017))

The following MRI sequences and techniques are clinically important:

- In T_1-weighted MRI (with and without gadolinium contrast), gray matter appears dark, white matter bright, and CSF very dark. T_1-weighted scans use a gradient-echo sequence with short T_E (echo delay time) and short T_R (repetition time). Together with T_2-weighted MRI, this is the most commonly used sequence. T_1-weighted images reflect anatomy well, whereas pathology is usually better seen on T_2-weighted imaging. Gadolinium contrast medium is used to enhance T_1-weighted images. Gadolinium enhancement of parenchymal lesions indicates blood–brain barrier damage, e.g., due to inflammation or malignancy.[1]
- With T_2-weighted MRI, gray matter is bright, white matter dark, and CSF very bright. T_2-weighted scans use a spin-echo sequence, with long T_E and long T_R. These sequences are more or less unaffected by inhomogeneities in the magnetic field. T_2-weighted imaging is sensitive to water and is therefore particularly well suited to detect edema. Leukoencephalopathy, demyelination, and edema appear as hyperintense signals.
- FLAIR suppresses CSF effects on the image, so as to better reveal hyperintense lesions. Thus, FLAIR is similar to T_2, but the CSF appears very dark, which is useful for identifying white matter lesions, e.g., subcortical ischemic infarcts, MS plaques, and vasogenic edemas.
- Gradient-echo sequences such as T_2*-weighted MRI (pronounced "T_2 star") and susceptibility-weighted imaging (SWI) are well suited to show hemosiderin deposits from old hemorrhages and vascular malformations that appear very dark on these images. Hemosiderin deposits are associated with blood from cerebral amyloid angiopathy, venous malformations, cavernomas, superficial CNS siderosis, hypertensive intracranial hemorrhages, and other cerebral vasculopathy.

---

[1] Following a lumbar puncture, diffuse meningeal contrast enhancement in the spine may be seen for days or weeks, and, although not pathological, this may lead to diagnostic confusion.

- DWI assesses the diffusion of water molecules in biological tissues. Cytotoxic edema due to acute ischemia is easily seen as a bright signal. It remains visible during the first 10 days after infarction. DWI has revolutionized imaging in acute stroke since the hyperintense signal change is more or less identical with the infarction core. It thereby helps to identify the patients who will likely benefit from intravenous thrombolysis (IVT) and/or mechanical revascularization and those who do not. Also, other cytotoxic edema appears as bright, e.g., cortical and basal ganglia hyperintense signal in CJD, cerebral abscesses, inflammatory lesions with infections, and autoimmune processes (e.g., MS, limbic encephalitis).
- Apparent diffusion coefficient (ADC) imaging is used to differentiate T_2-shine-through effects and other artifacts from real ischemic lesions and therefore complements DWI. ADC mapping can also distinguish old strokes from new ones as well as vasogenic from cytotoxic edema. The combination of MR DWI and ADC sequences may allow differentiating cerebral abscesses (black on ADC) from brain tumors (see Case 4.35 for illustration).
- Perfusion MRI involves administration of a tracer into the cerebral circulation, thereby facilitating monitoring of CBF. In acute stroke, the difference (mismatch) between the larger perfusion deficit and the smaller area of diffusion abnormality represents the ischemic penumbra. This is the potentially salvageable brain tissue. Perfusion/diffusion MRI already plays a major role in optimizing therapy of acute ischemic stroke.
- Short tau inversion recovery (STIR) images are T_1-weighted images following fat suppression. This is helpful in assessment of coronal orbital images or when visualizing cystic lesions or the course of larger peripheral nerves.
- Diffusion tensor imaging (DTI) allows mapping of fiber directions to assess the connectivity of different regions in the brain (called tractography) or to examine areas of neural degeneration and demyelination.

- Although still not quite as good as conventional angiography, MR angiography and venography are commonly used to demonstrate the cerebral vasculature. The advantages compared to conventional angiography are noninvasiveness and that it can be performed in one session together with acquisition of the other MR images. MR angiography can be performed with contrast enhancement or without (so-called time-of-flight (TOF) sequences).
- Functional MRI (fMRI) has revolutionized cortical mapping and neuropsychological studies. It demonstrates cortical activity by increase of blood flow in the relevant cerebral areas. When analyzing the data statistically, adjustment for multiple comparisons is crucial but unfortunately often disregarded.[2]
- MR spectroscopy is not structural imaging; rather, it is noninvasive spectral analysis of metabolites. Biochemical information is obtained from tissue in a so-called volume of interest, usually the cortex, white matter, or a brain lesion. Proton (or ^{1}H) magnetic resonance spectroscopy (MRS) can be used for prognostic purposes in, e.g., hypoxic brain damage and carbon monoxide poisoning. Increased levels of choline indicate damage of white matter, decreased N-acetyl aspartate levels suggest gray matter impairment, and lactate peaks reflect anaerobic metabolism.

---

[2]Simplified, if you perform a large number of tests, there is a statistical chance that some of the results will be false-positive simply *because* you have performed a large number of tests. Adjusting for multiple comparisons ensures that this "chance significance" is corrected for. The problem of unadjusted multiple comparisons when using fMRI has been elucidated elegantly by Bennet et al., who performed fMRI on a dead salmon. The fish was shown photos of people with different facial expressions and asked to guess the emotions they were having. Using standard acquisition, preprocessing, and analysis techniques, Bennett et al. (2009) showed that active voxel clusters could be observed in the dead salmon's brain when statistical thresholds remained uncorrected. Upon correction for multiple testing, the positive results disappeared.

5.2   Electroencephalography (EEG)

EEG reflects accumulated electrical activity caused by postsynaptic potentials of cortical neurons. It is cheap and noninvasive and, so far, remains the only routine method that offers real-time registration of neuronal activity. EEG is indicated for the study of epilepsy, sleep disorders, various encephalopathies (metabolic, infectious, ischemic, and traumatic), coma, and few rare diseases that can present with a pathognomonic EEG pattern (e.g., CJD, SSPE). In the drowsy patient, EEG helps to distinguish nonconvulsive status epilepticus from metabolic encephalopathy and psychogenic coma (catatonia). During surgical operations, EEG can be applied to monitor the depth of anesthesia, and it may serve as an indirect indicator of cerebral perfusion in CEA. EEG is also useful to distinguish coma of primary cortical dysfunction from coma due to disturbed brainstem regulation of cortical activity. Further, EEG is sometimes used to document electrical silence in the setting of brain death.

As stated above, EEG is critical in the diagnosis and monitoring of patients with epilepsy. Although a single, interictal EEG is abnormal in only 30–40% of patients with epilepsy, repeating the EEG once or twice increases the sensitivity to 60–80%. (Note that 2–4% of adults in the general population have epileptiform activity on EEG without having epilepsy.) EEG helps to classify seizure types, and this classification is essential for the choice of antiepileptic treatment. Video-EEG monitoring is very helpful to differentiate epilepsy from PNES and other events, and it is crucial in the assessment of the epilepsy surgery candidate. In the latter, subdural, sphenoid, or intracortical electrodes increase the diagnostic yield, as compared to scalp EEG. In addition, EEG can assist in decision making about treatment options in patients who have well-documented epileptic seizures. For instance, as stated above, in neurointensive care, the EEG can document "burst suppression" in the sedated patient with refractory status epilepticus, and it can be helpful in diagnosing NMDA receptor encephalitis by revealing "extreme delta brushes." In the outpatient clinic, it may assist in the decision to stop antiepileptic treatment in patients who have been seizure-free for a prolonged period.

Scalp EEG reveals electrical activity from cortical areas close to the skull bone, and for epileptic activity to be registered, it must arise from areas of 3–5 cm^2 or larger. Thus, EEG seldom reveals epileptic activity during focal motor status (too small an area), post-apoplectic epilepsy (too much cortical damage), and epileptic activity in the legs (because the leg area of the motor homunculus lies in the medial motor strip deep between the hemispheres). EEG can be affected by patient-related artifacts such as skin humidity, eye movements, and activities of the muscles of the head, the extremities, or the heart (the R wave from the QRS complex may be misdiagnosed as an epileptic spike, especially in the temporal leads), as well as technical disturbances.

The background activity decreases somewhat in the elderly, whereas benzodiazepines and barbiturates increase the frequency of the background activity. Drowsiness and sleep have characteristic patterns and must be distinguished from slowing of the EEG background seen with various encephalopathies. The EEG of the infant and child is very different from the adult EEG as the background activity of adults is usually fully established by the middle of the second decade. Gender differences of the EEG pattern have not been described.

EEG is analyzed by assessing the background activity and normal or pathological potentials (see below). Background activity is classified as slow (delta and theta activity), normal (alpha activity), or fast (beta activity).

- Delta activity has a frequency of <4 Hz. It may occur focally with subcortical lesions and in general distribution with diffuse lesions, metabolic encephalopathy, hydrocephalus, or deep midline lesions. Delta activity in the adult EEG during wakefulness is always pathological.
- Theta is the frequency range from 4 Hz to <8 Hz. Theta is seen as a normal feature in

young children and during drowsiness in older children and adults. It can also occur during meditation in people who have been practicing for many years. Excess theta for age represents abnormal activity, and it may occur as a focal disturbance due to subcortical (e.g., tumors, infarction) and epicortical lesions (e.g., subdural hemorrhages or hygromas). Generalized pathological theta activity is encountered in diffuse brain injury, metabolic encephalopathies, deep midline lesions, and hydrocephalus.

- Alpha frequency ranges from 8 to 13 Hz. It is best seen in the occipital leads; this is the so-called postcentral background activity. Occasionally, alpha is somewhat higher in amplitude on the dominant side. Alpha activity is elicited by closing the eyes and by relaxation, and it is blocked by eye opening or mental exertion. (In addition to the occipital alpha rhythm, there is another normal alpha rhythm: the mu rhythm. This is alpha range activity over the sensorimotor cortex that vanishes with movement of the contralateral arm.) Alpha activity is rarely abnormal. In the comatose patient, for instance, "alpha coma" refers to diffuse alpha activity that does not have the normal predilection for the occipital leads and that is not responsive to external stimuli. Alpha coma is associated with a poor prognosis. Diffuse abnormal alpha activity can also be seen in, e.g., pontine gliomas.

- Beta is the frequency range above 13 Hz. Beta activity is usually seen bilaterally in symmetrical distribution and is most evident in the frontal leads. It is the dominant rhythm in people who are alert and with eyes open. Increased beta activity can be induced by illicit drugs and various medications, especially benzodiazepines. Beta may be absent or reduced in areas of cortical damage.

There are several types of pathological activity:

- Pathological background activity, e.g., generalized theta and delta activity due to metabolic encephalopathies or neurodegenerative diseases.

- Locally decreased frequency, e.g., localized theta and delta activity due to a focal brain process such as a tumor or hemorrhage.
- Epileptiform activity, typically spikes and sharp waves. Spikes last for 20–70 ms and sharp waves typically for 70–200 ms. Paroxysmal activity is only classified as epileptiform if it clearly stands out from the background activity and is not an EEG mimic. Note that epileptiform activity can be absent in the EEG of patients who have epilepsy and that it occasionally can be present in people who do *not* have epilepsy. EEG mimics include, e.g., vertex waves during stage II sleep, benign epileptiform transients of sleep, wicket spikes, and 14- and 6-Hz positive bursts.
- Epileptic seizure activity is always pathological (in contrast to epileptiform activity, as stated above):
  - Generalized ictal patterns:
    The evolving discharge of a generalized tonic-clonic seizure is typically characterized by the rapid (>10 Hz) repetition of generalized spikes and polyspikes. The spikes usually increase in amplitude and decrease in frequency during the first 10 to 20 s of a generalized tonic-clonic seizure, corresponding to the tonic phase of the seizure. Subsequently, bursts of generalized high-amplitude spike and slow wave or polyspike discharges occur and are associated with clonic jerks. As the clonic jerks fade away toward the end of the seizure, a gradual tapering of the burst frequency is normally noted. The background activity is suppressed postictally, followed by widespread delta frequency slowing.

    The classic EEG during absence seizures is associated with generalized three-per-second spike and slow wave discharges that start and finish abruptly. Discharges may occur up to several hundreds of times a day and last only a few seconds. The patient usually stares unresponsively during these attacks and minor automatisms may occur, but electrographic seizure activity also can occur with preserved consciousness.

- Polyspikes and polyspike and wave discharges (4–5 Hz) are the cardinal feature of myoclonic seizures, e.g., occurring in JME, although they are occasionally seen in other generalized seizure types as well.
- Slow spike and wave discharges (2–3 Hz) are often observed in atypical absence seizures and may occur as part of the Lennox-Gastaut syndrome.

– Focal ictal patterns are manifold. As a rule, it is the rhythmicity and evolution of an EEG pattern that suggests that a focal pattern is ictal in nature:

- A focal epileptic seizure with secondary tonic-clonic generalization is seen on the EEG as a progressive seizure pattern, characterized by decreasing frequency and increasing amplitude, starting in one lead, and subsequently spreading to other leads. An isolated seizure usually lasts between 50 and 120 s (although frontal epileptic seizures, for instance, are typically much shorter).
- Lateralized periodic discharges (LPDs) and generalized periodic discharges (GPDs) may be seen in focal structural brain lesions such as stroke, tumor, or infectious encephalitis (e.g., temporal LPDs in herpes simplex encephalitis), as well as in anoxic brain injury. LPDs and GPDs were previously known as "periodic lateralized epileptiform discharges (PLEDs)" and "generalized lateralized epileptiform discharges," respectively, but this has been revised by the American Clinical Neurophysiology Society Critical Care Monitoring Committee in order to eliminate terms with clinical connotations (e.g., "epileptiform" suggests a propensity to seizures). In patients with brain injury and decreased consciousness, however, LPDs and GPDs with a dynamic character may indeed suggest nonconvulsive status epilepticus.

- Various EEG patterns may be seen in coma, e.g., nonconvulsive status epilepticus, generalized burst suppression, focal slowing suggesting a structural cause, alpha coma (less commonly beta, theta, or delta coma), and spindle coma with features that resemble those of normal sleep. Of note, recent technical advances have made continuous EEG (cEEG) monitoring feasible for an increasing number of surgical and nonsurgical patients in both general and neurointensive care departments. Quantitative EEG (qEEG) software programs allow the many hours of raw EEG data to be condensed into a few screenshots which can be assessed instantly. For instance, cEEG may assist in managing ICU patients with status epilepticus by showing a burst suppression pattern following sedation with propofol or barbiturates and by verifying that epileptic activity has ceased before a wake-up call is performed. In addition, cEEG monitoring following SAH can be used to detect an increased number of subclinical seizures, and it may predict delayed cerebral ischemia many hours in advance.

Finally, let us consider the most important electrophysiological principles of sleep. Sleep is either associated with rapid eye movements (REM sleep) or not (non-REM sleep). Non-REM sleep used to be divided into four stages, but following a revision by the American Academy of Sleep Medicine in 2007, only three stages remain (N1–N3):

- Stage N1 refers to the transition from alpha waves to theta waves. This stage is sometimes referred to as somnolence or drowsy sleep, in which muscle tone and conscious awareness of the external environment are decreasing. Myoclonic jerks often occur in this stage. Hypnagogic hallucinations can be due to narcolepsy but may also occur in healthy individuals.
- Stage N2 is characterized by sleep spindles, usually ranging from 11 to 14 Hz, and so-called K-complexes. Muscular activity decreases, and conscious awareness of the

external environment is lost. This stage corresponds to roughly 50% of total sleep in adults.

- Stage N3 (deep or slow-wave sleep) is characterized by the presence of at least 20% delta waves ranging from 0.5 to 2 Hz with a peak-to-peak amplitude of >75 µV. Night terrors, bed wetting, sleepwalking, and other parasomnias typically occur in stage N3.
- REM sleep accounts for 20–25% of total sleep time in most adults. Most dreaming that can be recalled after awakening occurs during REM sleep. Loss of muscle tone prevents people from physically acting out their dreams. The EEG is characterized by the background rhythm returning to what seems to be a drowsy state, with low-voltage theta and alpha frequency activity. Characteristically, the EEG reveals large amplitude eye movement artifacts. During routine EEG, REM sleep is rarely encountered, but if it occurs very rapidly ($\leq$10 min) after onset of drowsiness, the patient may have narcolepsy.

See Sect. 5.4.3 for polysomnography and other studies of sleep.

5.3 Electromyography (EMG) and Nerve Conduction Studies (NCS)

A general discussion of EMG and NCS is presented here, followed by a short overview of electrodiagnostic findings in selected neuromuscular disorders.

EMG and NCS are used:

- To localize lesions within the PNS: Is the lesion at the level of the spinal nerve root, plexus, peripheral nerve, neuromuscular junction, or muscle?
- For further differential diagnosis: Is it an axonal or a demyelinating neuropathy, a presynaptic or postsynaptic neuromuscular junction dysfunction, or an inflammatory or noninflammatory myopathic disorder?

- For assessing the severity of the disease, for monitoring therapeutic response, and for prognosis: For instance, is there sign of reinnervation after peripheral nerve trauma, is the lesion purely demyelinating, or are there secondary axonal features as well?

EMG and NCS may be regarded as extensions of the neurological bedside examination and must always be interpreted in light of the clinical data. When asking for a neurophysiological exam, make sure your questions are specific and precise; otherwise, you risk ending up with results that are difficult to interpret or even misleading.

5.3.1 EMG

EMG can distinguish neuropathic from myopathic weakness. In addition, it can differentiate between spinal root, plexus, and peripheral nerve disease by demonstrating the pattern of (clinical and subclinical) muscle involvement. EMG activity is recorded and evaluated during:

- Needle insertion.
  - Normal insertional activity in relaxed muscle is immediately followed by electrical silence.
  - Pathological insertional activity.
    Increased and prolonged insertional activity ($\geq$300–400 ms) may indicate membrane instability (usually due to neurogenic damage) but is often nonspecific.
    Decreased insertional activity may be seen, e.g., with muscle necrosis or replacement of muscle by connective tissue.
    Needle insertion may lead to myotonic or pseudomyotonic discharges. Myotonia refers to delayed muscle relaxation after contraction or needle insertion. Due to the waxing and waning amplitude of the motor units, it can be heard over the loudspeaker as the classic "dive bomber" noise. (Much of EMG pathology was described in the years following World War II.)

- Muscle relaxation.
  - Relaxed healthy muscle is electrically silent. Fasciculations are benign if weakness is absent. End-plate noise and spikes appear if the needle is close to the muscle end plate; these are normal and must not be confused with fibrillations.
  - Pathological spontaneous activity is a sign of muscle denervation and includes, e.g., fibrillations, fasciculations, and positive sharp waves.
    Fibrillations are involuntary contractions of single muscle fibers and invisible to the naked eye.
    Positive sharp waves are due to spontaneous discharges from groups of denervated muscle fibers.
    Myotonic discharges are also spontaneous potentials generated by single muscle fibers.
    Complex repetitive discharges represent the depolarization of a group of muscle fibers rather than a single fiber.
    Fasciculations. These represent involuntary firing of a single motor unit and all its muscle fibers; they are usually visible through the skin (without too much subcutaneous fat). Fasciculations are pathological if associated with weakness and atrophy.
    Similar to fasciculations, myokymic and neuromyotonic discharges are spontaneous potentials generated by motor neurons.
- Slight voluntary muscle contraction is used to analyze motor unit potentials (MUPs).
  - Neurogenic disorders are associated with MUPs of long duration and large amplitude. This is due to reinnervation of denervated muscle fibers leading to an increased number of fibers per motor unit. Neurogenic MUPs tend to be polyphasic.
  - Myopathic MUPs are normally of short duration and small amplitude due to loss of muscle fibers. They are usually polyphasic as well.

- Maximal voluntary muscle contraction is examined in order to evaluate the so-called recruitment pattern.
  - Neurogenic disorders show a dropout of motor units, which is seen on the EMG monitor as a picket fence appearance instead of a full interference pattern.
  - Myogenic disorders are associated with pathologically early recruitment of MUPs leading to a full interference pattern of low-amplitude potentials with minimal activation.

Single fiber EMG is a special examination technique used to demonstrate the phenomenon of increased "jitter," the difference in transmission of two individual muscle fibers belonging to the same motor unit. This helps to diagnose MG and is discussed below in more detail.

5.3.2 NCS

In NCS, the following electrophysiological measurements are essential:

- Motor conduction velocity (MCV). Motor NCS are performed by electrical stimulation of a peripheral nerve and recording from a muscle supplied by this nerve. MCV is assessed by stimulating the motor nerve at two or more different sites. Following this, MCV can be calculated by dividing the distance between the different stimulating electrodes with the differences in latencies. As a rule of thumb, normal MCV in the arms is ≥50 m/s and in the legs ≥40 m/s. MCV in demyelinating polyneuropathies is significantly decreased (>25% of normal), whereas in axonal polyneuropathies, MCV tends to be much less affected. This is because axonal polyneuropathies usually are associated with a large enough number of functioning axons to ensure a relatively high conduction velocity. In demyelinating neuropathies, in contrast, the myelin damage severely decreases the speed at which impulses propagate along the myelinated axon. Slowing of motor nerve conduction in the upper extremities to below 40 m/s and in the lower limbs to below 30 m/s cannot be explained by loss of fastest conducting fibers alone; thus, this is a neurophysiological sign of demyelination. Of course, in long-standing neuropathies, both secondary demyelinating and axonal changes may occur, which can obscure the electrophysiological picture.

- Distal motor latency is the time it takes for the electrical impulse to travel from the site of stimulation to the recording site (the muscle) and is measured in milliseconds.
- Compound muscle action potentials (CMAP or simply MAPs) are the muscle contraction resulting from stimulation of a motor nerve. The amplitude varies with the muscles studied but usually is ≥6 mV in the hand and ≥1 mV in the foot. The CMAP is called "compound" because both the muscle fibers and the motor nerve contribute to it; this is also why the amplitude is much larger than for sensory nerve action potentials (SNAPs) (see below). In axonal neuropathies, reduced CMAPs are due to loss of functioning motor axons in a given nerve.
- Sensory conduction velocity is comparable to MCV in the arms, but slightly slower in the legs (35 m/s). Sensory nerve conduction studies may be performed either antidromically or orthodromically. The former is generally preferred for technical reasons.
- SNAPs depend on the size of the nerve but are small (10–100 µV) compared to CMAP amplitudes. SNAPs reflect the simultaneous depolarization of all cutaneous sensory axons in a given nerve.
- Late responses. The F response and the H reflex are the two most commonly assessed late responses; they are "late" because they lag behind the CMAPs:
  - F waves. ("F" stands for foot because F waves were first recorded from intrinsic foot muscles). When stimulating a motor nerve, depolarization travels distally where it is recorded as part of the CMAP—and proximally to the anterior horn cells. Retrograde depolarization of some of these cells generates a new axon potential that

travels down the axon to the innervated muscle, where it is recorded as the F wave. F waves therefore allow evaluation of the proximal part of the motor axon. This is useful, for instance, in the assessment of proximal motor conduction failure as seen with GBS. (Normal CMAPs and absent F waves are highly suggestive of proximal demyelination and may be seen early in the course of the disorder.)
  - H reflex. ("H" stands for Johann Hoffmann, (German Neurologist, 1857–1919) who described the H reflex.) The H reflex is usually referred to as the neurophysiological equivalent of the Achilles reflex. Thus, it is a measure of the integrity of the S1 spinal stretch reflex. The tibial nerve is stimulated in the popliteal fossa, and the response is recorded from the soleus or gastrocnemius medius muscles. The absolute latency of the H reflex is increased in axonal and demyelinating polyneuropathies, and the reflex can also be absent. In the diagnosis of S1 radiculopathies, the H reflex must be performed bilaterally, and there is a greater than 1.5 ms difference from side to side. However, the clinical relevance of the H reflex is rather limited.
  - A waves are late responses only encountered in pathological conditions. They are rather nonspecific and may occur in any neuropathic process but are often seen with polyneuropathies and radiculopathies.

5.3.3 Electrodiagnostic Findings in Selected Neuromuscular Disorders

5.3.3.1 Spinal Radiculopathy

NCS and EMG can help to differentiate symptomatic radiculopathies from incidental spinal degeneration commonly found on MRI and CT of the spine. In radiculopathy, e.g., due to spinal disc herniation, the lesion is proximal to the dorsal root ganglion. This leaves the sensory nerve between the dorsal root ganglion and the innervated structure intact. Consequently, in pure nerve root lesions, *SNAPs are normal*, even when severe dermatomal sensory loss is present. In addition, nerve root compression may result in electrophysiological findings of motor axonal loss or focal demyelination. With lack of severe or multisegmental motor nerve root injury, however, motor nerve conduction studies, including F waves, are often normal.

The most sensitive electrophysiological sign of radiculopathy is when axonal denervation and reinnervation on needle EMG follow a *myotomal pattern*.[3] (Of course, the myotomal pattern may be complete or incomplete.) EMG is therefore well suited for differentiating cervical and lumbar root disease from lesions of the plexus or peripheral nerves. Additionally, most cervical radiculopathies occur above the C8–T1 myotomal level, which is the level commonly tested with routine NCS; thus, a radiculopathy at C8 or above will not reveal any abnormalities on routine NCS of the upper extremities. Abnormal spontaneous EMG activity such as fibrillations and positive sharp waves develops with a latency of 3–5 weeks following axonal injury. Reinnervation, which is marked by the development of long-duration MUP and a decrease in abnormal spontaneous activity, begins after approximately 12–16 weeks. Evaluation of *paraspinal muscles* is also important in distinguishing radiculopathy from plexopathy. This is because the dorsal branch of the spinal nerve, which innervates the paraspinal muscles, leaves the spinal nerve root proximal to the plexus. Thus, a plexus lesion is too distal to affect this nerve branch. An abnormal EMG sparing the paraspinal muscles, for instance, may point toward a lesion in the brachial plexus or the peripheral nerves, whereas with cervical radiculopathy, the

[3]For instance, a C8 nerve root lesion may lead to EMG abnormalities in the latissimus dorsi (thoracodorsal nerve), triceps, extensor digitorum communis, extensor indicis proprius (radial nerve), abductor pollicis brevis (median nerve), flexor carpi ulnaris, and flexor digitorum profundus muscles of the fourth and fifth digits (ulnar nerve), as well as in the small hand muscles (ulnar and median nerve). In contrast, an ulnar nerve lesion will leave the latissimus dorsi, triceps, extensor digitorum communis, extensor indicis proprius, and abductor pollicis brevis muscles intact.

first signs of acute denervation are in fact usually detected in the paraspinal muscles (approximately 7–10 days following the injury).

5.3.3.2 Plexus Lesions

Conventional electrodiagnostic studies can be insufficient for the evaluation of brachial plexus lesions. To improve the diagnostic yield, assessment should include the contralateral extremity, NCS of uncommonly studied nerves (e.g., medial and lateral antebrachial cutaneous nerves), and extensive needle EMG (in order to document that the *muscles involved do not follow a myotomal pattern or a peripheral nerve lesion*). Motor nerve root stimulation and SSEP (see below) can sometimes demonstrate involvement of more proximal structures as well. EMG shows denervation in the appropriate muscles. *Abnormal sensory potentials* and a *normal paraspinal muscle EMG* are characteristic for brachial plexus lesions and are precisely the opposite of what is normally found in spinal nerve root injury (see above). In plexus neuritis, there is predominant axonal involvement, as reflected by decreased amplitude of SNAPs and CMAPs. Although prognosis for plexus neuritis is usually good, persistent deficits can occur.

5.3.3.3 Axonal Polyneuropathy

Axonal neuropathies often leave the *MCV rather well preserved*. In contrast, CMAP amplitudes at both proximal and distal sites of stimulation are significantly reduced in axonal *large fiber polyneuropathies*. CMAP is a function of the motor axons of the stimulated nerve as well as of the innervated muscle from which the signal is registered. Thus, *CMAP reduction* reflects axonal loss, and the amount of the amplitude reduction from the normal or premorbid value is proportional to the amount of axonal loss. When all or most of the fastest conducting nerve fibers are affected, conduction velocity is slightly reduced but never to the extent of what is seen in demyelinating neuropathies (e.g., typically not more than 25% of the normal value). SNAPs are usually lower than normal in amplitude. The EMG shows denervation abnormalities early in axonal neuropathies but only late in demyelinating neuropathies (secondary axonal degeneration). Importantly, with *small fiber polyneuropathy*, neurophysiological findings are normal or rather uncharacteristic. Small fiber polyneuropathy is suggested clinically by a history of prominent pain and dysesthesias in the distal extremities, normal tendon reflexes, and posterior column function. Thermoregulatory sweat testing may be abnormal, and a skin biopsy may show a decreased small nerve fiber density.

5.3.3.4 Demyelinating Polyneuropathy

Nerve conduction studies in demyelinating neuropathies show moderate to *severe slowing of motor conduction*. As stated earlier, motor nerve conduction slowing in the upper extremities below 40 m/s and in the lower limbs below 30 m/s is an unequivocal sign of demyelination. CMAPs remain relatively preserved. Other signs of demyelinating neuropathy include *abnormal temporal dispersion* of the CMAP, *prolonged distal latencies*, *delayed or absent F waves* (suggesting demyelination of proximal nerve segments), and, importantly, *conduction block*. The latter is associated with a focal lesion of myelin. A conduction block is characterized by reduced proximal motor amplitude as compared to distal motor amplitude. In practice, a reduction of amplitude of $\geq 10\%$ or an increased duration of $\geq 15\%$, when occurring over short distances, is suggestive of conduction block. A block occurs in demyelinating neuropathies of various causes as well as with focal trauma or entrapment. However, conduction block and temporal dispersion are characteristic of *acquired* demyelinating polyneuropathy, and they are typically not seen in inherited neuropathies. Compared with acquired neuropathies, inherited demyelinating neuropathies such as CMT disease type 1 are usually characterized by diffuse and uniform conduction slowing. In other words, uniform slowing suggests that all myelinated fibers are affected in their entire length, in contrast to conduction blocks that occur due to patchy involvement of distinct nerve segments.

Common acquired demyelinating polyneuropathies include GBS, chronic demyelinating inflammatory polyradiculoneuropathy (CIDP),

MMN with conduction block, and polyneuropathy associated with anti-MAG IgM antibodies.

5.3.3.5 GBS (Acute Inflammatory Demyelinating Polyradiculoneuropathy, AIDP)

NCS reveal *predominant demyelinating features* such as severe slowing of proximal and distal motor conduction velocities, multifocal conduction block, and prolonged distal and F wave latencies. Slowing of motor nerve conduction and other signs of demyelination begin 3–7 days after symptom onset, and F wave slowing may be the earliest sign. In early GBS, EMG simply shows a reduction in motor unit firing, depending on the degree of paresis. After 14–21 days, spontaneous denervation activity may indicate *secondary axonal loss*. EMG is also useful for prognostic purposes since the degree of denervation is related to functional outcome and time to recovery.

5.3.3.6 CIDP

The electrophysiological findings for CIDP must meet three of the following four criteria:

- Reduced nerve conduction velocity in at least two nerves
- Partial conduction block in at least one nerve
- Prolonged distal latencies in at least two nerves
- Absent or prolonged F waves in at least two nerves

However, from a clinical point of view, CIDP is very likely when a patient has a chronic nongenetic polyneuropathy, which is progressive for at least 8 weeks and characterized by weakness in all four limbs, including proximal weakness in at least one limb, and by lack of a serum paraprotein (Koski et al. 2009).

5.3.3.7 Multifocal Motor Neuropathy with Conduction Block (MMNCB)

As the name suggests, NCS show *motor conduction blocks at multiple sites* that are *not* the usual sites of peripheral nerve entrapment (e.g., the wrist or the elbow). Other features of demyelination include prolonged F waves, slowed conduction velocities, and temporal dispersion of waveforms.

5.3.3.8 Polyneuropathy Associated with Anti-MAG IgM Antibodies

In the majority of patients with a polyneuropathy due to anti-myelin-associated glycoprotein (anti-MAG) antibodies, NCS show demyelinating features, although most will have signs of axonal degeneration as well. A characteristic electrophysiological pattern is disproportionate prolongation of distal motor latencies, indicating a length-dependent, distal demyelinating process. The so-called terminal latency index is useful to distinguish anti-MAG neuropathy from other acquired demyelinating neuropathies (Cocito et al. 2001).

5.3.3.9 MND (ALS)

Electrodiagnostic criteria (El Escorial criteria; Wilbourn 1998) for ALS include:

- Normal sensory nerve conduction studies
- Motor nerve conduction velocities being normal when recorded from unaffected muscles and ≥70% of the average normal value when recorded from severely affected muscles, reflecting axonal pathology
- Fibrillation and fasciculation potentials in muscles of the upper and lower extremities or in the muscles of the extremities and the head
- MUP reduced in number and increased in duration and amplitude

The revised El Escorial criteria for ALS require that the needle EMG examination shows active and chronic denervation in at least two out of four in the following regions: brainstem, cervical, thoracic, and lumbosacral regions.[4] However, it is not uncommon that a patient has clinically obvious ALS and does not (yet) meet the El Escorial criteria.

---

[4]Needle examination of the sternocleidomastoid muscles carries a sensitivity similar to examination of the tongue in patients with bulbar symptoms and may be better tolerated by the patient.

5.3.3.10 MG

Two major electrodiagnostic tests are available to evaluate the neuromuscular junction. *Repetitive nerve stimulation* involves repeated supramaximal stimulation of a peripheral nerve usually at a slow frequency of 2 or 3 Hz while recording the CMAPs from the appropriate muscle. Trains of 10 CMAPS are recorded. The first CMAP is compared to one of the later CMAPs to assess for decrease (decrement) or increase (increment) in size within each train. Myasthenic patients typically demonstrate *decrements* of more than 10–15%.

The second, more sophisticated test of neuromuscular junction function is *single fiber EMG*. A special EMG needle allows recording of single muscle fiber discharges. The variability in the time required for signal transmission across an individual neuromuscular junction can be measured by assessing the firing interval of single muscle fibers. This is known as *jitter*, which is considerably increased in MG and associated with intermittent blocking of neuromuscular transmission. Single fiber EMG is more sensitive than repetitive nerve stimulation in cases of mild generalized, ocular, or seronegative MG. Since jitter can also be increased in other neuromuscular diseases, the specificity of this technique is limited, however.

It should be noted that confirmation by electrophysiology is not necessary in patients with a typical clinical presentation of MG and a positive AChR antibody titer. Assessment with repetitive nerve stimulation and single fiber EMG can be reserved for patients with unusual phenotypes or lack of specific antibodies.

5.3.3.11 Lambert-Eaton Myasthenic Syndrome (LEMS)

Repetitive nerve stimulation (at much higher frequencies than what is used for evaluation of suspected MG) leads to an *increment* of greater than 100% in CMAPs. The incremental response in LEMS reflects postexercise facilitation. (At the bedside, a similar phenomenon can be observed during testing of the tendon reflexes; the reflexes become more active with each blow of the reflex hammer.) Electrophysiological tests cannot distinguish between paraneoplastic and nonparaneoplastic LEMS.

5.3.3.12 Inflammatory Myositis (Polymyositis, IBM)

EMG is more important to excluding neurogenic conditions than to confirming the diagnosis of inclusion-body myositis. (Muscle biopsy is the gold standard.) Inclusion-body myositis may be misdiagnosed as ALS because of normal sensation and asymmetric muscle weakness with atrophy. However, the pattern of muscle atrophy and weakness is very characteristic and involves the finger flexors and quadriceps muscles; dysphagia is also common and typically precedes dysarthria. The presence of myopathic potentials, especially if found in distal muscles such as the finger flexors, is suggestive of IBM. Although MUPs are usually myopathic, characterized by brief duration and small amplitude, neurogenic MUPs of long duration and increased amplitude are interspersed with myopathic MUPs in some patients. This pattern is also seen in patients with long-standing polymyositis. The inflammation may also cause neurogenic damage, thus leading to neuropathic MUPs. Increased spontaneous activity, characterized by positive sharp waves and fibrillation potentials, is present in both patients with IBM and polymyositis. Nerve conduction studies are normal. Reduction of spontaneous activity during serial EMG studies is considered a marker of treatment response in polymyositis.

5.3.3.13 Noninflammatory Myopathies

EMG findings in noninflammatory myopathies are variable. Fibrillations, positive sharp waves, and myotonic discharges are often encountered, although insertional activity can be normal and abnormal spontaneous activity absent. Myopathic motor units are recorded with voluntary contraction, especially with marked weakness.

5.4 Other Neuroelectrophysiological Investigations

5.4.1 Evoked Potentials

Evoked potentials are electrical potentials recorded from the CNS following the presentation of a stimulus. This is in contrast to spontaneous potentials as detected by EEG. In other words, evoked potentials record the time for a visual, auditory, or sensory stimulus to reach the cerebral cortex or, in case of motor evoked potentials (MEP), the time from stimulation of the motor pathways to a peripheral motor response.

Four kinds of evoked potentials are used routinely in clinical neurology:

- Visual evoked potentials (VEP) are caused by stimulation of a subject's visual field using a repetitive pattern stimulus such as a flickering checkerboard on a video screen. Of primary interest is the latency of a positive wave, the so-called P100, recorded at an occipital EEG electrode. VEP are mainly used to confirm previous optic neuritis in patients suspected of having MS. Ninety percent of patients with a history of definite optic neuritis have a unilaterally delayed P100. VEP can also be used for legal purposes in feigned blindness.
- Brainstem auditory evoked potentials (BAEP) can be used to trace the signal generated by a sound, from the cochlear nerve (wave I), through the cochlear nuclei (wave II), the superior olivary complex (wave III), the lateral lemniscus (wave IV), and inferior colliculus (wave V), to the medial geniculate nucleus (wave VI) and to the primary auditory cortex (wave VII). BAEP are useful to evaluate the integrity of the auditory pathways, especially in neonates and other patients who cannot cooperate with standard audiological testing. BAEP is also used to monitor brainstem function during posterior fossa surgery, thereby helping the surgeon to avoid damage to the nervous tissue.
- Somatosensory evoked potentials (SSEP) are recorded from the somatosensory cortex after electrical stimulation of peripheral nerves, most commonly the posterior tibial, median, and ulnar nerves. SSEP are useful in order to verify the organic nature of sensory complaints and to assess whether these have a central or peripheral origin. Similar to BAEP, SSEP can be used in neuromonitoring to help assess the function of the spinal cord during surgery. Increased latencies or decreased

amplitudes of the SSEP are indicators of neurological dysfunction. The so-called N20 refers to a negative peak at 20 ms recorded from the cortex when the median nerve is stimulated. Bilateral absence of the N20 in comatose patients following cardiac arrest is consistent with a dismal prognosis.

- Transcranial magnetic stimulation (TMS) involves stimulating the motor cortex or the spinal cord by applying a strong magnetic pulse and recording motor evoked potentials (MEP) in the activated muscles. This technique is used to examine the integrity of the motor pathways. Central motor conduction is the difference in MEP latencies with stimulation of the motor cortex and the spinal cord. A long central motor conduction implies dysfunction of the first motor neuron. This piece of information is important, for instance, in a patient who initially presents with widespread but isolated LMN dysfunction. It may suggest a diagnosis of ALS, if clinical UMN signs are still lacking.

5.4.2 Evaluation of the Autonomic Nervous System

Several tests are available that examine the function of the sympathetic and the parasympathetic systems, including Valsalva maneuver testing, heart rate recording, RR interval evaluation, tilt-table testing, microneurography, and thermoregulatory sweat testing. Detection of autonomic dysfunction is important in orthostatic hypotension, autonomic neuropathies, multiple system atrophy, and other parkinsonian syndromes, to name just a few examples. A skin biopsy can be useful in patients with symptoms suggestive of small fiber polyneuropathy.

5.4.3 Polysomnography and Other Studies of Sleep

Polysomnography is performed in a variety of sleep disorders, including obstructive sleep apnea, REM sleep behavior disorders, and periodic movements in sleep. It includes a limited EEG to measure sleep stages; assessment of respiratory parameters including oxygenation, chest excursion, and limb movements; a limited EMG (to assess muscle tone in REM and non-REM sleep stages); and an electrocardiogram.

The multiple sleep latency test (MLST) and maintenance of wakefulness tests are helpful in the evaluation of narcolepsy and other hypersomnias. MLST consists of four or five 20-min nap opportunities scheduled about 2 h apart. The test is often performed following an overnight polysomnography. Three or more sleep-onset REM periods combined with a mean sleep latency of less than 5 min is a finding that has high specificity and positive predictive value for narcolepsy. Nowadays, a clinical diagnosis of narcolepsy with cataplexy can also be confirmed by low CSF levels of hypocretin (also known as orexin).

5.5 Ultrasound of the Cerebral Vessels and the Heart

Extracranial and intracranial vessels can be examined noninvasively using ultrasound techniques, called Doppler ultrasonography and duplex ultrasonography. Doppler ultrasonography is based on a phenomenon described in 1843, by Christian Doppler, an Austrian mathematician and physicist.

The registered ultrasound frequency increases if the source (the erythrocytes reflecting the ultrasound waves) is moving toward the detector and decreases if the source is moving away from the detector. The Doppler signal can be converted to an audio signal or presented visually as a frequency-time spectrum. The most relevant parameter for the detection of stenosis is the maximal CBF velocity during systole and diastole. If the flow volume is constant, the speed of flow across a stenosis increases as the inverse square of the vascular diameter. Thus, the higher the grade of the stenosis, the greater is the flow velocity. The so-called B image ("B" stands for brightness) yields morphological information, thereby enabling the ultrasonographer to differentiate echo-dense tissues and to detect calcified atherosclerotic plaques. Duplex ultrasonography is the combination of B image with Doppler sonography, which offers both morphological and hemodynamic information. Color duplex ultrasonography involves the color-coded representation of flow velocity and direction superimposed on the B image. The color blue is used to represent blood moving away from the detector; red denotes blood moving toward the detector. The brighter the color, the greater the speed of flow.

The most common applications of Doppler and duplex ultrasound in neurology are:

- To look for moderate and high-grade stenosis of the ipsilateral carotid artery in anterior circulation cerebral infarction. Carotid stenosis is usually defined as moderate if the vessel lumen is decreased by 30–70% and as high grade if decreased by ≥70%. Every patient with an anterior circulation infarction who is potentially eligible for CEA should be screened for high-grade stenosis of the relevant carotid artery as soon as possible by Doppler sonography (or CT/MR angiography).[5] The sooner CEA is performed, the greater the likelihood to prevent a new stroke.
- To detect and monitor vasospasms of intracranial vessels following subarachnoidal hemorrhage using repeated intracranial ultrasound examinations. The ACA, MCA, and PCA can be evaluated through the temporal bone window; the intracranial segment of the vertebral artery and the basilar artery through the foramen magnum; and the ophthalmic artery through the orbital window.

Ultrasound of the heart can be performed as transthoracic echocardiography (TTE) and transesophageal echocardiography (TEE). Although the latter is minimally invasive, it is the preferred method to assess for possible emboli in the heart and aortic arch. Cardiac conditions with high risk of cerebral embolization include:

- Atrial fibrillation
- Mitral stenosis
- Left ventricular thrombus
- Infectious endocarditis
- Dilated cardiomyopathy
- Atrial myxoma
- Prosthetic heart valves
- Acute myocardial infarction
- Aneurysms of the atrial septum

The intravenous administration of ultrasonographic contrast medium is used to detect right-left shunts, such as a patent foramen ovale. The latter, especially when combined with a pseudoaneurysm of the atrial wall, may be a source for paradoxical emboli. (The embolus is paradoxical because it originates from the venous system and reaches the brain directly, bypassing the lungs).

5.6   Lumbar Puncture

Blood (150 mL), brain tissue (1400 mL), and CSF (150 mL) constitute the three components of the intracranial cavity. CSF is produced with a rate of 20 mL/h (=480 mL/24 h), which means that the CSF volume is replaced roughly three times per day.

Normal CSF is clear, colorless, and sterile. Normal values are as follows: protein 0.20–0.4 g/L (albumin <270 mg/L at age 30; <360 mg/L at age 65), glucose 50–75% of blood glucose, lactate 1.2–2.1 mmol/L, and cell count <5/mm^3 (mononuclear lymphocytes).

Physiological CSF pressure is 6–20-cm H_2O. When measuring CSF pressure during a spinal tap, make sure the patient is extending the legs as much as needed in order to decrease abdominal pressure and avoid compression of the jugular veins; otherwise, CSF pressure will be falsely increased. If there is free CSF flow through the ventricles and the subarachnoidal space and the patient is in the recumbent position, lumbar CSF pressure roughly reflects ICP.

Bloody CSF due to a traumatic tap clears in later tubes. The ratio of leukocytes/erythrocytes is the same as in the peripheral blood: 1/1000. (Thus, for every 1000 erythrocytes,

---

[5] In contrast to Doppler sonography, CT/MR angiography is more time-consuming but allows complete imaging of the intracranial and neck vessels, including the aortic arch, which is why CT/MR angiography can also detect carotid artery stenosis distally and proximally from the carotid artery bifurcation.

one more leukocyte may be present. In contrast, a significantly increased ratio suggests CSF pleocytosis.)

The albumin quote (CSF-albumin (mg/L)/S-albumin (g/L); normal ≤7–10) is a sensitive parameter for the integrity of the blood–brain barrier and varies with the patient's age and the laboratory.

The neurologist only rarely encounters patients with a polymorph CSF pleocytosis, since this is usually secondary to acute bacterial meningitis and thus the domain of the infectious disease specialist. Most neurological patients with a CSF inflammation will have a lymphocytic CSF pleocytosis. Noninfectious causes of a lymphocytic CSF pleocytosis include autoimmune inflammatory (e.g., MS, autoimmune encephalitis) and malignant conditions (e.g., meningeal carcinomatosis, CNS lymphoma). Infectious causes may be viral (e.g., enterovirus, herpes simplex I and II, HIV), bacterial (tuberculosis, neuroborreliosis, neurosyphilis, leptospirosis, listeriosis), fungal (cryptococcosis), and parasitic (toxoplasmosis).

- Bacterial meningitis is associated with increased ICP, polymorph pleocytosis (typically >> 1000 cells/mm^3; polymorphs >80%; but mononuclear predominance can be seen early in the disease), decreased glucose (<40% of blood glucose), increased protein (0.9–5 g/L), and increased lactate (>3 mmol/L). In meningitis due to *Listeria* and tuberculosis, polymorphs make up less than 50% of the white cell count. At very early stages, CSF abnormalities may be rather mild; if this is the case, another lumbar puncture is mandatory. As with other infective agents (virus, fungi), identification of the responsible pathogen is possible with direct microscopy, PCR, antibody analysis, or culture.
- Spirochetes diseases (neuroborreliosis, neurosyphilis) are characterized by CSF lymphocytosis and mild to moderate protein increase.
- In viral meningitis, there is normal or increased ICP, pleocytosis with mononuclear excess

(5–1000 cells/mm^3; polymorphs <50%; polymorph predominance possible in the first 48 h), normal glucose, and slightly increased protein (>0.4–0.9 g/L). At very early stages, CSF findings may be rather mild; consider a new lumbar puncture.
- Typical findings in fungal meningitis include normal or increased ICP, pleocytosis with 20–500 cells/mm^3 (polymorphs <50%), slight decrease of glucose (<75% of blood glucose), and increased protein (>0.4–5 g/L).
- Slow virus infections (e.g., JC virus leading to PML) and prion diseases (e.g., CJD) are typically associated with a normal CSF cell count and protein. CSF findings in CJD include increased 14-3-3 protein levels (although this has a rather low specificity and sensitivity) and a high total tau/phosphorylated tau protein ratio.
- If meningeal carcinomatosis or lymphomatosis are suspected, a large amount of CSF (2–10 mL) should be sent for cytology and flow cytometry; if negative, the tap should be repeated.
- GBS is associated with so-called albuminocytological dissociation. Increased protein (up to several g/L) occurs without pleocytosis or together with a minor increase of the cell count. High cell counts (≥50 cells/mm^3) should stimulate a search for an alternative diagnosis. During the first week of GBS, protein levels can be normal. If this is the case, another spinal tap should be performed during the second week in order to confirm the increase of protein content, consistent with an inflammatory polyradiculopathy.
- The great majority of patients with MS have increased IgG index and oligoclonal bands, which are signs of intrathecal immunoglobulin production. A mild pleocytosis is frequent, but more than 50 cells are considered a red flag.
- Neurodegenerative diseases are associated with markers of brain tissue damage and accumulation of pathological substrates. AD is associated with increased tau protein (both total tau and phosphorylated tau protein) and

low beta-amyloid.[6] Assessment of CSF biomarkers for AD is recommended in patients with cognitive impairment and diagnostic uncertainty (Simonsen et al. 2017; Herukka et al. 2017). Increased neurofilament (NFL) light protein is a useful diagnostic clue in ALS and atypical parkinsonism (in contrast, PD is associated with normal NFL levels).[7]

- Autoimmune encephalitis is associated with mild inflammatory CSF changes. An important exception is NMDA receptor encephalitis which frequently leads to a high CSF cell count, e.g., >200 cells/mm^3. As a rule of thumb, onconeural antibodies (e.g., anti-Ri, anti-Yo, anti-Ma2) occur in paraneoplastic conditions and bind to intracellular antigens, whereas surface antibodies (e.g., anti-NMDA receptor, anti-LGI1) bind to synaptic receptors and are only infrequently associated with malignancy (except for ovarial teratoma in women with NMDA receptor encephalitis). When autoimmune encephalitis is suspected, antibodies titers should always be measured in both plasma and CSF.

For post-lumbar puncture headache, see Chap. 3.

5.7 Neurogenetics

5.7.1 Basic Neurogenetics

The human genome comprises roughly 21,000 protein-coding genes encoded in the nuclear DNA. Of note, mitochondria have their own DNA. Hereditary neurological diseases are numerous, and the list of associated gene mutations is constantly increasing. There are excellent online databases available that provide comprehensive and up-to-date information of the human genetic disorders, e.g., Online Mendelian Inheritance in Man (OMIM). It is important to note that many features may obscure the inheritance pattern in a given pedigree; these include genetic mechanisms such as decreased penetrance, de novo mutations, and variable expression, as well as mechanisms unrelated to genetics (e.g., the lack of a reliable family history in a patient who was adopted as a child or whose biological father is different from the assumed).

The following section discusses inheritance patterns in nuclear gene disorders, mitochondrial disorders, and chromosomal syndromes.

Nuclear gene disorders are inherited according to Mendelian patterns:

- *Autosomal dominant disorders* affect both males and females and are typically inherited in a vertical fashion, i.e., they affect successive generations. The hallmark is male-to-male inheritance (thereby excluding X-linked transmission). Patients with an autosomal dominant condition are heterozygous. Therefore, their children have a 50% risk of inheriting the disease.
- In contrast, *autosomal recessive disorders* are typically transmitted in a horizontal fashion, i.e., they affect the children of clinically unaffected carrier patients. Consanguineous marriages increase the risk for autosomal recessive disease in the offspring. Males and females are equally likely to be affected. The risk for each child of carrier parents to receive both mutant alleles and become affected is 25%.
- The inheritance pattern for *X-linked disorders* is vertical, affecting multiple generations, but there is no male-to-male transmission (in contrast to autosomal dominant disease). X-linked disorders can have dominant or recessive inheritance patterns. If heterozygous females are consistently affected (a prime example being Rett syndrome), the pattern is X-linked dominant. If heterozygous females are unaffected or affected to a much slighter degree

---

[6]Tau proteins are abundant in the CNS and essential for stabilizations of microtubules in neurons. High total tau levels can be used as a marker of cortical axonal degeneration. Phosphorylation of tau is believed to be specific for AD and related tauopathies. Beta-amyloid is the main constituent of amyloid plaques in the brains of patients with AD. Since amyloid accumulates within the neurons and cerebral vessel, its amount in CSF is decreased in AD.

[7]Similar to tau protein, NFL light protein is an important component of neuronal axons. The CSF level of NFL light protein increases in disorders with neuronal damage and axonal degeneration and correlates with the amount of damage.

than males, the condition is X-linked recessive. Examples for the latter include Fabry disease and adrenoleukodystrophy: Whereas males tend to be severely affected early in life, females show no or only mild symptoms during adulthood. The risk for each child to inherit the mutation from a heterozygous mother is 50%. The risk for a daughter to inherit the mutation from an affected father is 100%; in contrast, the risk for a son is zero (because he receives the X chromosome from his unaffected mother).

Some hereditary neurodegenerative disorders are characterized by expansions of unstable nucleotide repeat sequences beyond their normal size, the so-called *DNA repeat disorders*. The repeating unit within the affected gene consists of three or more nucleotides. (Abnormal trinucleotide repeats are most common, e.g., CAG in HD, GAA in Friedreich's ataxia, and CAG in DRPLA.) Unstable DNA repeat disorders can be inherited in a dominant (e.g., HD, myotonic dystrophy type 1 and type 2), recessive (Friedreich's ataxia), or X-linked fashion (Kennedy's disease, fragile X syndrome). In many of these disorders, repeat size can increase with subsequent generations and may be associated with earlier and more severe manifestation of the disease, a phenomenon called *anticipation*. People are termed *premutation carriers*, if they have alleles with abnormal repeat numbers that are too low to cause the disease but that are unstable and may expand into the disease-causing range in the following generations. Importantly, however, some premutation carriers may nevertheless develop symptoms later in life, e.g., premutations related to the fragile X gene may lead to fragile X-associated tremor/ataxia syndrome (FXTAS). A typical patient with FXTAS would be a male above the age of 50 years with a history of cognitive deficits, intention tremor, gait ataxia, and a characteristic leukoencephalopathy on MRI (including the middle cerebellar peduncles) with a premutation repeat size in the order of <200 CGG repeats. This is quite different from the full-mutation disease-causing range of >200 repeats, leading to the classic fragile X syndrome, the most common inherited cause of intellectual disability and autism in boys, characterized by an elongated face, autistic behavior, and post-pubertal macro-orchidism. DNA repeat disorders include:

- Myotonic dystrophy type 1 (CTG; dystrophia myotonica-protein kinase gene (*DMPK*))
- Myotonic dystrophy type 2 (CCTG; CCHC-type zinc finger nucleic acid binding protein gene (*CNBP*))
- HD (CAG; huntingtin gene (*HTT*))
- Friedreich's ataxia (GAA; frataxin gene (*FXN*))
- Kennedy's disease/X-linked spinobulbar muscular atrophy (CAG; androgen receptor gene (*AR*))
- Fragile X syndrome (CGG; fragile X mental retardation gene 1 (*FMR1*))
- Spinocerebellar ataxias (e.g., ataxin 1 gene in spinocerebellar ataxia type 1 (*SCA1*))
- DRLPA (CAG; atrophin-1 protein (*ATN1*))
- Subtypes of ALS, FTD, or ALS/FTD (GGGGCC; C9orf72-gene (*C9orf72*))

Another important concept in Mendelian disorders (and chromosal abnormalities) is genomic imprinting. This process leads to silencing of the expression of a gene by alterations in chromatin. As a consequence, only the maternal or paternal copy of the gene is expressed.

Mitochondrial disorders differ from nuclear gene disorders because the mitochondrial DNA has unique characteristics. Since all mitochondria in the zygote are derived from the ovum, mitochondrial disorders are transmitted by the mother. Besides maternal inheritance, several features determine the degree of symptoms and the range of organ involvement, e.g., homoplasmy (which refers to the presence of all wild-type or all mutant mitochondrial DNA in a given person), as well as heteroplasmy and mitotic segregation (which both can alter the amount of mutant mitochondrial DNA, thereby leading to threshold effects). Chapter 4 discusses the common mitochondrial disorders.

Chromosomal syndromes are neurodevelopmental disorders due to structural, functional, or numerical abnormalities of chromosomes. Many of these disorders belong to the domain of pediatricians and are rarely encountered by the general neurologist (with the possible exception of Down syndrome). For instance, numerary chromosomal abnormalities include Down syndrome (resulting from three copies of the chromosome 21 or chromosomal rearrangements) and Klinefelter syndrome (47, XXY karyotype); microdeletion syndromes comprise DiGeorge syndrome (chromosome 22q11.2) and Williams syndrome (chromosome 7q11.23); genomic imprinting disorders encompass Prader-Willi syndrome (due to loss of the normally expressed paternal copy of the imprinted 15.q11.2 chromosome) and Angelman syndrome (due to loss of the maternal copy of the same chromosome region).

5.7.2 Genetic Testing

Accurate genetic diagnosis improves health outcome, even if the underlying disorder is not curable. Results may lead to initiation or change of disease modifying and/or symptomatic treatment. In addition, a genetic diagnosis has implications for reproductive counseling and family planning, and it may lead to identification of systemic involvement and comorbidities which need close surveillance (e.g., the possibility of a cardiomyopathy and cardiac conduction defects in a patient with myotonic dystrophy). Finally, an accurate genetic diagnosis helps with prognostication and may facilitate participation in clinical trials. However, a genetic diagnosis in late onset neurological conditions without cure is also associated with challenging ethical concerns.

Genetic testing may be done with the aim to establish or confirm a diagnosis in a patient with neurological symptoms (diagnostic testing) or in healthy family members of patients with a known familial disorder (presymptomatic testing). In both cases genetic testing should be preceded by genetic counseling and informed consent.

Careful guidance and information provided to the patient is of utmost importance in order to enable the patient to understand the impact of genetic testing on his life, including on the lives of the entire family. As a rule, presymptomatic genetic testing should follow the guidance from the International Huntington's Association (IHA 1994) and should not be performed in individuals below 18 years of age or unable to give informed consent.

The following methods for genetic diagnostic testing are currently available:

- Single-gene sequencing (Sanger sequencing). This is still the most common form of genetic testing in the clinical setting. The clinician orders testing according to a single differential diagnosis based on the clinical history and examination, e.g., testing for a *NOTCH 3* mutation in a young stroke patient with migraine-like headache and a family history of early-onset dementia, suggesting CADASIL.
- Multigene sequencing (panel testing, typically by next generation sequencing (NGS)). Genetic panels of variable sizes are available for testing multiple genes. This is usually performed when the clinical phenotype may be due to several different mutations, e.g., a patient with a CMT phenotype may be evaluated simultaneously for mutations in numerous genes.
- Chromosomal microarray analysis. This is an array-based form of comparative genomic hybridization (CGH array), enabling detection of clinically significant structural changes such as deletions or duplications in the genome (copy number variations). It may be particularly helpful in patients with unexplained developmental anomalies, including intellectual deficits. However, chromosomal microarray analysis cannot detect sequence variations.
- Multiplex ligation-dependent probe amplification (MLPA) is used to detect smaller deletions such as exon deletions/duplications.
- Clinical exome sequencing (CES). Clinical neurogenetics is likely to change dramatically in the near future due to the introduction of CES. Contrary to conventional methods, this state-of-the-art molecular diagnostic method is based on a massive parallel

analyzing strategy enabling rapid-scale sequencing of DNA at very much reduced costs. Indeed, the entire exome (i.e., the roughly 2% of the human genome representing the protein-coding regions) can now be sequenced, thereby significantly improving the diagnosis rate for suspected neurogenetic disorders. In the hands of experts, CES is particularly interesting in clinically heterogeneous phenotypes in both adults and children. However, prior to testing, expert evaluation with detailed clinical and family histories, as well as comprehensive neurological examination, including reasonable exclusion of common nongenetic differential diagnoses, is crucial to avoid diagnostic confusion because benign variants and polymorphisms, as well as incidental or secondary findings, are common. CES may have serious ethical implications, e.g., when incidentally finding a predisposition to cancer.

5.8 Other Tests

5.8.1 Blood and Urine Chemistry

The usual blood tests ordered for general medical conditions also provide important information in neurology. In addition, there are various other blood tests that are essential in specific neurological diseases, too many to include them all here. A few examples include serum copper and ceruloplasmin (as well as urinary copper levels) in Wilson's disease and copper deficiency myeloneuropathy, long-chain fatty acids in adrenoleukodystrophy, arylsulfatase A in metachromatic leukodystrophy, phytanic acid in Refsum disease, urinary and blood porphyrins in the porphyrias, and enzyme activity rates in hereditary metabolic diseases.

Autoantibodies relevant to clinical neurology are being detected at a breathtaking rate; some of the well known include:

- Anti-AChR and anti-MuSk in MG
- Anti-VGCC in LEMS
- Anti-GQ1b in Miller-Fisher syndrome
- Anti-endomysial and anti-gliadin encountered in neurological manifestations of celiac disease
- Anti-Ri, anti-Yo, anti-Hi, anti-Ma2, anti-amphiphysin, and various other onconeural antibodies occurring in paraneoplastic conditions (see Chap. 4)
- Anti-GAD65, anti-amphiphysin, anti-dipeptidyl-peptidase-like protein-6 (DPPX), anti-GABAa, anti-glycine receptor, and anti-glycine transporter 2 in stiff person syndrome
- Anti-aquaporin 4 in NMO and NMO spectrum disorders
- Anti-MOG in ADEM, relapsing and bilateral optic neuritis, and transverse myelitis
- Anti-NMDA receptor, anti-LGI1, anti-CASPR2, anti-AMPA receptor, anti-GABAb receptor, and many other antibodies in autoimmune encephalitis (as discussed in Chap. 4)
- Thyroid antibodies (anti-thyroglobulin, anti-TPO) in steroid-responsive encephalopathy associated with autoimmune thyroiditis (Hashimoto encephalopathy)

5.8.2 Tissue Biopsies

Whenever reasonable and safe, a biopsy can be obtained from the CNS and PNS and from non-nervous tissues (e.g., mediastinal lymph node biopsy in sarcoidosis, subcutaneous fat biopsy in amyloidosis) (Case 5.7). This adds the certainty of histopathology to the clinical study, and often a brain biopsy is the only way to establish the diagnosis (e.g., CNS lymphoma, high-grade astrocytoma) and guide therapy (e.g., radiation, chemotherapy). The threshold to perform a CNS biopsy varies considerably from hospital to hospital and from physician to physician, but in experienced hands, the complication rate is low (≈1% severe bleeding rate in stereotactic brain biopsy).

Brain biopsy may also be useful in rare and atypical cases of (rapidly) progressive dementia when a treatable condition cannot be excluded by other means. In a series of 90 biopsies performed in a tertiary referral center in London, UK, 57% were diagnostic (AD (18%), CJD (12%), and inflammatory disorders (9%)). Other diagnoses

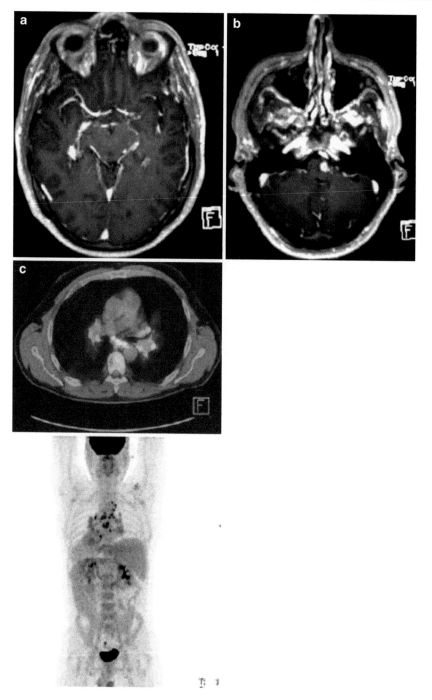

Case 5.7 Neurosarcoidosis. A 47-year-old male had a seizure with a rising epigastric sensation followed by oral automatisms and generalized tonic-clonic convulsions. Neurological examination a few hours later revealed slight dysarthria as well as hyperreflexia and a Babinski sign on the left side. Consistent with the clinical presentation, gadolinium-enhanced MRI showed lesions in the right mesial temporal lobe and the left side of the lower medulla oblongata (**a**, **b**). Hypermetabolic and enlarged bihilar lymph nodes were seen on a whole-body PET/CT (**c**). A mediastinal lymph node biopsy demonstrated non-caseating granulomas. A diagnosis of neurosarcoidosis was made. High-dose IV steroids were given, followed by oral prednisone and azathioprine. The patient made a complete recovery and follow-up MRI was normal. (PET images courtesy of Ian Law, Department of Clinical Physiology and Nuclear Medicine, Rigshospitalet, Copenhagen)

in individual patients included Pick's disease, CBD and other tauopathies, DLB, MS, Whipple's disease, PML, CADASIL, vasculopathies, and paraneoplastic encephalopathy. A raised CSF cell count was the only robust predictor of a potentially treatable (inflammatory) process at biopsy (Warren et al. 2005).

5.8.3 Formal Neuropsychological Examination

Patients in whom the bedside examination of cognitive functions is not sufficient may be referred to a formal neuropsychological examination. The role of the neuropsychologist is to examine and quantify the degree of cognitive impairment in each of several cognitive domains and to interpret the cognitive profile of the patient in relation to the (estimated) previous level of intellectual function. A formal neuropsychological examination may be useful for planning rehabilitation as well as for diagnostic decisions. Whenever ordering a neuropsychological test, make sure to ask a specific question. The importance of the cultural and educational background of the patient for interpretation of the test results cannot be overemphasized. Thus, the neuropsychological assessment usually starts with an estimation of the premorbid intelligence based on information on educational attainment and a test, such as the National Adult Reading Test (Nelson and Willison 1991). The neuropsychologist will then examine the current intelligence and a range of domain-specific tests in order to map the pattern of cognitive deficits. For each test, the neuropsychologist will compare with well-validated age-related national norms. For patients with severe cognitive impairment and those with current and ongoing drug or alcohol abuse, there is no (or little) added value of a formal neuropsychological examination. As is true for the clinical neurological examination performed by a neurologist, the experience and competence of the neuropsychologist and the cooperation of the patient influence the test results.

References and Suggested Reading

Albert MS, et al. The diagnosis of mild cognitive impairment due to Alzheimer's disease: recommendations from the National Institute on Aging-Alzheimer's association workgroups on diagnostic guidelines for Alzheimer's disease. Alzheimers Dement. 2011;7: 270–9.

McKhann GM, Knopman DS, Chertkow H, et al. The diagnosis of dementia due to Alzheimer's disease: recommendations from the National Institute on Aging-Alzheimer's Association workgroups on diagnostic guidelines for Alzheimer's disease. Alzheimers Dement. 2011;7:263–9.

Aminoff MJ. Aminoff's electrodiagnosis in clinical neurology. 6th ed. London: Saunders; 2012.

Bennett CM, Baird AA, Miller MB, Wolford GL. Neural correlates of interspecies perspective taking in the post-mortem atlantic salmon: an argument for proper multiple comparisons correction. In: 15th annual meeting of the Organization for Human Brain Mapping, San Francisco, 2009.

Cocito D, Isoardo G, Ciaramitaro P, et al. Terminal latency index in polyneuropathy with IgM paraproteinemia and anti-MAG antibody. Muscle Nerve. 2001;24:1278–82.

Douglass CP, Kandler RH, Shaw PJ, McDermott CJ. An evaluation of neurophysiological criteria used in the diagnosis of motor neuron disease. J Neurol Neurosurg Psychiatry. 2010;81:646–9.

Ebersole JS, Husain AM, Nordil Jr DR. Current practice of current electroencephalography. 4th ed. Alphen aan den Rijn, NL: Wolters Kluwer; 2014.

Fisch B. Fisch and Spehlmann's EEG primer: basic principles of digital and analog EEG. 3rd ed. Amsterdam: Elsevier; 1999.

Fogel BL, Satya-Murti S, Cohen BC. Clinical exome sequencing in neurologic disease. Neurol Clin Pract. 2016;6:164–76.

Gaspard N. ACNS critical care EEG terminology: value, limitations, and perspectives. J Clin Neurophysiol. 2015;32:452–5.

Herukka SK, Simonsen AH, Andreasen N, et al. Recommendations for CSF AD biomarkers in the diagnostic evaluation of MCI. Alzheimers Dement. 2017;13(3):285–295.

Hirsch L, Brenner R. Atlas of EEG in critical care. 1st ed. New Jersey, NJ: Wiley; 2010.

International Huntington Association (IHA) and the World Federation of Neurology (WFN) Research Group on Huntington's Chorea. Guidelines for the molecular genetics predictive test in Huntington's disease. Neurology. 1994;44:1533–6.

Kondziella D. The top 5 neurotransmitters from a clinical neurologist's perspective. Neurochem Res. 2016. In press.

Kondziella D, Friberg CK, Wellwood I, et al. Continuous EEG monitoring in subarachnoid hemorrhage: a systematic review. Neurocrit Care. 2015;22:450–61.

Koski CL, Baumgarten M, Magder LS, et al. Derivation and validation of diagnostic criteria for chronic inflammatory demyelinating polyneuropathy. J Neurol Sci. 2009;277:1–8.

LaRoche SM, editor. Handbook of ICU EEG monitoring. 1st ed. New York, NY: Demos Medical; 2012.

Nelson HE, Willison J, editors. National adult reading test. 2nd ed. NFER-Nelson; UK: Windsor; 1991.

Rumboldt Z, Castillo M, Huanq B, Rossi A. Brain imaging with MRI and CT: an image pattern approach. 1st ed. Cambridge: Cambridge University Press; 2012.

Simonsen AH, Herukka SK, Andreasen N, et al. Recommendations for CSF AD biomarkers in the diagnostic evaluation of dementia. Alzheimers Dement. 2017;13(3):274–284.

Sorbi S, Hort J, Erkinjuntti T, et al. Electromyography and neuromuscular disorders: clinical-electrophysiologic correlations. 2nd ed. Oxford: Butterworth-Heinemann; 2005.

Valdueza JM, Schreiber SJ, Roehl JE, Klinebiel R. Neurosonology and neuroimaging of stroke. 1st ed. Stuttgart: Thieme; 2008.

Warren JD, Schott JM, Fox NC, et al. Brain biopsy in dementia. Brain. 2005;128:2016–25.

Wilbourn AJ. Clinical neurophysiology in the diagnosis of amyotrophic lateral sclerosis: the Lambert and the El Escorial criteria. J Neurol Sci. 1998;160:S25–9.

Treatment of Neurological Disorders

6

Abstract

Not long ago, neurologists had hardly anything else to offer patients than a diagnosis and words of comfort. Indeed, the discrepancy between the elegance and precision of the clinical neurological diagnosis on one hand and the heartbreaking lack of any substantial therapeutic opportunities on the other was painfully clear to everyone. Fortunately, this situation has completely changed. Advances in our understanding of neurological disease due to modern neuroimaging, molecular neuroscience, and genetic testing, as well as more rigorous standards for the conduction of clinical trials, have translated into striking new therapeutic options. Apart from an ever-increasing drug arsenal, these include surgical therapies (e.g., deep brain stimulation for Parkinson's disease and hemicraniectomy for middle cerebral artery stroke), intravenous thrombolysis and mechanical thrombectomy for ischemic stroke, and a variety of immunomodulatory biological agents. Although many neurological diseases remain incurable, nowadays practically no disorder is untreatable. This chapter provides an overview of available medical and selected nonmedical treatment options in neurological diseases. Due to space limitations, the information is restricted to indications and, where feasible, suggestions for drug dosages. The treatment of cerebrovascular disorders and epilepsy, however, is covered in greater detail since it usually constitutes the largest and most urgent part of the workload for neurology residents on call. Many neurological disorders may have implications for driving and medicolegal issues. Specific rehabilitation programs may improve motor or cognitive functions significantly and are important for improving quality of life and for preventing functional decline. Counseling and regular follow-up should be an integral part of neurological management. Although not covered by this book, the neurologist should therefore be aware of local regulations and programs for medicolegal issues, neurorehabilitation, counseling, as well as primary prevention of neurological disorders and palliative end-of-life care.

© Springer International Publishing AG 2017
D. Kondziella, G. Waldemar, *Neurology at the Bedside*, DOI 10.1007/978-3-319-55991-9_6

Keywords

Deep brain stimulation • Drug treatment • Endovascular stroke treatment • Hemicraniectomy • Intravenous thrombolysis • Mechanical thrombectomy • Immunomodulatory therapy

In this chapter on treatment of neurological diseases, *every effort has been made to ensure the accuracy of the information, but medicine is an ever-changing science, and therefore neither the authors nor the publisher can take any responsibility for possible mistakes and their consequences* that may arise from the information in this chapter. For data on pharmacokinetics, pharmacodynamics, contraindications, precautions, and side effects, you are strongly urged to consult the usual references. Importantly, keep in mind that the treatment suggestions are, indeed, suggestions only. Despite the rise of evidence-based medicine, therapeutic decisions including the choice of drugs and dosages vary widely from country to country, from hospital to hospital, and from physician to physician. Checking with the national standard drug references, local protocols, and colleagues is always strongly recommended.

6.1   Coma and Acute Encephalopathies

Coma cocktail

- Thiamine 400 mg IV and vitamin B combinations IM (for possible Wernicke's encephalopathy).
- Dextrose 50% solution, 50 mL intravenously (IV) (for possible hypoglycemia, but do not administer glucose to a patient with suspicion of alcohol abuse without prior parenteral thiamine administration).
- Naloxone 0.4–2 mg IV may be repeated or given as continuous infusion, e.g., 0.8 mg/kg/h (for possible opiate intoxication, beware of withdrawal delirium and opiate rebound)
- Flumazenil 0.3 mg IV may be repeated (max 2–5 mg for possible benzodiazepine intoxication).

High ICP, general measures

- Elevation of the head to 30°, avoid lateral neck bending
- Maintenance of:
  - Normovolemia or mild hypervolemia
  - Adequate cerebral perfusion pressure (CPP) (e.g., >60 mmHg)[1]
  - Adequate oxygenation
  - Normothermia (e.g., acetaminophen 1000 mg every 6 h, surface cooling)
  - Normoglycemia
  - Adequate nutrition and pain management

High ICP, specific measures

- Controlled hyperventilation
- Intravenous osmotherapy
  - Hypertonic saline (3–10%) IV 1–2 mL/kg at 20 mL/min
  - Mannitol (20%); IV bolus 1 g/kg as needed or 0.5 g/kg every 4–6 h
- Ventriculostomy
- ICP monitoring devices (ventricular catheter, intraparenchymal probe, epidural transducer)
- Pharmacological coma (pentobarbital, thiopental, phenobarbital, propofol)
- Corticosteroids with tumors (e.g., dexamethasone 4–10 mg IV every 6 h, oral prednisolone 1 mg/kg once daily)
- Surgical decompression (hemicraniectomy with malignant MCA infarction, posterior fossa decompression with cerebellar infarction)
- Hypothermia after cardiac arrest

Idiopathic intracranial hypertension

- Acetazolamide 500–1000 mg ×2–4 p.o.

---

[1] CPP equals MAP minus ICP.

- Furosemide 40–160 mg/day
- Methylprednisolone (second choice due to negative impact on body weight)
- Dietary advice
- Serial lumbar punctures
- Ventriculoperitoneal shunt (or rarely, optic nerve sheath fenestration), in case of imminent visual impairment

Idiopathic and symptomatic intracranial hypotension (idiopathic or after lumbar puncture)

- Bed rest, fluids, and paracetamol.
- Blood patch.
- Caffeine 500 mg IV may be repeated once.
- Surgery if CSF leakage detected and operable.

Metabolic encephalopathies

- *Hepatic encephalopathy*
  - Low-protein diet
  - Bowel enemas
  - Lactulose 30–50 mL three times daily
  - Neomycin (up to) 1 g every 6 h (or metronidazole)
  - Treat dehydration and electrolyte abnormalities
  - Stop sedative and other CNS medications
  - Transjugular intrahepatic portosystemic shunt
- *Uremic encephalopathy*
  - Dialysis
  - Kidney transplantation
- *Electrolyte disturbances*
  - *Acute hyponatremia*: water restriction and saline IV (correction rate not to exceed 10 mM/24 h and 20 mM/48 h, monitor electrolytes every 2 h).
  - *Central pontine myelinolysis*: 1000 mL glucose 5% can decrease sodium plasma levels by 5 mmol/L and, only if given acutely, may sometimes reverse symptoms, when iatrogenic correction of hyponatremia has been too fast.
- *Wernicke's encephalopathy*
  - Thiamine 400 mg IV ×3 daily for 3 days and vitamin B combinations IM for 3 days, followed by p.o. substitution

- *Hypoglycemic coma*
  - 50% dextrose 50 mL IV (in malnourished patients 100 mg thiamine IV prior to glucose)
  - Glucagon 1 mg SC

Inflammatory encephalopathies (e.g., paraneoplastic and non-paraneoplastic autoimmune encephalitis, Hashimoto's encephalitis)

- Methylprednisolone 1 g/day for 3–5 days IV, then oral prednisolone taper
- IVIG 0.4 g/day for 5 days
- Plasma exchange (e.g., five to seven times in total, administered every other day)
- Treat underlying tumor, if present

Intoxication

- *Carbon monoxide*: hyperbaric oxygen
- *Cyanide*: hyperbaric oxygen, hydroxocobalamin
- *Organophosphate*: atropine, pralidoxime
- *Heavy metals*: dimercaprol, penicillamine
- *Opioids*: naloxone 0.2–0.8 mg IV as needed (beware of short half-life and opioid rebound)
- *Benzodiazepines*: flumazenil 0.2 mg IV as needed (beware of decreased seizure threshold)

Drug-induced encephalopathies

- *Neuroleptic malignant syndrome*
  - Withdraw neuroleptics, admit to ICU
  - Bromocriptine 2.5 mg p.o. test dose, increase to ×2–4 for 48 h
  - Dantrolene 25 mg p.o. or IV several times daily
  - Apomorphine SC with pretreatment with rectal domperidone may be an alternative
  - Electroconvulsive therapy
- *Neuroleptic malignant-like syndrome* (acute withdrawal of dopaminergic or GABAergic medication)
  - Reinstitution of dopaminergic (e.g., L-dopa) or GABAergic (e.g., baclofen) medication
  - Treatment in analogy to neuroleptic malignant syndrome
- *Serotonergic syndrome*
  - Withdraw offending drugs, admit to ICU

– Cyproheptadine (serotonin antagonist) 8 mg p.o., repeat after 2 h, if effective up to 8 mg every 6 h daily
– Benzodiazepines

Minimal conscious state following traumatic or anoxic-ischemic brain injury (arousal and alertness may improve following amantadine treatment)

• Amantadine 50 mg twice daily, increase to 100 mg twice daily after 3–7 days.
• If necessary, the dose can be increased to 200 mg twice daily.

6.2   Headache

Migraine (mild pain during attack)

• Paracetamol
• Nonsteroidal anti-inflammatory drugs (NSAID) (e.g., naproxen sodium 750 mg, not exceeding 1250 mg/24 h)

Migraine (moderate pain during attack)

• Triptans during early and mild pain following the aura (contraindicated in complicated migraine, heart disease, stroke, uncontrolled hypertension, and/or severe liver disease). There are various triptans, including almotriptan, eletriptan, frovatriptan, naratriptan, rizatriptan, sumatriptan, and zolmitriptan; they can be administered as:
– Nasal spray, e.g., zolmitriptan 2.5 mg or 5 mg; for second dose, wait 2 h, max. 10 mg/24 h
– Soluble tablets, e.g., zolmitriptan 2.5 mg or 5 mg; for second dose, wait 2 h, max. 10 mg/24 h
– Tablets, e.g., zolmitriptan (see zolmitriptan tablets); sumatriptan 50 or 100 mg, max. 200–300 mg/24 h; and almotriptan 12.5 mg, max. 25 mg/24 h Injection, sumatriptan 6 mg SC; for second dose wait 1 h, max. 12 mg/24 h
• Dihydroergotamine 1 mg/mL SC is rarely used as an alternative but is contraindicated in patients with ischemic cardiac disease (metoclopramide 10 mg IM should be given prior to dihydroergotamine to avoid nausea and vomiting).

Nausea

• Orally: prochlorperazine 5–10 mg ×3–4 daily; metoclopramide 10–20 mg ×3 daily
• Suppository: metoclopramide 20 mg ×3 daily
• Intravenously and intramuscularly: metoclopramide 10 mg ×1–3 daily

Status migrainosus

• Neuroleptics IV or IM, e.g., chlorpromazine 5–50 mg, haloperidol 5–10 mg, and prochlorperazine 5–10 mg

Migraine in pregnancy

• Pregnancy: paracetamol and caffeine (<300 mg, after first trimester)

Migraine (preventive treatment)

• Beta-blockers, metoprolol 100 mg once or twice daily or 200 mg once daily, and propranolol 20–80 mg once or twice daily
• Angiotensin II receptor blockers: candesartan 8–16 mg once daily
• Angiotensin-converting enzyme inhibitors: lisinopril 10–20 mg once daily
• Antiepileptics: topiramate 25 mg once daily (up to 50 mg twice daily), valproate 300–600 mg ×2–3 daily
• Calcium channel blockers: verapamil 120–180 mg twice daily, flunarizine 5–10 mg once daily
• TCA: amitriptyline 10–75 mg once daily
• Onabotulinum toxin A (for chronic migraine, defined as headaches occurring on 15 or more days each month, at least half of which have migrainous features)

Medication-overuse headache

• Headache diary, drug withdrawal, and patient education; headaches may get worse for 1–4 weeks during drug withdrawal.

- Transitional strategies for relief of withdrawal symptoms: promethazine 25 mg or levomepromazine 12.5–25 mg up to three times daily, in combination with antiemetics (e.g., domperidone 10 mg, metoclopramide 10 mg, or ondansetron suppositories 16 mg); alternatives include prednisolone 100 mg/day for 5 days and naproxen 750 mg once daily.
- Non-pharmacological measures (i.e., regulation of lifestyle, including regular meals, sleep and exercise, cessation of smoking and excessive alcohol consumption, limited caffeine consumption, and relaxation techniques).
- Comorbid depression and anxiety must be treated.
- Start preventive treatment, if needed.
- Close follow-up for 8–12 weeks.
- Most patients with medication-overuse headache can be managed on an outpatient basis, but those with significant psychological conditions, abuse of opioids or barbiturates, or earlier treatment failures may benefit from hospital admission and a multidisciplinary approach, including physiotherapy and psychological treatment.

Tension headache, acute treatment (medication should not be taken more than 2–3 times/week in order to avoid medication-overuse headache)

- Physical exercise
- Aspirin 500–1000 mg
- Paracetamol 1000 mg
- Ibuprofen 200–400 mg

Tension headache, chronic treatment

- Physical exercise
- Amitriptyline 25–75 mg/day (or imipramine 25–75 mg, less sedating) plus paracetamol

Cluster headache, acute treatment

- Inhalation of pure oxygen (e.g., 7–10 L/min for 10–15 min)

- Sumatriptan 6 mg SC, 20 mg intranasal, zolmitriptan 5 mg intranasal

Cluster headache, transitional treatment

- Prednisolone 60 mg/day p.o. for 3–5 days, taper by 10 mg every 3 days
- Ergotamine 1–2 mg, p.o. or as a suppository once or twice daily
- Methylprednisolone (120 mg) with lidocaine injected into the greater occipital nerve ipsilateral to the site of attack
- Avoidance of triggering factors, e.g., alcohol, daytime naps, and nitroglycerin

Cluster headache, maintenance treatment

- Verapamil (sustained release), start dose 120 mg twice daily, may be increased by 120 mg/week to 480 mg/day (or more).
- Lithium 600–900 mg (requires monitoring of serum levels, usually 0.4–0.8 mEq/L).
- Verapamil and lithium (300–600 mg daily) may be combined.
- Methysergide, corticosteroids, topiramate, and melatonin can be tried alternatively.
- Surgery (trigeminal nerve, autonomic pathways, hypothalamic DBS).

Paroxysmal hemicrania and hemicrania continua

- Indotest (indomethacin 25 mg ×3 daily for 3 days; if necessary, 50 mg ×3 daily for another 3 days).
- Maintenance up to 300 mg/day (often indefinite, but long-term remission possible) and 25–50 mg ×4 daily is usually effective.
- If indomethacin is not tolerated, preventive therapy as for cluster headache can be tried.

SUNCT

- Does not respond to indomethacin
- First choice: lamotrigine 100–200 mg/day
- Second choice: carbamazepine, topiramate, and gabapentin

Stabbing headache

- Does not usually require treatment but responds to indomethacin

Hypnic headache
Acute treatment: aspirin
Preventive treatment

- Lithium 300–600 mg/day at bedtime
- Indomethacin (25–75 mg at bedtime), flunarizine, caffeine (200 mg at bedtime)
- Verapamil (as for cluster headache)

Primary thunderclap headaches

- Cough headache: indomethacin 25–50 mg ×2–3 daily
- Headache associated with physical exertion/sexual activity (if acute, make sure to rule out subarachnoidal warning leak; if chronic, make sure to rule out arterial hypertension!).
- NSAIDs, e.g., indomethacin 25–75 mg 0.5–1 h prior to activity.
- Beta-blockers, e.g., propranolol 20–40 mg 0.5–1 h prior to activity or daily for a 3-month period.
- With orgasmic headache, a change of sex position is often helpful.

Giant cell arteritis
High-dose intravenous methylprednisolone in case of blindness, otherwise 60 mg/day p.o.; reduce to 20 mg over about 2 months, and thereafter reduce cautiously to 10 mg; mean treatment time 1.5–2 years; polymyalgia rheumatica without temporal arteritis can be treated with 5–10 mg/day.

Trigeminal neuralgia, related conditions, and atypical facial pain
See Sect. 6.11.

6.3 Cognitive Impairment and Dementia

For evidence-based reviews, see Hort et al. (2010), Sorbi et al. (2012), and Schmidt et al. (2015).

AD, DLB, and PD with dementia, symptomatic treatment with a modest effect on cognitive functions, activities of daily living, and behavioral symptoms.[2]

- Cholinesterase inhibitors (for mild to moderate AD, mixed AD, DLB, and PD with dementia)
  – Donepezil, tablets; starting dose 5 mg once daily, increase to 10 mg once daily after 4–6 weeks
  – Rivastigmine
    Capsules: 1.5 mg twice daily, may be increased to 6 mg twice daily (by 3 mg/2–4 weeks)
    Patch: 4.6 mg/24 h, after 4 weeks increase to 9.5/24 h
  – Galantamine, capsules, 8 mg once daily, may be increased to 24 mg once daily (stepwise by 8 mg/4–6 weeks)
- Glutamate (NMDA) antagonist (for moderate to severe AD): memantine, tablets, 5 mg once daily, increase to 20 mg once daily (stepwise by 5 mg/week)
- A combination of a cholinesterase inhibitor plus memantine may be given in patients with moderate to severe AD.

AD and other dementias, for severe behavioral disturbances and/or psychotic symptoms, where physical causes (e.g., infections) have been excluded or treated and where non-pharmacological interventions were not sufficient:

- If indicated and not already initiated: cholinesterase inhibitor and/or glutamate (NMDA) antagonist (as shown above).
- Atypical antipsychotics:
  – Risperidone 0.25 mg–0.5 mg p.o. once daily (before bedtime) may be increased to 1 mg p.o. once daily.
  – Olanzapine 2.5 mg p.o. once daily may be increased stepwise by 2.5 mg to 5 (−10)mg p.o. once daily.
  – Quetiapine 25 mg once daily may be increased stepwise by 25 mg, up to 50 mg ×2.

---

[2]Minor variations across countries exist regarding approved indications (concerning the severity and range of specific dementia syndromes).

- For patients with parkinsonian dementias: clozapine, start with 6.75 mg p.o. once daily, titrate by 6.75 mg every other day to 25 mg p.o. once daily.

There is insufficient evidence for the use of antipsychotics in patients with dementia. When prescribing antipsychotic treatments, always plan for a time-limited, short treatment period with regular review of treatment effect and side effects.

AD and other dementias, for depression, anxiety, stereotypical behavior, and sleep disturbance

- For depression in dementia, there is uncertain evidence for the efficacy of antidepressive treatment. A treatment trial of a SSRI, e.g., sertraline 50(−100) mg p.o. once daily (start with 25 mg), citalopram 10–20 mg p.o. once daily (start with 10 mg), or escitalopram 5–10 mg once daily (start with 5 mg) may be tried in patients with moderate to severe depression.
- Alternatively, try venlafaxine 37.5 mg p.o. once daily (may be increased to 75 mg once daily) or mirtazapine 15 mg p.o. once daily (may be increased to 30 mg p.o. once daily).
- Anxiety: appropriate care, calm environments, and non-pharmacological interventions should be initiated as a first priority. Treatment with benzodiazepines should generally be avoided but may be necessary in cases of severe anxiety for a very short period of time; oxazepam 7.5 mg p.o. once daily, may be increased to 15 mg p.o. ×2–3 daily.
- Stereotypical behavior in FTD: uncertain evidence, a SSRI may be tried (see above).
- Sleep disturbance and REM sleep behavior disorder: See Sect. 6.5 and treat for a short-time period if necessary.
- When possible, avoid psychopharmacological polypharmacia in patients with dementia.

Normal pressure hydrocephalus

- Ventriculoperitoneal shunt, as guided by lumbar perfusion test and/or tap test results

Vascular dementia

- Aggressive control of vascular risk factors (see Sect. 6.6).
- Cholinesterase inhibitors may be tried in the event of combined AD and vascular lesions.

Dementia associated with PD/DLB

- L-dopa and dopaminergic agonists can be tried to improve motor symptoms but may increase hallucinations and confusion.
- Cholinesterase inhibitors may be tried (for dosing see above).

Wernicke's encephalopathy, and *Korsakoff's syndrome*.
See Sect. 6.1.
Inflammatory encephalopathies (e.g., paraneoplastic and non-paraneoplastic limbic encephalitis, Hashimoto encephalitis).
See Sect. 6.1.

6.4 Epilepsy

6.4.1 General Aspects

AED that can be used as initial monotherapy (in alphabetical order, "*" denotes level A evidence as suggested by the "Updated ILAE Evidence Review for Initial Monotherapy") (Glauser et al. 2013):

- *Adults with partial-onset seizures*: carbamazepine*, gabapentin, lamotrigine, levetiracetam*, oxcarbazepine, phenobarbital, phenytoin*, topiramate, valproate, and zonisamide*
- *Children with partial-onset seizures*: carbamazepine, clobazam, clonazepam, lamotrigine, oxcarbazepine*, phenobarbital, phenytoin, topiramate, valproate, and zonisamide
- *Adults with generalized onset tonic-clonic seizures*: carbamazepine, gabapentin, lamotrigine, levetiracetam, oxcarbazepine, phenobarbital, phenytoin, topiramate, and valproate
- *Children with generalized onset tonic-clonic seizures*: carbamazepine, phenobarbital, phenytoin, topiramate, valproate, and oxcarbazepine

- *Children with absence seizures*: ethosuximide*, lamotrigine, and valproate*
- *JME*: clonazepam, lamotrigine (may occasionally worsen myoclonus), levetiracetam, phenobarbital, piracetam, topiramate, and valproate
- *Infantile spasms*: adrenocorticotropic hormone (ACTH), pyridoxine, valproate, and vigabatrin
- *Benign partial epilepsy syndromes in childhood* (e.g., benign partial epilepsy of childhood with centrotemporal spikes (BECTS)): if necessary, valproate and carbamazepine

New AED approved for the use as adjunctive treatment of partial-onset seizures

- Eslicarbazepine, lacosamide, retigabine, zonisamide, and rufinamide (Lennox-Gastaut syndrome)

Alcohol withdrawal period

Many different regimens have been proposed for the treatment and prevention of alcohol withdrawal seizures, including carbamazepine (200 mg three times daily for 5 days), clomethiazole (300 mg as needed), and phenobarbital (100 mg as needed). However, a task force group of the European Federation of Neurological Societies (EFNS) concluded in their guidelines on the diagnosis and management of alcohol-related seizures that "benzodiazepines are efficacious and safe for primary and secondary seizure prevention; diazepam or, if available, lorazepam, is recommended. The efficacy of other drugs is insufficiently documented [...] Benzodiazepines should be chosen for the treatment and prevention of recurrent alcohol withdrawal seizures" (Bråthen et al. 2005).

Uremic seizures

- Phenobarbital, phenytoin, and valproate

Postanoxic myoclonus

- Clonazepam, e.g., 2–3 mg IV or p.o. ×3 daily (however, if the patient is in coma following cardiac arrest and has myoclonic status epilepticus, the prognosis is usually very poor)

Eclampsia

- Magnesium sulfate 4 g IV and 10 mg IM, then 5 mg every 4 h as required

Contraception, pregnancy

- Decreased effects of oral contraceptive pill with hepatic enzyme inducers (e.g., barbiturates, carbamazepine, oxcarbazepine, phenytoin, primidone).
- Some data indicate that topiramate and lamotrigine may also decrease contraceptive efficacy to a certain degree via different mechanisms.
- Injectable contraceptives have usually no interactions with AEDs.
- Rescue contraception: First dose of the usual rescue pill should be doubled and a second single dose given 12 h later.
- Folic acid (5 mg/day) should be provided to all women of childbearing age to decrease the risk of neural tube defects.
- Aim for monotherapy!
- Generally, valproate is not recommended for fertile women due to its teratogenic effects and evidence that valproate during pregnancy can result in learning disabilities and decreased intelligence of the child.
- Contraceptive pills and pregnancy decrease serum levels of lamotrigine. Monitoring serum lamotrigine levels before, during, and after pregnancy (and adjusting the dosage) or initiation of contraception is useful.

Breast-feeding

Only ethosuximide, lamotrigine, levetiracetam, and phenobarbital are significantly released into breast milk; barbiturates and lamotrigine may lead to sedation of the infant.

Drug monitoring

As a rule, the steady state is reached after four to five half lives following initiation or change of antiepileptic drug therapy. Monitoring of serum levels can be useful in patients with signs of toxicity or lack of treatment response and if noncompliance is suspected.

- Carbamazepine (target level 20–40 µmol/L)
- Ethosuximide (300–700 µmol/L)
- Lamotrigine (10–60 µmol/L)
- Levetiracetam (35–120 µmol/L)
- Phenobarbital (60–120 µmol/L)
- Phenytoin (40–80 µmol/L or higher in case of status epilepticus)
- Valproate (300–700 µmol/L)

Pharmacokinetic drug interactions

- *Relevant drug interactions with another antiepileptic drug*: carbamazepine, ethosuximide, lamotrigine, oxcarbazepine, phenytoin, phenobarbital, topiramate, valproate, and zonisamide
- *Interactions with non-AED*: antibiotics, antidepressives, antifungal drugs, antihypertensive drugs, antipsychotics, cardiovascular drugs, theophylline, and warfarin
- *No clinically relevant drug interactions*: gabapentin, levetiracetam, and pregabalin

6.4.2 Status Epilepticus

- Lorazepam 4 mg IV (may be repeated once), diazepam 5–10 mg IV (may be repeated), and clonazepam 1–3 mg IV (may be repeated).[3]
- Fosphenytoin 15–20 mg PE/kg (not exceeding 100 mg PE/min); check serum phenytoin level after 2 h and, if necessary, give more (target level 80–100 µmol/L, do not forget to prescribe maintenance therapy); alternatively, valproate 1000–2000 mg IV, levetiracetam 2000 mg IV, or lacosamide 200–400 mg IV.
- General anesthesia (propofol, midazolam, thiopental); aim for burst suppression on EEG

monitoring; when seizures have been controlled for 12–24 h, withdraw sedation slowly (over 12 h); if seizures reoccur, another cycle of 12 h general anesthesia should be provided; and so on. Beware of the propofol infusion syndrome.[4]

6.4.3 Antiepileptic Drugs (AED)

The following AED are listed in alphabetical order:

Carbamazepine

- Start with 100 mg twice daily, then 200 mg twice daily; if necessary, increase with 200 mg/week until seizure control (target 200–400 mg twice daily, max. 800–1200 mg twice daily)
- Emergency loading 300–400 mg twice daily

Carbamazepine extended release

The extended-release formulation is preferred for long-term treatment because of more stable serum levels, thereby avoiding "high peak" concentrations.

- Initially 100 mg twice daily, then 200 mg twice daily, then increase with 200 mg/week until seizure control (target 400–600 mg twice daily)

Clonazepam

- Start with 0.5 mg at night, increase by 1–2 mg/week, maintenance 0.5–6 mg/day (occasionally, up to 8 mg daily), divided into two to three doses/day

Gabapentin

Gabapentin is the only AED that should be given three times a day because of the short half-life:

---

[3]For subjects in status epilepticus, intramuscular midazolam is at least as safe and effective as intravenous lorazepam for *prehospital* seizures (Silbergleit et al. 2012).

[4]Propofol infusion syndrome is a rare, but potentially fatal, complication of prolonged administration (≥48 h) of high doses of propofol (≥4 mg/kg/h). It leads to metabolic acidosis, hypertriglyceridemia, rhabdomyolysis, cardiac arrhythmias, and multiorgan failure.

- First day 300 mg once daily, second day twice daily, and third day three times daily
- Increase by 300 mg/day until seizure control (target dose 900–1200 mg, max. 3600 mg)

Lamotrigine
Monotherapy:

- 25 mg once daily during first 2 weeks, followed by 50 mg once daily during the next 2 weeks
- Then increase with 50 mg every week or every second week until seizure control (target 50–100 mg twice daily, max. 500 mg/day)

In combination with valproate:
Valproate prolongs lamotrigine clearance by roughly 100%:

- 25 mg once daily every other day (!) for 2 weeks, followed by 25 mg once daily for next 2 weeks.
- Then increase with 25 mg every week or every second week until seizure control (target 50–100 mg twice daily, max. 500 mg/day).

In combination with carbamazepine, phenytoin, phenobarbital, primidone, or other inducing drugs:

- 50 mg once daily for 2 weeks, followed by 50 mg twice daily for next 2 weeks
- Then increase with 100 mg every or every second week until seizure control (target 100–200 mg twice daily, max. 500 mg/day)

Levetiracetam
Monotherapy:

- 250 mg twice daily for 1–2 weeks (or less), then 500 mg twice daily (target dose; if required, faster titration is usually well tolerated)
- If necessary, increase with 500 mg every few days until seizure control (max. 3000 mg/day)

In combination with other AEDs:

- 500 mg twice daily (target level)

- If necessary, increase with 1000 mg every few days until seizure control (max. 3000 mg/day)

Oxcarbazepine

- 300 mg twice daily (target dose 600–1200 mg/day)
- If necessary, increase with 600 mg every week until seizure control (max. 2400 mg/day)

Pregabalin

- 75 mg twice daily for 1 week
- If necessary, increase to 150 mg twice daily
- If necessary, increase to 300 mg twice daily after another week (target dose 150–600 mg/day)

Topiramate
Monotherapy:

- 25 mg once daily in the evening for 1 week
- Then 25 mg twice daily, increase with 25 mg every week
- Target dose 50 mg twice daily (max. 500 mg/day)

In combination with other AEDs:

- 50 mg once daily (evening) for 1 week
- Then 50 mg twice daily, increase with 50 mg every or every other week
- Target dose 100 mg–200 mg twice daily (max. 1000 mg/day)

Valproate

- Start with 300 mg twice daily
- Fast increase possible, maintenance 600–3000 mg/day

Valproate extended release
Extended-release formulation is preferred for long-term treatment because of more stable serum levels:

- Initially 600 mg/day–1500 mg/day, e.g., 300 mg twice daily or 500 mg twice daily

- Fast increase possible, maintenance 1200–3000 mg/day

Rational polytherapy

Rational polytherapy is the combined use of two or more AEDs with favorable pharmacokinetic interactions and/or different mechanisms, e.g., a sodium channel blocker and a drug with GABAergic properties.

- Valproate with lamotrigine for partial-onset and generalized seizures.
- Valproate with ethosuximide for absence seizures.
- Lamotrigine with topiramate for a range of seizure types.
- Levetiracetam, which has a unique mechanism and no known drug interactions, can theoretically be combined with any AED.

6.4.4 Epilepsy and Mood Disorders

Depression and related depressive disorders are highly prevalent in patients with epilepsy. The lifetime incidence of depression among patients with chronic epilepsy is 30%, and its prevalence in patients admitted to a tertiary epilepsy center may be as high as 50% (Kanner 2003; Boylan et al. 2004). Yet depression in these patients remains underdiagnosed and undertreated. This is particularly worrisome as depression is associated with poor seizure control, and the risk of suicide in patients with epilepsy is greatly increased (Baker 2006; Pompili et al. 2006). Reluctance to treat depression results from the traditional belief that antidepressants decrease seizure threshold. However, there is growing evidence that many antidepressants have anticonvulsant effects instead and that modern antidepressants may indeed reduce seizure frequency in patients with pharmacoresistant epilepsy. When adhering to the usual precautions, treatment with selective reuptake inhibitors of serotonin (SSRI, e.g., citalopram 20 mg once daily, escitalopram 10 mg once daily, sertralin

50 mg once daily) in patients with epilepsy and depression is safe and should not be withheld.

6.4.5 Options for Patients with Medically Refractory Seizures

Despite the continuous introduction of new AEDs, approximately one-third of patients with epilepsy do not become seizure-free. Options for these patients include:

- Epilepsy surgery
- Vagus nerve stimulation
- Ketogenic diet
- Deep brain stimulation (DBS); see below

6.4.5.1 Epilepsy Surgery

Resection of epileptogenic tissue can have a tremendous effect both in regard to seizure control and quality of life. As a rule, a patient should be referred to a tertiary epilepsy clinic if two proper antiepileptic drug trials have failed. The following criteria have to be fulfilled prior to epilepsy surgery:

- The diagnosis of epilepsy is verified.
- A focal epileptogenic area is identified (by using MRI, video-EEG monitoring, and perhaps invasive EEG recording, ictal and interictal SPECT, magnetoencephalography, and neuropsychological testing).
- It is reasonably certain that resection of the epileptogenic area will not lead to unacceptable neurological deficits.

Temporal lobe resection is the most commonly performed epilepsy surgery and is generally associated with the best results. However, if seizure control cannot be obtained by medical treatment, resection of epileptogenic areas outside the temporal lobe can lead to satisfactory seizure control as well. Occasionally, callosotomy or hemispherectomy may be necessary.

6.4.5.2 Vagus Nerve Stimulation

Vagus nerve stimulation is another option for some patients with refractory epilepsy, especially those who are not suitable for epilepsy surgery or who have had insufficient benefit from surgery. Vagus nerve stimulation reduces seizure frequency with ≥50% in one-third of patients. It has few side effects and may have antidepressive properties.

6.4.5.3 Ketogenic Diet

Several studies have shown beneficial effects of the ketogenic diet in patients with pharmacoresistant epilepsy, especially in children. In a recent study on ketogenic diet for treatment of childhood epilepsy, after 3 months of ketogenic diet, the mean percentage of baseline seizures had decreased by 75% in the diet group compared to the controls (Neal et al. 2008). Energy from a ketogenic diet is largely derived from fat. The composition is traditionally 80% fat and 20% proteins and carbohydrates, but some studies have shown similar success with the modified Atkins diet.

6.4.5.4 Deep Brain Stimulation (DBS)

DBS has not yet been widely used for the treatment of epilepsy, although some data suggest that, e.g., bilateral stimulation of the anterior nucleus of the thalamus may have beneficial effects for patients with partial seizures with or without secondary generalization.

6.5   Sleep Disorders

Obstructive sleep apnea

- Lifestyle adjustments, weight loss
- Continuous positive airway pressure treatment at night
- Modafinil during daytime for excessive sleepiness

Narcolepsy

- Lifestyle adjustments (e.g., short naps during daytime, avoidance of heavy meals)
- Modafinil
  - Start with 100 mg twice daily (morning and lunchtime).
  - Increase to 200 mg twice daily if necessary.
- Dexamphetamine
  - 5–10 mg ×3 daily (duration of action roughly 2 h).
  - Increase up to 15–20 mg ×3 daily if necessary.
- Methylphenidate
  - Start with 5–10 mg once daily.
  - Increase by 10 mg/week, two or three doses per day, max. 60 mg/day.
  - Switch to extended-release form (same daily dose, once daily, e.g., methylphenidate 10 mg twice daily = methylphenidate extended release 20 mg once daily).
- Selegiline (5–10 mg twice daily, morning and lunchtime)
- Gamma-hydroxybutyrate liquid preparation, e.g., taken before bed and second dose 4 h after initial sleep (4.5–9 g per night)

Cataplexy

- Fluoxetine 20–60 mg once daily
- Clomipramine 25–50 mg once daily, increase to 50 mg twice daily if necessary during first week
- Venlafaxine 75 mg once daily, increase by 75 mg/week if necessary, max. 300 mg/day
- Gamma-hydroxybutyrate (see above)

Poor sleep

- Good sleep hygiene is crucial. Avoid heavy meals, alcohol, coffee, and other stimulating beverages before bedtimes as well as a large fluid intake during evening hours; a regular daily schedule is important; no sleeping in on weekends and daytime naps should be avoided; optimization of bedroom temperature, air quality, darkness, and sound; no reading or watching television in bed; a short walk and other forms of light (in contrast to exhaustive) exercise in the evening can be beneficial; consider psychotherapeutical measures, e.g., writing a diary before going to bed, and if unable to sleep, leave the bedroom but avoid stimulating activities and try again after a while.

- Zopiclone 3.75 mg once at bedtime (may be increased to 7.5 mg).

Jet lag, delayed sleep phase syndrome, night shift, and others

- Melatonin 2 mg 1–2 h before sleep
- Light therapy
- Caffeine
- Modafinil

REM sleep behavior disorder

- Clonazepam 0.25–1 mg at bedtime
- Melatonin 2 mg once before sleep, may be increased to 6 mg
- Anecdotal success with levodopa, carbamazepine, and gabapentin

6.6 Cerebrovascular Disorders

Patients with acute stroke or TIA should be evaluated and treated as soon as possible in *dedicated stroke units*. One out of 12 patients is saved from death or disability simply by being cared for in a stroke unit as compared to a general medical ward or mobile stroke teams. This effect is irrespective of age, gender, and stroke severity. (In comparison, the simple administration of aspirin within 48 h after stroke prevents death or disability in just 1 out of 100 patients.) Perhaps even more impressive is the fact that emergent diagnostic evaluation and initiation of secondary prevention in TIA patients at specialist stroke centers is associated with an 80% risk reduction for a new cerebral ischemic event (Lavallée et al. 2007). Also, dedicated stroke centers allow for early initiation of multidisciplinary rehabilitation.

6.6.1 Intravenous Thrombolysis (IVT)

IVT, using alteplase (a recombinant tissue plasminogen activator, rt.-PA), is the first treatment with documented effect in acute ischemic stroke. It was approved in the USA in 1996 and has been widely adapted in Europe since 2003. For every eight patients, IVT increases the number of stroke survivors who are neurologically intact after 3 months from two to three. Of course, also patients without complete resolution of neurological deficits can benefit from IVT. The number needed to treat for significant neurological improvement is 3.6 for patients treated within 90 min, 4.3 for treatment within 91 and 180 min, and 5.9 for treatment within 181 and 270 min. The number needed to harm (i.e., to induce a significant intracranial and/or extracranial hemorrhage) is 65, 38, and 30 for the corresponding time intervals. This translates into a net benefit of IVT of 1 in 3.8 patients, if treatment can be initiated within 90 min, 4.9 between 91 and 180 min, and 7.4 between 181 and 270 min (Lansberg et al. 2009). Thus, the earlier IVT is initiated, the more effective and safer it is.

Indications and inclusion criteria for IVT comprise the following:

- Ischemic cerebral infarction, if treatment can be initiated within the time window of 4.5 h from symptom onset (at the time of writing, IVT given after 3 h is off-label in the USA).
- Neurological deficits as measured by the NIHSS ≤25. Higher NIHSS values indicate a larger volume of ischemic tissue with possibly reduced effect of IVT and higher risk of secondary hemorrhage. IVT can also be given for subtle neurological deficits if there is risk for significant handicap (e.g., a patient with isolated dysphasia only has an NIHSS score of ≤3).
- CT of the brain has excluded intracranial hemorrhage and extensive infarction (≥1/3 of MCA territory, ≥1/2 of ACA territory).
- Age ≥18 years. IVT can be administered with or without reduced dosage in adolescents and children but is then off-label.

Contraindications (absolute or relative) to IVT include:

- Inclusion criteria are not fulfilled, e.g., CT of the brain shows intracranial hemorrhage or an established infarction of >1/3 of MCA territory, or the patient is outside the time window.

- Large stroke volume with stroke-related impairment of consciousness.
- Uncontrolled arterial hypertension (systolic ≥185 mmHg, diastolic ≥110 mmHg).
- Increased bleeding risk. The beneficial effects of IVT must always be weighed against the risks for an intracranial or systemic hemorrhage in patients prone to bleeding.
  - Intracranial bleeding risk, e.g.:
    Previous (non-lacunar) stroke or serious head injury ≤3 months
    History of intracerebral hemorrhage or vascular malformation (if bleeding source has not been identified and eliminated)
    Symptoms suggestive of subarachnoidal hemorrhage
    Diabetes mellitus and a history of prior stroke
  - Increased systemic bleeding risk, e.g.:
    An international normalized ratio (INR) ≥1.5 is an absolute contraindication. However, the INR level should be assessed before the decision is made to withhold IVT. Many patients on warfarin present with an acute ischemic stroke because they are below the therapeutic INR interval (usually INR 2–3) and then they might be IVT candidates nevertheless.
    Platelets ≤100,000/mm^3 (relative, depending on the degree of thrombocytopenia).
    Hereditary coagulopathies (relative, depending on the kind and degree of the coagulation disorder).
    Major surgery, trauma (e.g., due to a fall at stroke onset), or delivery ≤14 days.
    Gastrointestinal or urinary tract bleeding ≤21 days (if bleeding source has not been eliminated).
    Active pancreatitis, active GI ulcer.
    Symptoms suggestive of endocarditis or aortic dissection (but not carotid or vertebral artery dissection).
    Arterial puncture at noncompressible sites ≤7 days (relative).
- Terminal malignancy or other critical illness.
- Poor premorbid function (modified Rankin Scale ≥3).

- Stroke mimics. Obvious stroke mimics should not be treated with IVT. However, the diagnosis of a stroke mimic as compared to an ischemic cerebrovascular event can be challenging in the emergency room, and therefore, it is important to be aware of a recent report in which 69 out of 512 (14%) patients were ultimately diagnosed as having a stroke mimic (the most common being epileptic seizures, migraine headaches, and functional disorders), yet intracranial hemorrhage or other significant side effects did not occur in any of these patients (Chernyshev et al. 2010). Thus, when contraindications are ruled out, it is better to give IVT than to withhold it.

Alteplase is given intravenously (0.9 mg/kg); the maximal dosage is 90 mg. Ten percent is given as a bolus, the rest as a continuous infusion over 60 min. Immediately prior to bolus injection, confirm that the patient still has significant neurological deficits. If systolic blood pressure is ≥185 mmHg or diastolic blood pressure is ≥110 mmHg, labetalol may be administered (e.g., 5–20 mg ×1–2). Do not give IVT if blood pressure values remain above the upper limits. Evaluate neurological deficits using the NIHSS at initial assessment and 2 and 24 h following IVT (Chap. 3). Neurological performance and vital parameters must be carefully monitored at least during the initial 24 h. Insertion of a nasogastric tube, urinary catheter, intra-arterial lines, and similar procedures should be performed prior to IVT, if necessary, and avoided for at least 3 h after IVT.

The main predictors of a clinically significant intracranial hemorrhage following IVT are old age, severe neurological deficits, arterial hypertension, hyperglycemia, early signal changes on CT of the brain, a large infarct volume, and a high degree of small vessel disease (as assessed by cerebral atrophy and periventricular leukoaraiosis on CT or white matter signal change on T_2-weighted MRI). Symptomatic ICH usually occurs within 24 h after thrombolysis. Intracranial hemorrhage after 36 h is considered unrelated to IVT. In the initial National Institute of Neurological Disorders and Stroke (NINDS) trial, alteplase treatment was associated with a rate of symptomatic intracranial bleeding of 6.4% compared with 0.6% in the placebo group (The National Institute of Neurological Disorders and Stroke rt.-PA Stroke Study Group 1995). The mortality rate in cases of symptomatic ICH was roughly 50%, but the global mortality rate was nevertheless lower in the rt.-PA group than in the placebo group (The National Institute of Neurological Disorders and Stroke rt.-PA Stroke Study Group 1995). In case of severe headache, vomiting, hypertension, and worsening of neurological deficits occurring during IVT, alteplase infusion should be stopped and a CT of the brain performed immediately. If CT reveals hemorrhage, one possible approach is to administer 1 g intravenously of the antifibrinolytic agent tranexamic acid, followed by fresh frozen plasma 10 mL/kg body weight. Administration of cryoprecipitate to increase the levels of fibrinogen and factor VIII in addition to 6–8 units of platelets is another option. Immediate neurosurgical evaluation is necessary.

If CT of the brain 24 h following IVT has excluded a hemorrhage transformation or primary intracranial bleeding, antiplatelet therapy should be initiated. Unless there are contraindications, patients with both chronic and paroxysmal atrial fibrillation should be on an anticoagulant (one of the new generation anticoagulants or warfarin), but when to initiate treatment depends on the volume of infarcted brain tissue and the presence of absence of intracranial hemorrhage. There are no established time criteria, but a patient with a TIA or minor cerebral infarction (as assessed by neuroimaging, e.g., MR DWI) can probably be started on full anticoagulation with minimal delay, whereas patients with a moderate infarct size will have to wait for 7 or more days and patients with an intracranial hemorrhage and/or large ischemic infarct should have a new CT of the brain after at least 14 days showing resolution of intracranial hemorrhage before anticoagulation can be prescribed.

Deep vein thrombosis prophylaxis with subcutaneous low-molecular heparin is usually safe 24 h after IVT, even in the presence of intracranial hemorrhage. Of note, intermittent pneumatic compression is an effective method of reducing the risk of deep vein thrombosis, possibly improving survival in patients who are immobile after stroke (CLOTS (Clots in Legs Or sTockings after Stroke) Trials Collaboration 2013).

6.6.2 Endovascular Therapy (EVT) for Acute Ischemic Stroke

Unfortunately, IVT only has a modest effect in proximal cerebral vessel occlusions. In acute MCA stroke, for instance, IVT has nearly no potential to recanalize occluded vessels if thrombus length exceeds 8 mm (Riedel et al. 2011). Even if recanalization is achieved, there remains a high risk of reocclusion. The patient group for which immediate recanalization would be the best option is therefore also least likely to benefit from IVT alone. In addition, patients with stroke because of cholesterol and calcified emboli or atherosclerotic stenosis may respond poorly to IVT. EVT is therefore indicated in ischemic stroke due to proximal occlusions of large cerebral vessels, and 10–15% of all presenting stroke patients may be eligible for EVT. Recanalization is achieved more frequently, more rapidly, and more reliably due to direct thrombolytic drug delivery into the clot, mechanical clot retrieval, and/or angioplasty. In 2015, results of five randomized trials (MR CLEAN, EXTEND-1A, ESCAPE, SWIFT PRIME, and REVASCAT), involving nearly 1300 patients, convincingly demonstrated the clinical effectiveness of EVT. In each of these trials, functional independence at 90 days following stroke (mRS 0–2) occurred significantly more often in the EVT groups as compared to iv thrombolysis alone. Improved neuroimaging-based patient selection and new-generation "stent-retrievers" are generally credited for these benefits (Case 6.1).

EVT options include:

- Intra-arterial (i.a.) thrombolysis
- Mechanical clot removal (thrombectomy, e.g., using self-expandable, retrievable stents, or suction devices)

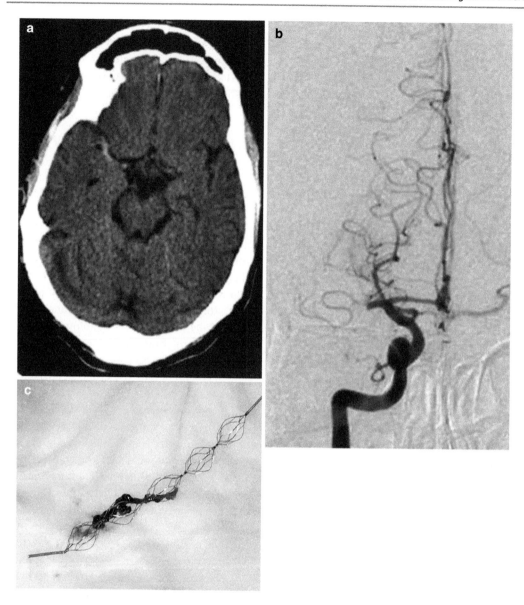

Case 6.1 Thrombectomy for middle cerebral artery occlusion. A 55-year-old male presented with sudden onset of left hemiplegia, hemianopia, gaze paresis, and neglect (NIHSS 19). CT of the brain revealed a dense MCA artery sign on the right (**a**). IVT was started 2.5 h after onset, and the patient was referred for EVT. Complete occlusion of the right M1 MCA was seen on the cerebral angiography (**b**). Thrombus material was extracted using a stent-retriever (Eric 6x44 microvention) (**c**). Final angiogram 4.5 h after symptom onset showed full recanalization of the MCA (TICI 3; **d**). Although a subcortical right hemisphere infarct was noticed on the CT the next day (**e**), the NIHSS score had decreased to four. Subsequently, the patient returned to work, and at the 3-month follow-up, only subtle left-sided weakness remained (NIHSS 2, mRS 1) (adapted with permission from Kondziella et al. (2013))

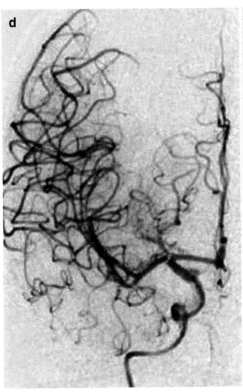

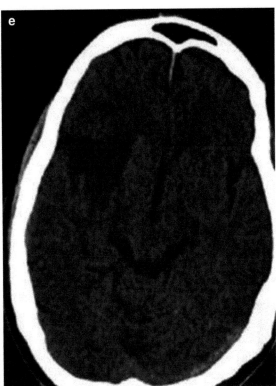

Case 6.1 (continued)

- Endovascular angioplasty (balloon dilatation and permanent stenting)

The combination of these options is termed multimodal reperfusion therapy. Mechanical thrombectomy using stent retrievers and suction devices is currently the method of choice.

Indications and contraindications for EVT in acute ischemic stroke are listed in Table 6.1. EVT is often performed in general anesthesia because it is technically less challenging; however, conscious sedation is faster, avoids arterial hypotension, and is associated with a more favorable oucome. Therefore, conscious sedation is preferable to general anesthesia. Periprocedural complications are rare and include direct vascular trauma because of dissection, perforation, or spasm of vessels as well as embolization of thrombi into previously unaffected, usually more distal vessels. EVT is available only at highly specialized centers, and a 24-h service requires a sufficient number of interventionists, anesthetists,

and stroke neurologists. Transport from peripheral hospitals and preparation of the patient in the angiography suite may delay treatment, but these effects can be overcome by initiating IVT prior to referral ("bridging" or "drip-and-ship" approach).

Predictors of unfavorable outcome following EVT include old age, arterial hypertension, high baseline NIHSS score, large infarct volume (>70 cm^3), a history of previous stroke, long procedure duration, absence of collateral vessels on CT angiogram, and ICA occlusion. The most important variable predicting good outcome is successful and early recanalization (Baker et al. 2011).

6.6.3 Surgical Decompression for Space-Occupying Ischemic Stroke

Decompressive hemicraniectomy is the removal of a large part of the skull and incision of the

Table 6.1 Indications and contraindications for EVT in acute ischemic stroke

	Anterior circulation	Posterior circulation
Indications	Significant neurological deficits (NIHSS ≥10, but lower with, e.g., isolated nonfluent aphasia)	Significant neurological deficits or risk of developing such deficits[a]
	Occlusion or stenosis of proximal large intracranial vessels[b]	BA occlusion or stenosis
	Presenting within the time window[c]	
	If IVT is contraindicated, did not have effect, or is likely not to have effect	
Contraindications[d]	Established infarction of more than 1/3 of MCA territory or 1/2 of ACA territory on CT of the brain	BA thrombosis with coma (Glasgow Coma Scale <9) and widespread manifest brainstem infarction on MR DWI or CT
	Lack of relevant large vessel occlusion on CT or MR angiogram	Other contraindications as for anterior circulation
	Uncontrolled hypertension (>185/110 mmHg)	
	Compromised cardiorespiratory function and other significant medical disease interfering with EVT or general anesthesia	
	Poor premorbid function (modified Rankin Scale ≥3)	

Reprinted with permission from Kondziella et al. (2013)

[a]In posterior circulation stroke, the time window is 12–24 h and beyond; the larger time window is due to the often more protracted and fluctuating course of posterior compared to anterior circulation ischemia and the grave prognosis (90–95% mortality) without successful BA recanalization (16, 17)

[b]Occasionally, patients with more distal vessel occlusions (e.g., M2 MCA) may also be considered for EVT if the remainder of the criteria is fulfilled

[c]The time window for anterior circulation stroke is 6–8 h but may be longer in case of fluctuating symptoms, corresponding perfusion-diffusion mismatch on MRI, and good collateral pial circulation (15)

[d]Of note, increased bleeding tendency (e.g., postoperative state, thrombocytopenia, international normalized ratio >1.5) is not necessarily a contraindication

restrictive dura over the ipsilateral hemisphere to relieve ICP and brain tissue shifts (Case 6.2). In 2007, a meta-analysis of DECIMAL (*decompressive craniectomy in mal*ignant middle cerebral artery infarction) (Vahedi et al. 2007a), DESTINY (*de*compressive *s*urgery for the *t*reatment of malignant *in*farction of the middle cerebral artery) (Jüttler et al. 2007), and HAMLET (*hemicraniectomy after middle cerebral artery infarction with life-threatening edema trial*) (Hofmeijer et al. 2009) showed that patients below the age of 60 years randomized within 48 h of stroke onset to surgical decompression had a significantly better outcome in terms of survival (78% vs. 29%, pooled absolute risk reduction 50% [33–67%]) as well as functional status (mRS ≤3, 43% vs. 21%, risk reduction 23% [5–41%]). Numbers needed to treat was 2 for overall survival and 4 for survival with mRS ≤3 (moderate disability with an ability to walk unassisted or better) (Vahedi et al. 2007b). The side of the lesion did not represent an independent prognostic factor for the resulting functional handicap. Quality of life following decompressive craniectomy appears to be good; 83% of hemicraniectomy patients in a recent study reported that their life was satisfying or rather satisfying (Skoglund et al. 2008).

- Three randomized controlled trials (DESTINY, DECIMAL, and HAMLET) showed that hemicraniectomy for malignant MCA

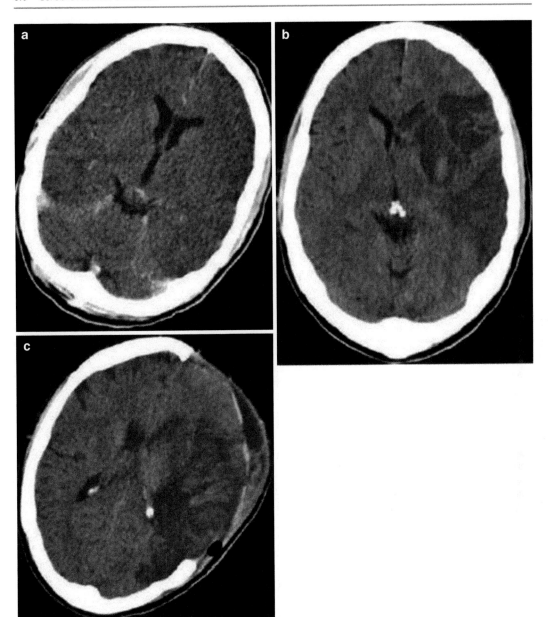

Case 6.2 Hemicraniectomy for malignant middle cerebral artery infarction. A 47-year-old male underwent acute percutaneous coronary intervention for myocardial infarction when he suddenly developed right-sided hemiparesis and aphasia (NIHSS 21). CT of the brain revealed an embolic occlusion of the left ICA and M1 MCA and lack of early ischemic signs (not shown). Despite mechanical thrombectomy 3.5 h after stroke onset, CT following the procedure showed early hypodense signal change in the MCA territory (**a**, also note head turning to the side of the lesion). Thirty-six hours after stroke onset, decline of consciousness developed, and the CT showed mass effect and obliteration of the left lateral ventricle (**b**). An emergency hemicraniectomy was performed resulting in resolution of midline shift (**c**). The bone defect was closed 2 months later using a titanium mesh. At 1-year follow-up, the patient remained severely dysphasic with a right-sided hemiparesis but was able to walk using a cane (mRS 3) (adapted with permission from Kondziella et al. (2013))

infarction increases survival and improves outcome in patients younger than 60 years and if surgery is performed within 48 h of stroke onset. (Yet clinical deterioration due to midline shift and cerebral edema often develops after that period.) DESTINY II revealed that early hemicraniectomy in patients older than 60 years of age with malignant MCA infarcts also leads to increased survival rates, but functional outcome is less convincing. Obviously, the decision to perform decompressive surgery must be made on an individual basis.

- The bone defect should be replaced as soon as the brain tissue is back within the skull circumference to avoid hydrocephalus and/or paradoxical herniation, the so-called sinking skin flap syndrome. This syndrome affects one-fourth of patients 3–5 months after hemicraniectomy for malignant MCA infarction and occurs when atmospheric pressure exceeds ICP.
- Although no randomized controlled trials have investigated decompressive craniectomy in cerebellar infarction, clinical experience clearly indicates a benefit. In general, cerebellar hemispherectomy is not associated with significantly reduced neurological function in the long term. In case of concomitant hydrocephalus, external ventricular drainage may be necessary in addition to craniectomy. The level of consciousness prior to operation is the most powerful predictor of outcome. Importantly, good outcome can also be seen in patients older than 60 years of age (Case 6.3).

6.6.4 Arterial Dissection

The choice is between anticoagulation (with heparin and warfarin) and antithrombotic treatment (e.g., aspirin, clopidogrel, or both in combination), and local treatment traditions vary widely. At the time of writing, there are no data indicating that one approach is superior to the other, but studies are underway. As a rule of thumb, anticoagulation should be given if embolic episodes occur despite antithrombotic treatment, but in uncomplicated cases and with intracranial dissections, antithrombotic treatment is often prescribed because of the relatively lower incidence of hemorrhage compared to anticoagulation.

6.6.5 Symptomatic Treatment of Ischemic Stroke

- Blood sugar levels should be kept within normal levels.
- Hyperthermia is detrimental, and if body temperature exceeds 37.5 °C, paracetamol 1000 mg every 6 h should be prescribed.
- The SCAST study (Sandset et al. 2012) showed that acute blood pressure lowering in the first days is not associated with better outcome in patients with established ischemic stroke, but most patients will need antihypertensive drug treatment later (see below).
- Screening for dysphagia is mandatory to decrease the rate of aspiration pneumonia; a nasogastric tube should be inserted if the swallowing is judged to be unsafe.
- Early mobilization is important to decrease the risk for deep venous thrombosis and aspiration pneumonia, and physiotherapy and occupational therapy are part of neurorehabilitation that should begin as soon as possible.
- As stated above, intermittent pneumatic compression reduces the risk of deep vein thrombosis and may improve survival in immobile stroke patients (CLOTS Trials Collaboration 2013). Low-molecular heparin for prophylaxis of deep vein thrombosis should be prescribed if the patient is not fully mobilized. Thigh-length graduated compression stockings are ineffective (CLOTS Trials Collaboration 2009).
- All stroke patients should be informed about the high risk of poststroke depression. Depression affects at least one-third of all patients with stroke, has detrimental effects on neurorehabilitation, and should be treated immediately. In addition to their antidepressive effects, antidepressants such as SSRI, e.g., citalopram 20–40 mg once daily, have been shown to improve motor recovery (Chollet et al. 2011), and they may prolong survival.

Case 6.3 Surgical decompression for space-occupying cerebellar stroke. A 62-year-old male with a history of atrial fibrillation developed acute onset of headache, vertigo, and gait ataxia. A CT 6 h later showed an ischemic infarct of the right cerebellar hemisphere (**a**). Two days later, he became confused and began to vomit; shortly thereafter, his level of consciousness decreased. A CT revealed obliteration of the basal cisterns and obstructive hydrocephalus (**b**). Immediate cerebellar decompression (**c**) and ventriculostomy (**d**) were performed. A CT a week later showed decreasing ventriculomegaly and cerebellar edema (**e**). On follow-up 3 months later, moderate right-sided ataxia of the extremities was noticed, but the patient remained mostly independent in his activities of daily living (mRS 2) (adapted with permission from Kondziella et al. (2013))

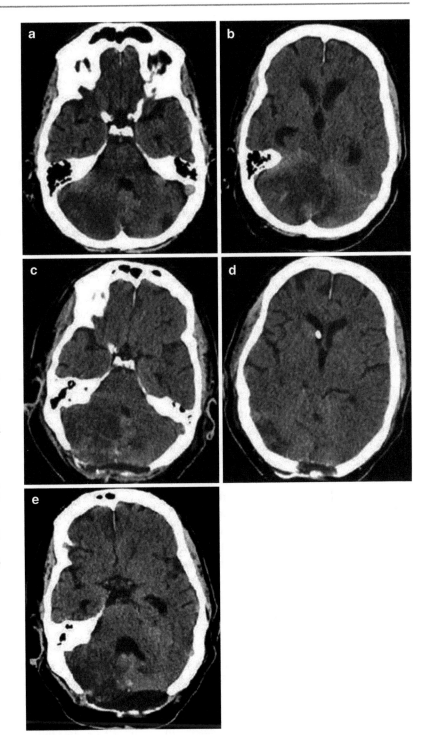

monoclonal antibodies (natalizumab, alemtuzumab, and daclizumab). In Europe, treatments for relapsing-remitting MS are divided into first-line therapies that are considered more safe (the "old injectables" interferon-β 1a/1b and glatiramer acetate, as well as the oral drugs teriflunomide and dimethyl fumarate) and second-line therapies that are considered more risky, albeit also more efficacious (the monoclonal antibodies, and fingolimod).

Of particular concern is the possibility of JC-virus reactivation leading to PML, most frequently observed with natalizumab. Risk stratification is necessary and based on JC virus antibody titers, length of therapy, as well as the presence or absence of previous immunosuppression. The most important adverse effect associated with alemtuzumab is secondary autoimmunity with a delayed onset (e.g., thyroid disorders and immune thrombocytopenia), whereas fingolimod requires, among other precautions, cardiac monitoring for possible grade 2 atrioventricular conduction block. Mitoxantrone is no longer recommended for routine use in patients with relapsing-remitting MS due to its serious adverse effects (mainly related to cardiotoxicity).

The impressive drug arsenal, as well as the potential for severe adverse advents, requires that MS patients are treated by neurologists experienced in the disease and its therapies. As a rule, patients are offered treatment based on a benefit-risk approach, taking into account their disease profile (aggressive or mild) and preferences with respect to side effects (e.g., need for contraception with potentially teratogenic drugs). Patients with relatively milder disease activity might be offered first-line therapies, while patients with a more aggressive course (or those who failed to respond adequately to first-line therapies) may choose from second-line therapies as the initial treatment.

At the time of writing, a fourth monoclonal antibody, ocrelizumab, is expected to enter the market soon. Given its efficacy and favorable safety profile (at least as far as can be concluded from the pre-marketing trials), ocrelizumab is likely to be approved as first-line treatment, which

would change current treatment algorithms significantly. In the future, we are very likely to see many more novel drugs with similar (or even better) efficacy and safety profiles. For a recent review on safety concerns, risk management, and treatment algorithms, see Sorensen 2016.

MS relapse with significant neurological deficit (including optic neuritis and transverse myelitis): methylprednisolone IV 1 g/day for 3–5 days, possibly with oral taper.

Disease-modifying drugs for relapsing-remitting MS

- Patients with less than average disease activity
  - Interferon-β 1a, 30 μg IM once per week
  - Interferon-β 1a, 22 μg or 44 μg SC ×3 weekly
  - Pegylated IFN-β 1a, 125 μg SC once every 2 weeks
  - Interferon-β 1b, 250 μg SC every 48 h
  - Glatiramer acetate 20 μg SC once daily
  - Teriflunomide 14 mg p.o. once daily
  - Dimethyl fumarate 120 mg p.o. twice daily for 7 days, thereafter 240 mg twice daily
- Patients with more aggressive MS and those without adequate response to first-line therapies
  - Natalizumab 300 mg IV every 4 weeks
  - Alemtuzumab 12 mg IV once daily for 5 days, followed 12 months later by 12 mg IV once daily for 3 days
  - Daclizumab 150 mg SC once every month
  - Ocrelizumab (expected approval in 2017)
  - Fingolimod 0.5 mg p.o. once daily
- Off-line therapies
  - Rituximab
  - Ofatumumab
  - Autologous hematopoietic stem cell transplantation

Other off-line treatments, including regimes occasionally used for secondary progressive MS

- Long-term IV steroids, e.g., 1 g/month, or with overlying relapse
- Oral chemotherapeutics

- Azathioprine, increase weekly by 25 mg ×2 to 2.5 mg/kg/day
- Cyclophosphamide 1–2 mg/kg p.o. daily
- Methotrexate 7.5–20 mg p.o. once a week
- Mitoxantrone 12 mg/m² IV every 3 months (maximum cumulative dose 100–140 mg/m²)
- Cyclophosphamide 800 mg/m² monthly bolus infusion

Symptomatic treatment for chronic MS

- Incontinence with urgency and frequent but incomplete emptying
  - Anticholinergics (after post-void bladder assessment using ultrasound), e.g., tolterodine 2 mg once or twice daily, tolterodine retard 4 mg once daily, and oxybutynin 2.5–15 mg/day
  - Desmopressin, p.o. 60–240 μg once daily at night or prior to social activity
  - Desmopressin, nasal spray 10–40 μg once daily at night or once daily daytime prior to social activity
  - Botulinum toxin injection into detrusor muscle
  - Prophylactic antiseptic: nitrofurantoin 50–100 mg at night
  - Self-catheterization
- Erectile dysfunction
  - Sildenafil, 25–100 mg once daily (1 h prior activity)
  - Tadalafil, 10–20 mg (at least 0.5 h prior activity)
  - Vardenafil, 5–10 mg (0.25–1 h prior activity)
- Fatigue
  - Amantadine 100 mg ×2–3 daily
  - Modafinil, start with 100 mg ×2 daily (morning and lunchtime), increase to 200 mg ×2 daily, if necessary
  - Methylphenidate 5–20 mg/day
- Gait difficulties: Fampridine 10 mg twice daily
- Spasticity
  - Baclofen p.o., e.g., 20–100 mg/day (increase slowly)
  - Tizanidine, start with 2 mg at night, increase slowly to 16–20 mg/day

- Baclofen, intrathecally via a pump system with a programmable reservoir
- Botulinum toxin IM, in selected muscles
- Physiotherapy

Episodes of acute deficits due to other inflammatory CNS disorders (e.g., acute demyelinating encephalomyelitis, NMO, Behçet disease, CNS vasculitis)

- Methylprednisolone IV 1 g/day for 3–5 days, with or without oral taper
- Plasmapheresis (e.g., ×5–7; administered every other day)
- IVIG 0.4 mg/kg for 5 days
- Cytotoxic chemotherapy, p.o./IV

Autoimmune encephalitis, paraneoplastic, and non-paraneoplastic

- Methylprednisolone 1 g/day for 3 days IV, then oral prednisolone taper
- IVIG 0.4 g/day for 5 days
- Plasma exchange (e.g., ×5–7; administered every other day)
- Treat underlying tumor, if present
- Second-line treatment (for NMDA receptor encephalitis): rituximab, cyclophosphamide

Adverse effects of steroids, short-term

- High blood sugar: initiate insulin therapy.
- Psychosis, mania, depression, and insomnia: stop steroids and seek psychiatric expertise.

Adverse effects of steroids, long-term

- Diabetes mellitus: insulin therapy.
- Arterial hypertension: antihypertensive agents.
- Ventricular ulcers: proton-pump inhibitors.
- Osteoporosis: patients on steroid therapy should receive calcium and vitamin D supplements (with or without bisphosphonates, whether or not the patient has manifest osteoporosis).
- Cataracts: regular ophthalmological evaluation.

- Increased risk of infections and poor wound healing.
- Beware of adrenal insufficiency with acute stress (surgery, infections) and steroid withdrawal.

6.8   Infectious Diseases

Adult bacterial meningitis, empirical intravenous drug therapy (always check with local protocols).

According to the recent EFNS guidelines on the management of community-acquired bacterial meningitis,

> "parenteral therapy with a third-generation cephalosporin is the initial antibiotics of choice in the absence of penicillin allergy and bacterial resistance; amoxicillin should be used in addition if meningitis because of Listeria monocytogenes is suspected. Vancomycin is the preferred antibiotic for penicillin-resistant pneumococcal meningitis. Dexamethasone should be administered both in adults and in children with or shortly before the first dose of antibiotic in suspected cases of Streptococcus pneumoniae and H. influenzae meningitis. In patients presenting with rapidly evolving petechial skin rash, antibiotic therapy must be initiated immediately on suspicion of Neisseria meningitidis infection with parenteral benzyl penicillin in the absence of known history of penicillin allergy." (Chaudhuri et al. 2008).

Possible dosing options for adults are as follows (again, local protocols may be significantly different!):

- Cefotaxime—2 g IV every 4–8 h
- Ceftriaxone—2 g IV every 12 h
- Vancomycin—750–1000 mg IV every 12 h or 10–15 mg/kg IV every 12 h
- Ampicillin/Amoxicillin 2 g IV every 4 h if Listeria is suspected
- Meropenem 2 g IV every 8 h
- Benzylpenicillin 250,000 U/kg/day (equivalent to 2.4 g every 4 h)
- Steroid therapy: dexamethasone, 0.15 mg/kg every 6 h for 2–4 days

Shunt-associated meningitis

- Intrathecal antibiotics (e.g., vancomycin 5–20 mg daily) can be given to patients with nosocomial meningitis (e.g., ventricular shunt-associated meningitis) that does not respond to IV antibiotics.

Mollaret's meningitis

- Aciclovir if HSV2, indomethacin

Amoebic meningitis

- Amphotericin B IV for 2–4 weeks

Tuberculous meningitis

- Isoniazid (+ pyridoxine 10–20 mg once daily) plus rifampicin plus pyrazinamide plus ethambutol (or streptomycin) plus dexamethasone

Cryptococcal meningitis

- Amphotericin, flucytosine, and fluconazole

Brain abscess

- According to likely focus but include cefotaxime and metronidazole; if traumatic abscess, add vancomycin. Most cerebral abscesses require neurosurgical intervention.

Syphilis

- Penicillin G 2–4 mU IV ×6 for 14 days (if the patient is allergic to penicillin, doxycycline 200 mg every 6 h p.o. for 28 days may be prescribed).

Viral encephalitis due to HSV-1

- Aciclovir 10 mg/kg IV every 6 h for 14–21 days

Herpes zoster

- Valaciclovir 1 g ×3 daily for 7 days or aciclovir IV

PML due to HIV

- HAART, cidofovir 5 mg/kg IV once weekly; mirtazapine

Cerebral malaria

- Artesunate, quinine, and quinidine

Schistosomiasis and cysticercosis

- Praziquantel

Toxoplasmosis

- Sulfadiazine plus pyrimethamine, trimethoprim–sulfamethoxazole, and pyrimethamine plus azithromycin

Borrelia burgdorferi

- Doxycycline 100–200 mg p.o. twice daily for 14–21 days
- Penicillin 1000 mg ×3 daily 7–10 days
- Benzylpenicillin 2.4 g IV every 6 h for 10 days
- Ceftriaxone 2 g/day IV

Diphtheria

- Benzylpenicillin 2.4 g IV ×4 daily for 10 days
- Erythromycin 50 mg/kg/day IV for 10–14 days
- Diphtheria antitoxin IV or IM

6.9 Parkinson's Disease

Initial monotherapy.
Dopamine replacement therapy should be started when symptoms are severe enough to affect activities of daily living, walking, and/or employment. Motor symptoms with less functional impairment may be treated initially with dopamine agonists or monoamine B (MAO-B) inhibitors only. Although controversial, initial monotherapy using dopamine agonists may delay complications of levodopa therapy in younger patients (i.e., motor fluctuations and dyskinesias).

- Young age: dopamine agonist or MAO-B inhibitors can be considered (the latter only if symptoms are mild); however, if fast effect is needed, start with levodopa for 4–6 weeks and then add a dopamine agonist and decrease levodopa as much as possible.
- Medium age: dopamine agonist or levodopa.
- Old age: levodopa.

Levodopa

- Benserazide/levodopa 12.5/50 mg, 25/100 mg; carbidopa/levodopa 10/100 mg, 12.5/50 mg, 25/100 mg.
- Start with 50–100 mg levodopa once or twice daily; increase by 50–100 mg every 3 days.
- Maintenance: 300–600 mg daily, divided by 3–4 doses (or more in patients with "wearing off" fluctuations).
- If daily dose exceeds 600 mg, a dopamine agonist should be added.
- Depot preparations can be given once a night to prevent nocturnal immobility; quick-release preparations can be given during daytime if required.

Dopamine agonists (non-ergot)

- Pramipexole: 0.088 mg ×3 daily during first week, 0.18 mg ×3 daily during second week, and 0.36 mg ×3 daily during third week; thereafter, increase by 0.54 mg weekly as needed to max. 3.3 mg daily.
- Ropinirole: 0.25 mg ×3 daily during first week; thereafter, increase by 0.25 mg three times daily per week; maintenance dose 3–16 mg (or more) daily.
- Ropinirole, sustained release form: 2 mg once daily during first week, increase by 2 mg/ week, maintenance 6–24 mg once daily.
- Rotigotine (transdermal patch): 2 mg/24 h, increase by 2 mg/week, maintenance 6–16 mg daily.
- Apomorphine, SC injection as rescue medication (pretreatment with domperidone for 3 days is necessary to prevent vomiting and hypotension). Requires careful titration, maintenance 2–7 mg ×1–10 times daily, max. 100 mg/day; with more than six injections/ day, continuous subcutaneous infusion of apomorphine by a pump system is preferable.

MAO-B inhibitors
MAO-B inhibitors may be given initially as monotherapy in patients with mild symptoms or to increase "on time" in fluctuating patients

- Rasagiline 1 mg once daily
- Selegiline 5–10 mg once daily

Catechol-O-methyltransferase (COMT) inhibitors
Increases CNS delivery of levodopa by retarding its degradation; thus, it is always given in combination with levodopa.

- Entacapone: 200 mg together with every dose of levodopa

Amantadine
Although not a first choice, this glutamate receptor antagonist can be beneficial in patients with tremor, particularly in early disease, and in more advanced disease, it may reduce dyskinesia.

- 100 mg once daily, increase by 100 mg every 3 days, max. 400 mg/day

Treatment options with advanced PD
In long-standing patients with severe motor fluctuations and dyskinesia, a variety of advanced treatment options exist.

- DBS (only useful if there still is some response to levodopa therapy)
  - Nucleus subthalamicus
  - Globus pallidus, pars interna
- Jejunal infusion of levodopa and carbidopa, dispersed as a viscous gel, using a patient-operated portable pump (Duodopa therapy)
- Amantadine continuous subcutaneous infusion using a patient-operated portable pump

Treatment of nonmotor symptoms

- *Psychosis*: optimize medication list. Quetiapine, olanzapine, or clozapine may be used in low doses for a short period of time (see Sect. 6.3).
- *Dementia*: acetylcholinesterase inhibitors (donepezil, galantamine, rivastigmine; see Sect. 6.3).
- *Drooling*:
  - Botulinum toxin injection into parotid gland

  - Sublingual atropine, 1 drop ×2 of 1.0% ophthalmic solution
  - Scopolamine, transdermal (patch)
- *Nausea*: domperidone 10–20 mg ×1–3 daily.
- *Hypotension*: optimize medication list, e.g., discontinue antihypertensive drugs and MAO-B inhibitors.
  - Fludrocortisone 0.1 mg once or twice daily (up to 1 mg/day), taken in the morning or at bedtime
  - Dihydroergotamine 2.5 mg or 5 mg twice daily
  - Midodrine 2.5–5 mg three times daily

6.10   Non-parkinsonian Movement Disorders

Dystonia
Acute dystonic reactions

- Biperiden 2.5–5 mg IV or IM, followed by biperiden p.o., 2 mg ×1–4 for 7 days

Dopa-responsive dystonia (hereditary progressive dystonia with diurnal fluctuation, also known as Segawa disease or DYT5 dystonia):

- Low doses of levodopa

Tardive dystonia and dyskinesia

- Withdraw offending drug, if necessary switch to atypical antipsychotics
- Botulinum injections
- Tetrabenazine

Adult-onset focal dystonia

- Botulinum toxin

Idiopathic generalized dystonia

- In young patients, a diagnostic trial of levodopa (400–600 mg) is needed to exclude dopa-responsive dystonia (see above).
- Medical treatment, often in combination: anticholinergics (e.g., trihexyphenidyl 2 mg ×1 a

day, increase stepwise up to 20 mg/day), tetrabenazine, baclofen, clonazepam, and dopamine antagonist.
- DBS (globus pallidus, bilateral).

Chorea and hemiballismus

- Chorea and ballismus: tetrabenazine (slowly titrated with 6.25 mg every 4–7 days up to 70 mg three times daily).
- Carbamazepine and valproate as second-line therapy (first line in Sydenham chorea).
- Benzodiazepine and/or atypical antipsychotics may reduce anxiety and behavioral symptoms.

HD

- Chorea: tetrabenazine, sulpiride 100–200 mg twice daily, or olanzapine

Wilson's disease

- Low-copper diet (<1 mg/day)
- Penicillamine 1–2 g/day, in 2–4 divided doses
- Trientine 1.2–2.4 g/day, in 2–4 divided doses
- Zinc acetate 50 mg three times daily
- Tetrathiomolybdate
- Ultimately, liver transplantation

Myoclonus

- Cortical myoclonus: piracetam, valproate, primidone, and clonazepam
- Subcortical myoclonus: clonazepam
- Hiccups: valproate, baclofen, gabapentin, and chlorpromazine, vagus nerve stimulation

Essential tremor

- First-line agents
  - Beta-blockers
    Propranolol 10 mg twice daily initially, maintenance 60–120 mg twice daily
  - Primidone: starting dose 25 mg at night, usual maintenance dose 50 mg at night or twice daily; if necessary, titration up to 250 mg and above is possible

- Second-line agents
  - Antiepileptics
    Gabapentin 300–600 mg two or three times daily
    Topiramate 25–200 mg twice daily
  - Benzodiazepines (clonazepam)
  - Mirtazapine
- Nonmedical treatment options
  - DBS (thalamic, ventral intermediate nucleus; bilateral)
  - Stereotactic thalamotomy
  - Botulinum toxin
  - Wrist weights

Dystonic tremor

- Botulinum toxin.
- Anticholinergics, primidone, and gabapentin occasionally are helpful.

Primary orthostatic tremor

- Clonazepam
- Primidone and gabapentin

Tics

- Dopamine antagonists, including atypical and typical antipsychotics (e.g., aripiprazole, pimozide, risperidone, tetrabenazine, pergolide, haloperidol)
- Botulinum toxin (rarely)
- Cognitive behavioral therapy and other psychotherapeutic programs

Restless legs

- Check for and treat possible causes, e.g., neuropathy, iron deficiency, and renal failure.
- Strong evidence supports use of pramipexole (0.18–0.54 mg bedtime), rotigotine, cabergoline, and gabapentin.
- Moderate evidence exists for ropinirole (0.25–4 mg bedtime), pregabalin, and IV ferric carboxymaltose.
- There is only low evidence for levodopa (50–200 mg bedtime; cave: augmentation).

- In patients on hemodialysis with secondary RLS, vitamin C and E supplementation can be subscribed together with ropinirole.

6.11   Cranial Neuropathies and Related Conditions

Giant cell arteritis

- With visual symptoms: 1000 mg methylprednisolone IV for 3 days; thereafter, 1 mg/kg body weight/day (e.g., 60–100 mg daily) prednisolone p.o. until symptom relief.
- Without visual symptoms: 60–100 mg/day prednisolone p.o. for 2 weeks after complete recovery.
- Reduce prednisolone cautiously, e.g., by 5 mg every 2 weeks up to 20 mg/day, thereafter 2.5 mg every 2 weeks until 10 mg/day and 1.25 mg every 4 weeks.
- Upon relapse, increase again to least effective dose (2 years of treatment usually necessary).
- Prophylaxis for osteoporosis is mandatory (see above).

Tolosa-Hunt disease

- Prednisolone 60–100 mg once daily.
- Low-dose radiation therapy of the affected sinus cavernosus may be an alternative option.

Nutritional/toxic optic neuropathy

- Remove toxins
- Hydroxocobalamin 1 mg IM per week, oral vitamin B, and folate

Superior oblique myokymia: carbamazepine (dosage as for trigeminal neuralgia)

Trigeminal and glossopharyngeal neuralgia

- Carbamazepine (600–2000 mg daily)
- Second line: gabapentin (2400–3600 mg/day), valproate (1500–2000 mg/day), phenytoin (300–400 mg/day), topiramate (100–200 mg/day), baclofen (20–100 mg/day), and clonazepam (6–8 mg/day).
- Phenytoin/fosphenytoin IV (dosage as for status epilepticus) is very effective as rescue medication.
- Botulinum toxin (trigeminal neuralgia).
- Surgical: microvascular decompression or destructive procedures (balloon compression, glycerol injection into trigeminal cistern, radio frequency ablation of trigeminal ganglion, stereotactic gamma knife surgery).

Atypical facial pain

- Antidepressants, baclofen; behavioral therapy

Bell's palsy

- 50 mg prednisolone once daily for 7–10 days (but only if treatment can be initiated within the first 72 h)
- Artificial tears: 1–2 drops in each eye ×3 daily or more
- Eye protection at night
- In case of suspected Borrelia infection and CSF pleocytosis: doxycycline 200 mg once daily for 2 weeks or 400 mg once daily for 10 days

Hemifacial spasm

- Botulinum toxin
- Carbamazepine (dosage as for trigeminal neuralgia)
- Posterior fossa microvascular decompression

Facial myokymia

- Botulinum toxin

Gustatory sweating

- Botulinum toxin

Ramsay Hunt syndrome (reactivation syndrome of herpes zoster in the geniculate ganglion)

- Aciclovir 800 mg ×5 for 1 week
- Prednisolone 40–60 mg once daily for 1 week
- Symptomatic vertigo treatment

Acute vertigo

The following medication should be given only during a short period in order not to interfere with central compensation mechanisms.

- Dopamine antagonists (prochlorperazine, metoclopramide, domperidone)
- Meclizine 25 mg once or twice daily
- Benzodiazepines (e.g., diazepam 2 mg two to three times daily)

Typewriter tinnitus

- Carbamazepine (dosage as for trigeminal neuralgia)

Spasmodic dysphonia

- Botulinum toxin

6.12 Autonomic Dysreflexia with Spinal Cord Injury

In spinal cord trauma above TH6, painful or other stimuli below the transection level may lead to acute massive vasoconstriction including the mesenteric vessels and arterial hypertension. (The patient is "cold and pale" below the lesion and "red and hot" above). Since patients with chronic injury to the cervical or upper thoracic spinal cord usually have very low blood pressure, even blood pressure readings with apparently normal values (e.g., 130/80 mmHg) may be associated with life-threatening hypertensive encephalopathy:

- Let the patient sit upright.
- Remove tight clothing.
- Monitor blood pressure every 2–5 min.
- Perform intermittent catheterization or check indwelling catheter for obstruction. Bladder distension is the most common cause of autonomic dysreflexia.

- If blood pressure remains ≥150 mmHg, give, e.g., glyceryl nitrate sublingual 2.5–5 mg (can be spit out by the patient in case of hypotension) or nifedipine 10 mg (bite and swallow).
- If symptoms persist, disimpact bowel (bowel problems are the second most common cause of autonomic dysreflexia) and search for other stimuli normally associated with pain, e.g., decubital wounds.

6.13 Neuromuscular Disorders

6.13.1 Motor Neuron Diseases and Peripheral Neuropathies

6.13.1.1 Amyotrophic Lateral Sclerosis

- *Sodium channel blocker*: riluzole 50 mg twice daily, prolongs survival by 2 months on average
- *Salivation and drooling*
  - Atropine 0.25–0.75 mg oral
  - Amitriptyline 10–25 mg
  - Hyoscine patches 1 mg/72 h
  - Botulinum toxin
- *Tenacious secretions*: acetylcysteine 200 mg two or three times daily, fluids p.o.
- *Pain, spasticity, and cramps*
  - Levetiracetam
  - Baclofen
  - Morphine
- *Nutrition*: percutaneous endoscopic gastrostomy
- *Emotional incontinence and depression*
  - SSRI (citalopram 20–40 mg once daily)
  - Tricyclic antidepressant (amitriptyline 25–100 mg at night)
- *Dyspnea*
  - Home ventilation, CPAP, cough assistant
  - Morphine 2.5–5 mg every 6 h
- *Anxiety*
  - Benzodiazepines (lorazepam, diazepam, oxazepam)
  - Counseling

6.13.1.2 Peripheral Nerve Disorders

- *Corticosteroids* (for vasculitic neuropathy and CIDP, but not GBS): start oral prednisolone

1 mg/kg/day for 2–5 weeks depending on treatment response and then decrease slowly over many weeks; maintenance dosage as low as possible.

- *Azathioprine*: start with 2.5 mg/kg/day until clinical benefit, then maintenance with, e.g., 1 mg/kg/day.
- *Cyclophosphamide*: 2 mg/kg p.o. daily for 3 months.
- *Plasma exchange*: 5- or 7-day courses, 50 mL plasma/kg exchanged every other day; low-dose heparin.
- *IVIG*: 0.4 g/kg once daily for 5 days; prior to IVIG treatment, order serum electrophoresis and exclude IgA deficiency to avoid anaphylactic reactions. Most authorities suggest that in patients with GBS, IVIG treatment is initiated when symptoms are severe enough as to affect gait.

6.13.1.3   Peripheral Neuropathic Pain
- AED
  - Gabapentin 900–3600 mg
  - Pregabalin 75–600 mg
  - Carbamazepine 200–600 mg
  - Lamotrigine 300–400 mg
- Antidepressants
  - Nortriptyline, start with 10 mg three times daily; if necessary, increase by 10 mg every 2–3 days to 25–50 mg three times daily
  - Amitriptyline 25–100 mg (probably less efficient than nortriptyline and imipramine)
  - Imipramine (20–)100–200 mg/day, e.g., start with 10–25 mg once or twice daily, increasing by 25 mg every second day
  - Duloxetine 20–120 mg
  - Venlafaxine 150–220 mg
  - Paroxetine 40 mg
  - Citalopram 40 mg
- Opioids should be used cautiously in chronic pain. As a rule, mild analgesics should be tried prior to opiods and short-lasting opiods prior to patches.
  - Tramadol 50–400 mg
  - Oxycodone 40–60 mg
- Capsaicin patch (8%), locally

- Acute neuropathic pain: regional nerve blockade (local injections of anesthetic agents, e.g., lidocaine)
- Surgical, e.g., dorsal root entry zone lesioning

6.13.1.4   Central Neuropathic Pain
For the sake of convenience, central neuropathic pain is discussed here together with the more common peripheral neuropathic pain.

- Spinal cord injury pain: lidocaine IV, alfentanil IV, propofol IV, morphine plus clonidine intrathecally, and baclofen intrathecally
- MS: carbamazepine, phenytoin, valproate (paroxysms), and TCA (non-paroxysmal pain)
- Central poststroke pain: amitriptyline and lamotrigine
- Transepidermal nerve stimulation (TENS)
- Spinal cord stimulation
- DBS
- Surface stimulation of motor cortex

6.13.2 Neuromuscular Junction Disorders and Myopathies

6.13.2.1   Myasthenia Gravis (MG)
MG, tensilon test
  See Chap. 3.
  MG, symptomatic treatment

- *Anticholinesterase therapy*
  - Pyridostigmine: start with 30–60 mg every 6 h and gradually titrate as necessary to 60–120 mg every 4–6 h; 180 mg timed-release pyridostigmine can be given at night in case of severe weakness upon awakening. With appropriate immunomodulatory therapy (see below), patients rarely need more than 120 mg pyridostigmine ×5/day.
  - Neostigmine IV or SC: if a patient is transferred from oral Mestinon to intravenous neostigmine (e.g., because of a surgical procedure), it is important to remember that the dosage difference is roughly 30:1 (thus, 30 mg Mestinon p.o. = 1 mg neostigmine IV).

- *Anticholinergics* (given for muscarinergic side effects): atropine
- *Potassium substitution* (aim for high-normal or slightly elevated potassium plasma levels).
  - Potassium
  - Spironolactone 50–100 mg once daily

MG, immunosuppressive treatment

- Prednisolone
  - Depending on the severity of the symptoms, one may either choose a "start low, go slow" approach (e.g., 10–25 mg once daily) or a high-dose regimen (e.g., 1 mg/kg or 60–100 mg once daily, but beware of temporary worsening weakness; often combined with IVIG or plasma exchange). Patients should soon be started on azathioprine or another steroid-sparing therapy, in order to decrease maintenance prednisolone as much as possible.
- Azathioprine
  - Start with 50 mg once or 25 mg twice daily
  - Increase by 25 mg/day until 2.5 mg/kg/day
- Thymectomy: Thymectomy is performed in every patient with a suspicion of thymoma on CT of the chest but also MG patients without thymoma can benefit, especially young women with severe generalized symptoms and who are acetylcholine receptor antibody positive
- IVIG 0.4 g/day for 5 days (effective for up to 2 months)
- Plasma exchange (effective for up to 2 months; if given prior to steroids, it may prevent temporary decline and, thus, possibly need for respirator treatment)
- Others: mycophenolate, cyclophosphamide, cyclosporine, etanercept, and rituximab

6.13.2.2 Lambert-Eaton Myasthenic Syndrome (LEMS)
- 3,4-Diaminopyridine (DAP) 4–12 mg ×3–4 daily (max. 100 mg)
- Pyridostigmine
- Prednisolone 30–60 mg

- Azathioprine 2.5 mg/kg
- IVIG 0.4 g/day for 5 days (often less effective than in MG)
- Plasma exchange (often less effective than in MG)
- Removal of underlying tumor (usually a SCLC), if present

6.13.2.3 Neuromyotonia (*Isaacs Syndrome*)
Carbamazepine, lamotrigine, phenytoin, valproate, and gabapentin; immunomodulatory treatment.

6.13.2.4 Muscle Cramps
Muscle stretching exercises; medical treatment is only rarely needed (quinine, carbamazepine, lamotrigine, and gabapentin).

6.13.2.5 Myopathies
- *Duchenne muscular dystrophy*: prednisolone, cardiac drugs (angiotensin-converting enzyme inhibitors, beta-blockers, diuretics, digoxin, anticoagulants)
- *Myotonic dystrophy*: modafinil for excessive daytime sleepiness, mexiletine for myotonia
- *Hyperkalemic and normokalemic periodic paralysis*: salbutamol inhaler (attacks), low-potassium diet, thiazide diuretics, acetazolamide, and lamotrigine
- *Hypokalemic periodic paralysis*: oral potassium (avoid intravenous potassium); low-carbohydrate, low-sodium diet; and acetazolamide.
- *Myotonia congenita*: mexiletine (start with 50 mg once daily, increase up 200 mg ×2–4 daily)
- *Myotonia*: quinine (kinin 100, 250 mg), 300–600 mg ×2–3 daily
- *Malignant hyperthermia*: dantrolene 2.5 mg/kg IV, repeat up to total dose of 10 mg/kg
- *Acute myositis*: prednisolone (titrate according to clinical response and plasma creatine kinase levels), azathioprine, methotrexate, cyclosporine A, and mycophenolate; if severe: plasmapheresis and IVIG

References and Suggested Reading

Baker GA. Depression and suicide in adolescents with epilepsy. Neurology. 2006;66(Suppl):S5–12.

Baker WL, Colby JA, Tongbram V. Neurothrombectomy devices for the treatment of acute ischemic stroke: state of the evidence. Ann Intern Med. 2011;154:243–52.

Berkhemer OA, Fransen PS, Beumer D, et al. A randomized trial of intraarterial treatment for acute ischemic stroke. N Engl J Med. 2015;372:11–20.

Boylan LS, Flint LA, Labovitz DL, et al. Depression but not seizure frequency predicts quality of life in treatment resistant epilepsy. Neurology. 2004;62:258–61.

Bråthen G, Ben-Menachem E, Brodtkorb E, et al. EFNS Task Force on Diagnosis and Treatment of Alcohol-Related Seizures. EFNS guideline on the diagnosis and management of alcohol-related seizures: report of an EFNS task force. Eur J Neurol. 2005;12:575–81.

Burns A, editor. Standards in dementia care. London: Taylor & Francis; 2005.

Calabresi PA, Radue EW, Goodin D, et al. Safety and efficacy of fingolimod in patients with relapsing-remitting multiple sclerosis (FREEDOMS II): a double-blind, randomised, placebo-controlled, phase 3 trial. Lancet Neurol. 2014;13:545–56.

Campbell BC, Mitchell PJ, Kleinig TJ, et al. Endovascular therapy for ischemic stroke with perfusion-imaging selection. N Engl J Med. 2015;372:1009–18.

Chaudhuri A, Martinez-Martin P, Kennedy PG, et al. EFNS Task Force. EFNS guideline on the management of community-acquired bacterial meningitis: report of an EFNS Task Force on acute bacterial meningitis in older children and adults. Eur J Neurol. 2008;15:649–59.

Chernyshev OY, Martin-Schild S, Albright KC, et al. Safety of tPA in stroke mimics and neuroimaging-negative cerebral ischemia. Neurology. 2010;74:1340–5.

Chimowitz MI, Lynn MJ, Derdeyn CP, et al. Stenting versus aggressive medical therapy for intracranial arterial stenosis. N Engl J Med. 2011;365:993–1003.

Chollet F, Tardy J, Albucher JF, et al. Fluoxetine for motor recovery after acute ischaemic stroke (FLAME): a randomised placebo-controlled trial. Lancet Neurol. 2011;10:123–30.

CLOTS (Clots in Legs Or sTockings after Stroke) Trials Collaboration. Effectiveness of intermittent pneumatic compression in reduction of risk of deep vein thrombosis in patients who have had a stroke (CLOTS 3): a multicentre randomised controlled trial. Lancet. 2013;382:516–24.

CLOTS Trials Collaboration, Dennis M, Sandercock PA, et al. Effectiveness of thigh-length graduated compression stockings to reduce the risk of deep vein thrombosis after stroke (CLOTS trial 1): a multicentre, randomised controlled trial. Lancet. 2009; 373(9679):1958–65.

Compter A, van der Worp HB, Schonewille WJ, et al. Stenting versus medical treatment in patients with symptomatic vertebral artery stenosis: a randomised open-label phase 2 trial. Lancet Neurol. 2015; 14:606–14.

Confavreux C, O'Connor P, Comi G, et al. Oral teriflunomide for patients with relapsing-remitting multiple sclerosis (TOWER): a randomized, double-blind, placebo-controlled, phase 3 trial. Lancet Neurol. 2014;13:247–56.

Diener HC, Bogousslavsky J, Brass LM, et al. Aspirin and clopidogrel compared with clopidogrel alone after recent ischaemic stroke or transient ischaemic attack in high-risk patients (MATCH): randomised, double-blind, placebo-controlled trial. Lancet. 2004; 364(9431):331–7.

Etminan N, Brown Jr RD, Breseoglo K, et al. The unruptured intracranial aneurysm treatment score: a multidisciplinary consensus. Neurology. 2015;85:881–9.

European Heart Rhythm Association; European Association for Cardio-Thoracic Surgery, Camm AJ, et al. ESC Committee for Practice Guidelines. Guidelines for the management of atrial fibrillation: the Task Force for the Management of Atrial Fibrillation of the European Society of Cardiology (ESC). Europace. 2010;12:1360–420.

Glauser T, Ben-Menachem E, Bourgeois B, et al. Updated ILAE evidence review of antiepileptic drug efficacy and effectiveness as initial monotherapy for epileptic seizures and syndromes. Epilepsia. 2013;54:551–63.

Goyal M, Demchuk AM, Menon BK, et al. Randomized assessment of rapid endovascular treatment of ischemic stroke. N Engl J Med. 2015;372:1019–30.

Hemphill JC, Greenberg SM, Anderson CS, et al. Guidelines for the management of spontaneous intracerebral hemorrhage: a guideline for healthcare professionals from the American Heart Association/American Stroke Association. Stroke. 2015;46:2032–60.

Hofmeijer J, Kappelle LJ, Algra A, et al. Surgical decompression for space-occupying cerebral infarction (the Hemicraniectomy After Middle Cerebral Artery infarction with Life-threatening Edema Trial [HAMLET]): a multicentre, open, randomised trial. Lancet Neurol. 2009;8:326–33.

Hort J, O'Brien JT, Gainotti G, et al. EFNS guidelines for the diagnosis and management of Alzheimer's disease. Eur J Neurol. 2010;17:1236–48.

Jovin TG, Chamorro A, Cobo E, et al. Thrombectomy within 8 hours after symptom onset in ischemic stroke. N Engl J Med. 2015;372:2296–306.

Jüttler E, Schwab S, Schmiedek P, et al. Decompressive surgery for the treatment of malignant infarction of the middle cerebral artery (DESTINY): a randomized, controlled trial. Stroke. 2007;38:2518–25.

Jüttler E, Unterberg A, Woitzik J, et al. Hemicraniectomy in older patients with extensive middle-cerebral-artery stroke. N Engl J Med. 2014;279:1091–100.

Kanner AM. Depression in epilepsy: prevalence, clinical semiology, pathogenic mechanisms, and treatment. Biol Psychiatry. 2003;54:388–98.

Kondziella D, Cortsen M, Eskesen V, Hansen K, Holtmannspötter M, Højgaard J, Stavngaard T, Søndergaard H, Wagner A, Welling KL. Update on acute endovascular and surgical stroke treatment. Acta Neurol Scand. 2013;127:1–9.

Lansberg MG, Schrooten M, Bluhmki E, Thijs VN, Saver JL. Treatment time-specific number needed to treat estimates for tissue plasminogen activator therapy in acute stroke based on shifts over the entire range of the modified Rankin Scale. Stroke. 2009;40:2079–84.

Lavallée PC, Meseguer E, Abboud H, et al. A transient ischaemic attack clinic with round-the-clock access (SOS-TIA): feasibility and effects. Lancet Neurol. 2007;6:953–60.

Lip GY. Using the CHA2DS2-VASc score for stroke risk stratification in atrial fibrillation: a clinical perspective. Expert Rev Cardiovasc Ther. 2013;11:259–62.

Mendelow AD, Gregson BA, Fernandes HM, et al. Early surgery versus initial conservative treatment in patients with spontaneous supratentorial intracerebral haematomas in the International Surgical Trial in Intracerebral Haemorrhage (STICH): a randomised trial. Lancet. 2005;365:387–97.

Mohr JP, Parides MK, Stapf C, et al. Medical management with or without interventional therapy for unruptured brain arteriovenous malformations (ARUBA): a multicentre, non-blinded, randomised trial. Lancet. 2014;383:614–21.

Neal EG, Chaffe H, Schwartz RH, et al. The ketogenic diet for the treatment of childhood epilepsy: a randomised controlled trial. Lancet Neurol. 2008; 7(6):500.

Pisters R, Lane DA, Nieuwlaat R, et al. A novel user-friendly score (HAS-BLED) to assess one-year risk of major bleeding in patients with atrial fibrillation: the Euro Heart Survey. Chest. 2010;138:1093–100.

Pompili M, Girardi P, Tatarelli R. Death from suicide versus mortality from epilepsy in the epilepsies: a meta-analysis. Epilepsy Behav. 2006;9:641–8.

Powers WJ, Clarke WR, Grubb Jr RL, et al. Extracranial-intracranial bypass surgery for stroke prevention in hemodynamic cerebral ischemia: the Carotid Occlusion Surgery Study randomized trial. JAMA. 2011;306:1983–92.

Rhea J, Saver JL. The impact of recanalization on ischemic stroke outcome: a meta-analysis. Stroke. 2007;38:967–73.

Riedel CH, Zimmermann P, Jensen-Kondering U, et al. The importance of size: successful recanalization by intravenous thrombolysis in acute anterior stroke. Stroke. 2011;42:1775–7.

Samuels MA, Ropper AH. Samuels's manual of neurologic therapeutics. 8th ed. Philadelphia: Lippincott Williams & Wilkins; 2010.

Sandset EC, Murray GD, Bath PM, et al. Scandinavian Candesartan Acute Stroke Trial (SCAST) Study Group. Relation between change in blood pressure in acute stroke and risk of early adverse events and poor outcome. Stroke. 2012;43:2108–14.

Saver JL, Goyal M, Bonafe A, et al. Stent-retriever thrombectomy after intravenous t-PA vs. t-PA alone in stroke. N Engl J Med. 2015;372:2285–95.

Schmidt R, Hofer E, Bouwman FH, et al. EFNS-ENS/EAN Guideline on concomitant use of cholinesterase inhibitors and memantine in moderate to severe Alzheimer's disease. Eur J Neurol. 2015;22:889–98.

Silbergleit R, Durkalski V, Lowenstein D, et al. Intramuscular versus intravenous therapy for prehospital status epilepticus. N Engl J Med. 2012;366:591–600.

Skoglund TS, Eriksson-Ritzén C, Sörbo A, et al. Health status and life satisfaction after decompressive craniectomy for malignant middle cerebral artery infarction. Acta Neurol Scand. 2008;117:305–10.

Sorbi S, Hort J, Erkinjuntti T, Fladby T, et al. EFNS-ENS Guidelines on the diagnosis and management of disorders associated with dementia. Eur J Neurol. 2012;19:1159–79.

Sorensen PS. Safety concerns and risk management of multiple sclerosis therapies. Acta Neurol Scand. 2016; doi:10.1111/ane.12712.

The National Institute of Neurological Disorders and Stroke rt-PA Stroke Study Group. Tissue plasminogen activator for acute ischemic stroke. N Engl J Med. 1995;333:1581–7.

Vahedi K, Vicaut E, Mateo J, et al. Sequential-design, multicenter, randomized, controlled trial of early decompressive craniectomy in malignant middle cerebral artery infarction (DECIMAL Trial). Stroke. 2007a;38:2506–17.

Vahedi K, Hofmeijer J, Juettler E, et al. Early decompressive surgery in malignant infarction of the middle cerebral artery: a pooled analysis of three randomized controlled trials. Lancet Neurol. 2007b;6:215–22.

Wang Y, Zhao X, Liu L, et al. Clopidogrel with aspirin in acute minor stroke or transient ischemic attack. N Engl J Med. 2013;369:11–9.

Index